The Power of Psychiatry

The Power of Psychiatry

Edited by

Peter Miller and Nikolas Rose

Polity Press

© Polity Press, 1986
First published 1986 by Polity Press, Cambridge, in association
with Basil Blackwell, Oxford.

Editorial Office:
Polity Press, Dales Brewery, Gwydir Street, Cambridge CB1 2LJ,
UK.

Basil Blackwell Ltd, 108 Cowley Road, Oxford OX4 1JF, UK.

Basil Blackwell Inc., 432 Park Avenue South, Suite 1503, New
York, NY 10016, USA.

British Library Cataloguing in Publication Data
The Power of psychiatry.
  1. Psychiatry
  I. Miller, Peter B.   II. Rose, Nikolas
  616.89   RC454

ISBN 0–7456–0235–5
ISBN 0–7456–0236–3 Pbk

Typset by Photo·Graphics, Honiton, Devon
Printed in Great Britain by Billing and Sons Ltd, Worcester

Contents

List of contributors

Hilary Allen, BSc, RMN, PhD   Engaged in research on the disproportionate psychiatrization of women within the criminal justice system. In addition to teaching sociology at Brunel University, has worked in both hospital and community psychiatric services, and has published articles on clinical, organizational and socio-legal aspects of psychiatry and lectured and published on various aspects of feminist politics.

Pat Carlen, BA, PhD   Senior Lecturer in Criminology at the University of Keele; Author of *Magistrates' Justice* (Oxford, Martin Robertson, 1976) and *Women's Imprisonment* (London, Routledge & Kegan Paul, 1983); co-author (with F. Burton) of *Official Discourse* (London, Routledge & Kegan Paul, 1979); co-editor and co-author (with D. Christina, J. Hicks, J. O'Dwyer and C. Tchaikowsky) of *Criminal Women* (Cambridge, Polity Press, 1985); editor of *The Sociology of Law* (University of Keele, 1976) and, (with M. Collinson) of *Radical Issues in Criminology* (Oxford, Martin Robertson, 1980). Author of articles on courts, penal politics, law and psychiatry and member of editorial advisory groups of *Law in Context* and *The Howard Journal of Criminal Justice*.

Colin Gordon, BA   Editor and co-translator of (Brighton, Harvester, 1980) *Power/Knowledge*, a collection of Michel Foucault's essays and interviews. Member of editorial group of *Radical Philosophy* (1976–9) and of *Ideology and Consciousness* (now *I & C*) since 1978. Has contributed to these journals, and also to *Times Literary Supplement* and to *Magazine littéraire*, on the work of Foucault and related authors, and on questions of philosophy, social-political theory and the politics of psychiatry. Co-editor, translator and contributor to *The Foucault Effect: Studies in the History of Government*

Rationality (Brighton, Harvester, 1985); other contributions will appear in S. Lash and S. Whimster (eds), *Max Weber: Studies in Rationality and Irrationality* (London, Allen & Unwin, forthcoming) and in *Radical Philosophy Reader* (London, New Left Books, forthcoming).

Kobena Mercer, BA PhD research student in Sociology at Goldsmiths College, University of London working on British racism in the 1960s. Also working for the Centre for Caribbean Studies, based at Goldsmiths' College. Formerly member of Black Health Workers and Patients Group, a campaigning group whose work on race and psychiatry has been published in *Race and Class* and *International Journal of Social Psychiatry*. Has also been involved in a black community mental health project – Afro Caribbean Mental Health Association – based in the London Borough of Lambeth.

Peter Miller, BSc, PhD Lecturer in the School of Management and of Economic Studies, University of Sheffield. Visiting Lecturer, London Graduate School of Business Studies, University Extension Lecturer, London University. On the editorial board of *I & C*. Published work covers psychiatry and social theory. Most recently: a critical analysis of theories of power. *Domination and Power* (London, Routledge & Kegan Paul, forthcoming, 1986).

Shulamit Ramon BA, MA, PhD Lecturer in Social Work in the Department of Social Administration at the London School of Economics. Most recent published work is a book on attitudes and decisions on psychiatry taken by politicians and professionals in Britain during the 1920s and 1950s: *Psychiatry in Britain: Meaning and Policy* (London, Croom Helm, 1985).

Nikolas Rose BA, MSc, PhD Lecturer in the Department of Human Sciences at Brunel University. Formerly member of editoral boards of *I & C* and *Politics and Power*. Published articles on psychology, psychiatry, politics, social policy and social theory – most recently *The Psychological Complex* (London, Routledge & Kegan Paul, 1985), a study of the development and role of 'applied psychology' in England. Has been practically involved in policy formation on community psychiatric services in London.

Introduction

Peter Miller and Nikolas Rose

The power of psychiatry is, once more, in the forefront of social debate. In Britain, arguments about psychiatric ideologies and practices have been given urgency by proposals for the closure of large psychiatric hospitals, the planning of community psychiatric services and the reform of mental-health legislation. Similar debates are occurring everywhere where the dominance of the mental hospital over mental-health services is coming under question – in the process of sectorization in France, the establishment of a network of community mental-health centres in Italy and other countries of the European community, and in the USA.

Since the early 1960s, critiques of psychiatry have been a major influence on the way such issues have been posed and their policy implications worked out. Criticisms of psychiatry as a repressive and custodial project for the control of social deviance have been influential in the move away from the segregation of the mentally distressed, and in the proposals that carceral psychiatry be replaced by a prophylactic and therapeutic endeavour co-extensive with the community itself. Criticisms of psychiatry for its failure to live up to its promise of alleviating mental troubles have tended to identify this failure with excessive reliance upon medical expertise, the institution of the hospital and the notion of mental illness. Such criticism has supported proposals for the establishment of comprehensive and multidisciplinary mental-health services, and for the development of such services in the territory of daily existence – the family, the neighbourhood, the school and the workplace.

Whilst the contributors to this volume have no unitary perspective – political, theoretical or practical – they nonetheless share a certain unease about such critiques and the alternatives they propose. By way of introduction, it may prove useful to draw out some common themes that might form the basis of a rather different analysis of the power of contemporary psychiatry. Such an analysis would not view power as some kind of monolithic and malign presence, to which we must oppose ourselves and which we must strive to abolish. Rather, it would analyse the power of psychiatry in terms of what it makes thinkable and possible, the new objectives to which it allows us to aspire, the new types of problem it allows us to conceive, the new types of solution it inserts into our reality. This broadens the focus of analysis from a concentration upon medicine and the mental hospital to a consideration of the development of techniques of social regulation animated by psychiatric themes, the adjustment of institutional practices in the light of psychiatric considerations, and the instrumentalization of social relations in the service of psychiatric objectives – the minimization of mental pathology and the promotion of mental health. It also implies a different perspective from that common to most contemporary critiques of psychiatry.

The most powerful challenge to psychiatry over the last twenty years came from that set of loosely allied arguments known as anti-psychiatry. Central to the anti-psychiatric critique of psychiatry was an epistemological thesis, the assertion that the object of psychiatric knowledge and technique – 'mental illness' – either did not exist as an objective phenomenon or did not exist as an illness appropriate for medical attention. Whilst developments in critical psychiatry since the 1960s have been more prepared to acknowledge that severe and crippling mental distress has a reality and an anthropological generality that is not grasped by the notions of labelling and social construction, these writings have similarly tended to suggest that a critique of psychiatry should begin from an alternative account of the reality of such distress, of its true nature and origins. No doubt the question of the truth of mental disorders, how they may be understood conceptually and responded to therapeutically, must remain a key issue in debates over psychiatry. But we would argue that an analysis of the reality of mental distress cannot serve to establish what psychiatry is, or where it could or should go. A knowledge of the social functioning of psychiatry cannot be derived from a critique of its theoretical inadequacies – not least because, as these essays show, such theoretical and therapeutic disputes are internal elements in the history and actuality of psychiatry. Rather than seeking to base our criticism of psychiatry upon the truth of madness, these studies reverse the direction of investigation; they suggest that it is more productive to take the reality of psychiatry rather than the reality of mental distress as the point of departure for our inquiries.

But the reality of psychiatry is rather different from the image painted in most critiques. Critical challenges to psychiatry since the 1960s have taken as their target the 'hard' end of medical and institutional psychiatry – the asylum, custodialism, psycho-surgery, electro-convulsive therapy and the use of drugs. They have offered, explicitly or implicitly, a remodelled, 'softer' psychiatry – in therapeutic communities, in 'the community', using family therapy, psychotherapy or other talking cures – as an alternative and a solution to the problems of psychiatry. These essays dispute this diagram of psychiatry as radically divided between a repressive medicalized sector and a life-enhancing psychotherapeutic alternative. A rather different set of contours for psychiatry is sketched out, one that seeks to take account both of what psychiatry is as a body of professional expertise and techniques, and of what it informs and enables within a wider set of practices for the regulation of behaviour. This contemporary psychiatric system extends far beyond the medicalized institution. It comprises a widespread but loosely related assemblage of practices that seek to regulate individual subjectivities and manage personal and social relations in the name of the minimization of mental disorder and the promotion of mental health.

Within such a psychiatric system, the relations between psychiatry and psychology are particularly significant. Whilst they clearly have distinct professional characteristics, theoretical systems and technologies of normalization, these essays draw attention to the dependencies, interrelations and collaborations that have existed and continue to exist between them. This interplay of the psychiatric and the psychological would itself be sufficient to reveal the limitations of critiques based upon a straightforward opposition to medical expertise. Once it is also recognized that medical psychiatry has long accepted a role for social and psychological factors in the precipitation and prevention of mental disorder, and has actively solicited alliances with non-medical professions in establishing the new territory of psychiatry, it becomes clear that the reality of the psychiatric system cannot be understood in terms of the conceptions of 'the medical model' and 'medical imperialism' that animate much of the critical literature.

Similarly, the contemporary psychiatric system does not operate as implied by the sociological notions of social control. The elements of this system are not all connected in origin or inspiration; although they necessarily function alongside one another, their relations are as much those of contingency as of complicity – they intersect, aid, hinder, compete and contradict. The notion of social control also misleads us in seeking to understand what is distinctive about this system. This lies in the emergence of mental health as an objective and of strategies for the regulation of individuals, families, institutions and populations in relation to such an objective. Even if one wished to argue that this was a form of 'control', it would be necessary to understand it in terms of the radically new set of relations between state and civil society that have taken shape in the second half of the twentieth century. In this new nexus the state is not the fundamental source or locus of social power. Psychiatry, in the sense of discipline, a technology and a way of thinking, is a constitutive feature of these new power relations, enabling mental health to be seen as a national asset, an economic advantage, a social necessity and a personal desire.

The essays in this volume develop a number of new and somewhat different themes for the analysis of the power of contemporary psychiatry. In the first, Peter Miller locates recent critiques of psychiatry in relation to transformations of the psychiatric system itself, and the wider political context that has enabled psychiatry to become a public issue. This analysis shows that critiques of psychiatry – whether directed at the institutional existence of psychiatry, its theoretical codes, its juridical legitimacy or its technological efficacy – have been of crucial significance in strategies for its modernization and transformation, whether these are failed or successful. Political and radical critiques of psychiatry, even those that have sought to pose fundamental questions of what psychiatry is, have ended up inspiring programmes for the technical reorganization and extension of psychiatry.

At least one element in the failure of these radical challenges to psychiatry to achieve their goal has been their inability to grasp the nature of the contemporary psychiatric system. In order to evaluate their critique, and the alternatives that are proposed, it is necessary first to describe this system. In his survey of aspects of the recent history of psychiatry in Britain, Nikolas Rose dispels the belief that 'the community' as the territory for psychiatric activity is a recent invention. The emergence of this territory has little to do with the myth of community as a spontaneous network of supportive relations of personal intimacy and social cohesion. But, conversely, the language of community should not be seen merely as either a rationalization for a strategy designed to minimize the welfare expenditure of a state in fiscal crisis, or a legitimation for an extension of the control apparatus of the state. The development of a psychiatry of the community is linked to a transformation in the rationale of government and the social vocation of psychiatry, in which a whole range of social ills come to be seen as flowing not so much from major mental pathologies as from minor and remediable failures of individual subjectivities to function at their optimally adjusted level. The contemporary psychiatric system seeks not merely to eliminate mental illness, but to manage all aspects of life with the aim of producing and maintaining mentally healthy citizens. The promotion of socially competent and trouble-free psyches has become central to institutional efficiency, social tranquillity and personal happiness. The power of psychiatry today must be understood in relation to these positive aspirations of psychiatry, and interrogated in relation to the proliferation of strategies for the social management of personal capacities in the name of mental health.

One significant set of critiques of both institutional psychiatry and community psychiatry has come from within feminism. With respect to the contemporary reorganization of psychiatry, it has been argued that the closure of institutions in the name of the community is one element in a strategy that seeks to transfer the burden of caring for the bulk of the mentally distressed into the private domain, which means on to wives and mothers. Whilst there is, no doubt, much truth in this argument, the essays in this volume suggest that the decarceration of psychiatry must be understood also in terms of its positive aspirations. Whilst the promotion of mental health has been added to the domestic responsibilities of women, the psychiatric community would ideally incorporate the 'private' domain of the home and family into the field of social management by professional expertise.

The critique of psychiatric sexism has been directed to the heart of psychiatric knowledge and practice itself. Women are more likely than men to be the recipients of the ministrations of psychiatry, no matter whether one is considering the doling out of tranquillizers by general practitioners or admissions to psychiatric hospitals. It has been argued that psychiatry is sexist and that it reflects and supports a patriarchal system. Psychiatry is accused of branding as mentally ill those who are casualities of an oppressive social order and of utilizing stereotypes of sexually appropriate behaviour, pathologizing and, hence, policing those who deviate from them. Further, psychiatry has been criticized on the grounds that it seeks neither to cure the conditions that women suffer, nor to challenge their causes but merely to patch up the victims and enable them to cope with the demands made upon them by a patriarchal society.

In her discussion of some of these issues, Hilary Allen questions the notion that contemporary psychiatry is constitutively sexist, and shows how such a position makes it impossible to understand the specific ways in which psychiatry encounters women. Indeed in contemporary psychiatry there is no significant attention to the relation between gender and mental health, and psychiatry is reluctant to intervene when gender-role deviation is the main 'symptom'. Whilst psychiatry, like other social practices, echoes conventional expectations of gender, gender-role maintenance is not fundamental, but incidental to psychiatric practice. Ironically, it is within feminist therapy that one finds a constitutive 'psychiatry' of the feminine in which women's troubles are seen as arising from their psychical condition as women. Such a psychiatry of the feminine does not challenge the psychiatric system but, paradoxically, extends its remit, potentially, to all women.

One significant development within psychiatry in recent years has been its confrontation with the question of race. Against what we might refer to as a latent racism of psychiatric expertise and competence, there has recently emerged an attempt to relativize cultural difference. The name given to this is transcultural psychiatry. Kobena Mercer questions the concepts of 'culture' and 'ethnicity' that are central to such an enterprise. The emphasis within transcultural psychiatry upon the education of professionals in the characteristics of cultural diversity, in focusing our attention upon the problem of communication between doctor and patient, limits our analysis of how black people encounter the institutional workings of the psychiatric system. What the transculturalist option effects is a transformation of race into a phenomenon that may be utilized with psychiatric knowledge, and an expansion of the potential points of psychiatric surveillance and intervention to the ways in which different ethnic groups organize their familial and kinship relations, their gender and sexual relations and their modes of child-rearing. Simultaneously, it transforms racism into a problem that can be dealt with at the level of psychiatric practice and technique. Transculturalism within psychiatry can thus be seen as one of a range of related practices for the government of cultural diversity within the contemporary welfare state.

Within a broadened definition of what constitutes the terrain of psychiatry, crucial issues may be seen to arise in the intersection of concerns over mental health with the world of employment and unemployment. What is at issue here is the relationship between the economic and the psychological. To operate on the latter is to enhance the former. Such a strategy depends not just on remedying the ill-effects of the economic machine, but on optimizing the level of functioning of the psychological machine and, thereby, enhancing the economic returns. A similar concern arises in relation to the unemployed, although the concern there is primarily with questions of motivation and morale. In his examination of these issues, Peter Miller shows how contemporary developments emphasize the bonding of individuals to their labour by means of a psychological commitment rather than by a wage, full employment now being conceived as a condition of both economic and psychological health. Similarly, in the proliferation of interventions aimed at the unemployed, one sees the emergence of a rationale that would seek to make unemployment a simulacrum of employment, lacking only the wage relation. As we move towards a final dominance of the psychological principle of work over the economic principle, it is appropriate to question this prioritization of the subjective dimensions of employment and unemployment over their economic dimensions.

Since the mid-1970s, first in the USA and later in Britain, one influential group of mental-health reformers have sought to use the law to promote their aims. They have posed their demands in terms of rights – both the rights of the mentally ill to services and treatment, and rights that would protect individuals from illegitimate confinement in hospital and from the forced administration of so-called treatments. Drawing heavily upon radical critiques of the scientific pretensions, objectivity and effectiveness of psychiatric diagnosis and treatment, they have sought to make the judicial instance the arbiter of the exercise of psychiatric power. Nikolas Rose analyses this strategy and identifies its fundamental limitations. Not only are such strategies unlikely to achieve substantive improvements in the position of mentally distressed individuals, but the language of rights effectively depoliticizes debate over the nature and organization of psychiatry. Rights strategies are mistaken in their analyses of psychiatric power and of the effects of legal mechanisms; paradoxically they are entirely consistent with the direction of psychiatric modernization. Despite their apparent opposition, contemporary psychiatry and rights-mindedness are based upon the same disputable notions of citizenship and personal autonomy, and share a rationale for the contractualization of subjectivity.

One other category that has been central to the relations of the legal and the psychiatric is that of psychopathy. This category, which in its modern form dates only from the Second World War, appears simultaneously uneasy and necessary for both psychiatry and the law. What it effects is a working relationship between these two great instances of social power in the regulation of a-social and anti-social behaviour which might seem, at face value, to be neither criminal enough to warrant prolonged confinement in prison nor mad enough to justify the compulsory attention of psychiatry. Shulamit Ramon's essay addresses these questions, describing the attempts of different professional groups, policy makers and legislators to either appropriate the category of psychopathy or to distance themselves from it. Whilst the status of the category remains problematic, and many of its aspirations have been disappointed, it nonetheless enables the state to accomplish the social management of a group of troublesome individuals, and enables psychiatry to sustain its mandate over socially undesirable conduct that falls outside the ambit of the system of criminal justice.

Of course, psychiatry has a presence within the criminal justice system itself. Over the past fifty years the psychiatric element in punishment has become increasingly evident. The role of psychiatry is varied, ranging from the preparation of psychiatric court reports to the routine administration of psychoactive drugs to prisoners, from the regimes of special hospitals and secure units to those in prison therapeutic communities. Much secrecy has previously surrounded the operation of the Prison Medical Service, with information coming to light principally in the form of occasional scandals, the autobiographies of ex-prisoners, or the radical critiques of those who denounce the complicity of psychiatry with a brutal system of criminal justice. In response, the Prison Medical Service has justified its role in terms of the need to treat psychiatrically disturbed prisoners, and the progressive part that can be played in reformatory regimes by a psychiatric knowledge of therapeutic milieux. Against such a justification must be placed the increasing recognition of the pathogenic psychiatric consequences of imprisonment itself. In an attempt to dispel the doubts and suspicions surrounding prison psychiatry, the Prison Medical Service and prison psychiatrists granted Pat Carlen extensive interviews, and her discussion of psychiatry in prisons is based also upon visits to many psychiatric facilities in prisons and much experience of prison research. This essay thus begins the long overdue investigation of the penal function of psychiatry. On the basis of a detailed discussion and judicious analysis of the reality of psychiatry in the prison system, Carlen argues that while the criminal has been psychiatrized the prison itself has withstood psychiatrization. The promises of psychiatry have been insufficient to establish it as the dominant power within the prison; instead it has been assimilated and refashioned within the power of the prison system itself.

Each of these essays raises, in one way or another, the issue of psychiatry's connection with political and social processes. In his reflections on this question, Colin Gordon considers the extent to which the social status and political ramifications of psychiatry arise from its character as a distinctive product –

and problem – of modern democracy. Psychiatry is intimately linked to the question of citizenship; in a bourgeois polity it is faced with the twin demands of participating in the preservation of norms of social conduct without violating constitutional propriety, and of restoring afflicted persons to their proper status as competent citizens. Such concerns should neither be seen as masking a project of political control nor as resolvable through some innovation of social policy: they are central to the existence of psychiatry as a political science. Whilst we need to treat the present language of community with vigilance and caution, this analysis directs our attention to a prospect of community that should not be confused either with a problem of individual liberty or with the reorganization of techniques for the professional and administrative management of high-risk sectors of the social body.

What lessons can be learned from these studies concerning the contemporary politics of mental health? Perhaps only a questioning of the assumption that what we need is a genuine community psychiatry, a comprehensive discipline of mental health. It is understandable that we should be attracted by the belief that mental disorders are conditions arising from social existence rather than biological processes, and the correlative hope that the miseries engendered by unemployment, sexual incompatability, infertility, bad housing, poverty, urban decay, violence, troublesome children and so forth might be solved or ameliorated by psychiatric knowledge and expertise. But rather than extending the remit of psychiatry to the manifold problems of social and personal life, should we not ask of psychiatry that it takes as its rationale the problem of cure rather than the project of normalization?

These essays suggest that we might pause before evaluating our personal lives, our experiences of labour and our social relationships in psychiatric terms. The pursuit of a contentment conceived in terms of mental health, a happiness conceived in terms of subjective liberation, or a quality of life conceived in terms of psychlogical fulfillment, both inaugurates an interminable quest for an unrealizable goal and inspires a continual expansion of psychiatric expertise. We should exercise caution before encouraging the proliferation of devices for the regulation of subjectivity, and the transformation of the self into an object for inspection and rectification in the name of mental health.

1

Critiques of psychiatry and critical sociologies of madness

Peter Miller

Central to those practices that have constituted psychiatry over the past century and a half is the process of critique. Throughout its existence psychiatry has been subjected to a series of fundamental attacks. It has been accused of being excessively repressive and carceral. It has also been accused of being insufficiently supervisory and insufficiently curative of those individuals prone to potential insane acts. The former has predominated in recent years, with sociology and historiography significant contributors to this critique. The aim of this essay is to examine this process of critique, the sociological analyses that have been a part of it, and the links that can be identified between these critiques and the modernizations of psychiatry's functioning. I begin by looking at critiques of psychiatry in the nineteenth century, and then continue by addressing the range of critiques that have emerged in this century with a view to registering the different strategies that have developed for the modernization of psychiatry. Next, I examine the recent Anglo-American sociological and historical literature that is critical of psychiatry. I then discuss a separate tradition of historiography – that associated with the works of Michel Foucault and Robert Castel – and argue that it has significant advantages over that of the Anglo-American approach.

The principal arguments of this essay can be summarized as follows. First, far from being a new phenomenon, critiques of psychiatry date almost from its inception, they are an integral and constitutive part of psychiatry's institutional, therapeutic, juridical and professional practice. Psychiatry is inconceivable without such critiques, which range from limited ones internal to the profession to wholesale denunciations from outside. Critiques of psychiatry have had such a vigorous existence for nearly a century and a half that one is entitled to talk of 'anti-psychiatries' in the plural rather than 'anti-psychiatry' in the singular. We should, however, distinguish between those critiques of psychiatry that have been limited to issues such as different therapeutic devices, and those that mount a fundamental challenge to its authority.

Critiques of psychiatry are not wholly external to its functioning. They can be related to what we can term modernizations of the psychiatric apparatus, as well as to failed strategies for its reform. The history of psychiatry is a history of fundamental transformations of its institutional, theoretical, professional and juridical existence. The critiques mounted against psychiatry, both from inside and outside, are a significant element in this process of modernization and transformation. We can, for instance, relate the critique of the asylum coming from anti-psychiatry to the emergence in the 1960s of a move in a number of countries away from the asylum as the administrative and institutional basis for psychiatry. This is not to suggest that we can explain the emergence of 'community psychiatry' by exclusive reference to anti-psychiatry. But, nonetheless, anti-psychiatry provided support for an anti-institutional lobby both within and on the margins of the psychiatric apparatus.

Second, I identify the different levels at which critiques of psychiatry have been mounted. I refer to four different levels: institutional, theoretical, juridical, and technological. The institutional critique has focused on both the asylum and also its absence. The theoretical critique has been addressed to particular theoretical categories psychiatry uses in its attempt to explain mental illness; it has also been directed at the very concept of mental illness itself. The juridical critique has had a number of dimensions, sometimes concerning the rights of patients, sometimes the modes of supervision and regulation of internment, and sometimes the legal status of the insane person as a citizen. Irrespective of its level, however, we are entitled to suggest that the juridical critique is the visible dimension of a profound series of interchanges between two distinct strategies for the regulation of asocial behaviours. Such interchanges, I argue, are a central and constitutive aspect of psychiatry's existence. The critique of the technological level of psychiatry refers to a level of functioning mid-way beween a theoretical category and a 'mere' technical operation. The 'moral treatment' of the nineteenth century is an example of this technological dimension, in that it brought together the doctor and the patient in a particular environment – the asylum – and with a particular notion of treatment. A displacement of one of these elements would have brought about a disruption to the very practice of moral treatment.

Third, I argue that what has been called anti-psychiatry has bequeathed to us a set of notions that hinder our understanding of psychiatry and also the process of critique. These notions form a triptych – that psychiatry is predominantly an affair of the asylum, madness and medicalization – that continues to inform historical analysis and contemporary critique. This focus holds out the hope that we might be able to ground a critique of psychiatry on the basis of the residual reality of madness. If we could only establish what madness is, then psychiatry's claims to pronounce on it and to treat it could be evaluated.

My argument is that we will do better if we turn the question around and *take psychiatry rather than madness* as the starting point of our enquiries, and then proceed to look at the range of behaviours it addresses. Madness as the constitutive object of psychiatry's existence is only a transitory phenomenon. For more than half a century now, the focus of psychiatry's concern has been shifting from madness to the less severe forms of behavioural disturbances and personal distress. In taking madness as the central point of a critique of psychiatry, what is obscured by sociologists is the fundamental reorganization of psychiatry that has taken place since the First World War. The central concern today of any critical confrontation with psychiatry should no longer be to denounce psychiatry's medicalizing of personal distress, and the asylum as the institutional embodiment of the power of the psychiatrist. We should be paying closer attention to psychiatry's *social vocation*, its increasing distance from an absolute segregative model of treatment. The dominant model of contemporary psychiatry is not the isolated and deranged individual, but the mildly distressed individual in the family and in the community.

Fourth, I propose some elements of an alternative mode of

explanation and understanding of psychiatry, one that owes much to the works of Michel Foucault and Robert Castel.[1] In general terms such an approach refuses to explain psychiatry's existence by reference to baldly stated exigencies of social control or the requirements of capitalist economic production relations. This is not because psychiatry is seen to be entirely independent of such phenomena. It is, rather, a result of a different interpretation of this interrelation, one in which psychiatry is seen to be implicated in capitalist social relations in a constitutive and positive role. Psychiatry as an institution needs to be understood in its intersection and competition with a range of other social practices, including the judicial apparatus. Attention needs to be directed at the process of psychiatrization, the means by which specific behavioural characteristics ranging from insanity to everyday unhappiness become constituted as psychiatry's legitimate and often exclusive concern. We need also to address the question of what institutional psychiatry comprises.

My argument is that to understand contemporary psychiatry we need to understand the heterogeneity of psychiatric practice, the different therapeutic, institutional and professional resources it has at its disposal. The term 'psychiatric system' is a way of designating this heterogeneity and coherence. It refers to an ensemble of diverse theoretical categories, therapeutic practices, institutional sites, and legal codifications, which are to a significant extent interdependent. Understood like this psychiatry is no one thing, but a loosely assembled set of practices that extends from the 'hard' core represented by the asylum and electro-shock, passes through the recent and emergent community mental-health moves, and extends to the 'soft' end that takes the form of various psychotherapies. The history of psychiatry is a history of reorganizations and transformations of this 'system'.

Critiques of psychiatry in the nineteenth century

The nineteenth century was a period in which the insane, having been separated from the criminal classes and the indigent, became the privileged object for a specific type of internment, one that had therapeutic ambitions, however attenuated these proved to be in reality. This was, as one author has remarked, psychiatry's 'golden age'.[2] It was a period in which a degree of coherence and articulation was attained between the asylum as an institutional site for psychiatry's operation, a theoretical account of mental illness, a legal code for the regulation of psychiatry, and a technology that helped to effect the articulation of these different elements. The nineteenth century was, however, also a period in which all of these elements were attacked. There were profound and fundamental challenges to psychiatry's ability to intervene on the insane person towards a curative or therapeutic end. Psychiatry's ambition to provide a curative machine in the shape of the asylum, and a theoretical code for the understanding of mental disturbances was attacked at every level.

The first level of critique concerned psychiatry's institutional apparatus – the asylum. It is the most striking of the critiques directed at nineteenth-century psychiatry as well as the most resounding in terms of the echoes that remain after more than a century. In countries as different as Britain, France and the USA, the asylum was attacked for a wide range of reasons.[3] There was a general attack on the conditions in which people were incarcerated and the brutality and deprivations of the environment. Institutions were described as deficient in every comfort, as dirty, and providing the most appalling living environment.

Psychiatry's institutional apparatus was already viewed in the mid-nineteenth century as predominantly carceral rather than curative and there soon emerged a critique of the principle of isolation itself. It is important to recall that isolation from one's everyday social environment in an asylum was generally seen as having therapeutic effects. Prompt removal of the insane person from his/her home environment, or 'community', was viewed as an important condition for the recovery of his/her sanity. In France, as early as 1860, this principle of isolation as a curative mechanism was opened up to criticism. A commission representing the most prominent alienists of the time was dispatched to inspect the Belgian village of Gheel where the insane lived in a state of semi-liberty amongst the peasants.[4] This was only the beginnings of what was to emerge as a sustained attack on the principle of isolation as a general requirement for the treatment of mental distress. In Britain there was a similar movement of opinion around the same time, the first reports appearing in British journals in 1857.[5]

There were mixed reports on what took place at Gheel, but the conclusions are less important than the way it functioned as a model for an alternative mode of care of the insane. Instead of segregation and isolation, what Gheel offered was care based on a domestic principle of familial-community support.

The critique of the asylum was a critique also of its capacity to operate as the properly medical and curative environment it aspired to be. The asylums were faced with an increasing tide of heterogeneous individuals, including lunatics, idiots, epileptics, paralytics, the elderly and the physically infirm. As asylums grew in size during the middle decades of the nineteenth century there emerged increasingly vociferous statements that suggested that the asylum was incapable of operating as a medical institution, that it was becoming a place in which an undifferentiated mixture of individuals were gathered together, whose common feature was simply that they were shut away. Critics were to argue that the organized monotony of the asylum was simply a device for maintaining order rather than effecting a cure.

The second level of critique concerned psychiatry's theoretical framework. Throughout its history psychiatry has opted for a degree of eclecticism in the analysis of mental disorders, particularly with regard to the causal role attributed to social and moral factors. Today the dominant model is one in which organic and genetic factors are viewed as underlying causes, whilst social, familial and environmental pressures function as the 'trigger'.[6] In the early decades of the nineteenth century the situation was different. A psychological model was dominant, within which the notion of 'moral treatment' occupied a central place.[7] 'Moral', as used here, was not a critical label but referred to a space distinct from the nerves, the fibres, the ducts of the body and their contents. Emotions, daily routines, the enjoyment of luxury figured in this explanatory schema. In the second half of the nineteenth century this dominant psychological model was displaced by means of a critique that centred on psychiatry's aspiration to secure as its theoretical basis a fully medical model of mental disorder that would place it closer to general medicine. If madness was really a mental illness, it should be possible to explain it by reference to a causal mechanism. Mental disturbance was no longer seen as exclusively moral, but the link between morality and madness was not broken. Morality was, rather, redistributed according to a schema that distinguished predisposing and exciting causes.

The critique was effective and the displacement that occurred in the second half of the nineteenth century entailed a demand for an aetiology based on hidden causal mechanisms rather than a description or classification of signs. This was to be of the same order as the aetiology of general medicine: it was to seek to identify a specific and constitutive lesion. As one author has put it, a move away from a 'social phenomenology of disorder',[8] and toward general medicine. But we should be careful when interpreting this shift, for it was not a question of a simple inversion, a capture of the theoretical knowledge of insanity by organicist medicine. It was, rather, a shift that had the effect of producing a combined medico-psychological account of mental illness. A somatic aetiology gained an increasingly central position within psychiatric knowledge, but this was never to completely disperse the psychological model. And, in so far as the psychological model provided a direct link to a moral conception of insanity, the continuation of this connection was assured.

The third level of critique was directed at the legal codification of psychiatry's existence. Central here was the issue of internments, which had two dimensions. One of these was the supervision of the world of internment itself. The other concerned access to the asylum – the legal regulation of the internment process. As I have suggested already, psychiatry's relationship with the law consists of a series of interchanges between two distinct strategies of social regulation. With regard to internment we can characterize this interrelationship as one in which the judicial apparatus makes constant attempts to actively intervene in the process of access to the asylum, to establish itself as arbiter of the legitimacy of a psychiatric internment'.[9] As with the other levels of critique this again is one of long standing and is not specific to Britain. In France the law of 1838, which is still in force, made psychiatrists the deciding authority in matters of internment. As early as the 1860s, however, there was a government commission investigating the functioning of the law, and in 1870 proposals for the constitution of a jury that would have exclusive power to decide on admissions.[10] These proposals for reform were unsuccessful, but their very existence over one hundred years ago suggests that more is at issue than a simple matter of legal safeguards.

In Britain, the nature of attempts to get the law to take an active role in psychiatric internments was different. It consisted principally of moves to provide legal supervision of the powers of psychiatrists rather than to wholly displace them. Two pieces of legislation had accorded psychiatrists their power over the carceral world of the asylum. The first of these was the Madhouse Act of 1828, which introduced legal requirements for medical attendance in an asylum. Arrangements had to be made for a doctor to visit patients at least once a week and to sign a register weekly. It also provided for a commission to licence and supervise lunatic asylums, although the activities of the commission were confined to the Metropolitan area. The 1845 Lunatics Act extended such legal regulation. A bill providing for extensive and detailed inspection of all asylums in the country was introduced and passed in 1842. This was formalized in two related pieces of legislation in 1845, which established a permanent national Lunacy Commission with powers to inspect all types of asylums, and which introduced a principle of compulsion into the erection of county and borough asylums for pauper lunatics.

Various writers have interpreted this legislation as the medical profession securing an almost exclusive prerogative to control the treatment of the insane.[11] However, whilst it is true that this legislation provided a mandate for the medical profession, this was not an unconditional and perpetual one. It was rather one that established that the boundary between the legal and medical regulation of asocial behaviours is potentially a fluid one. To the extent that psychiatry was recognized as a medical enterprise it was open to the intrusion of legal forms of regulation of its functioning, both with regard to admissions and the internal world of the asylum.

The fourth and final level of critique refers to what I have called the 'technological' dimension of psychiatry's functioning. In the nineteenth century moral treatment provides the best example of this. One way of interpreting the stakes surrounding its role is to view it as part of a binary struggle to establish a medical as opposed to a non-medical model for the treatment of insanity.[12] I am, however, attracted by a different interpretation, one that locates moral treatment within its strategic role in the emergence of carceral psychiatry.

In the mid-nineteenth century psychiatry was not in a strong position to entrench itself as the unquestioned arbiter of the world of unreason. It had very weak curative credentials. It lacked a strong conceptual basis on which to establish an organic aetiology of mental illness. It also lacked a secure professional structure. Most importantly, however, it lacked the means by which it could function outside the asylum. The critique of moral treatment was not just a critique of its non-medical basis. In Morel's formulations it was a critique also of psychiatry's inability to move beyond the walls of the asylum and to join forces with a preventive hygienic strategy of social regulation that was at issue.[13] As Morel was to state: 'We are no longer confronted with an isolated individual, but in the presence of a society, and the power of the means of action should be appropriate to the objective.'[14] From the critique of moral treatment reforms could proceed in two directions:that of making the asylum a more strongly medicalized environment, or that of a social-hygienic strategy of preventive interventions directed at the individual in his/her social milieu. Schematically, we can say that in Britain the former strategy was pursued in the second half of the nineteenth century. As Rose argues in chapter 2, the latter strategy emerged in Britain in the 1920s and 1930s. Community mental-health centres, which in Britain are still only in an embryonic stage, can be viewed as an attempt to devise an administrative framework that incorporates both dimensions, as well as many other intermediary operations within its interstices.

It is difficult to summarize what was at stake in all these different levels of critique mounted against psychiatry in the nineteenth century. But it is, nonetheless, clear that *psychiatry's carceral apparatus provides a strong linking thread across them all.* The critique of the conditions of internment, the modes of access to the asylum, the conceptual basis for psychiatric internments, and the legal regulation of psychiatry's functioning all took as their target the asylum. What resulted from this series of interchanges was not a medicalization of madness but an attempt to medicalize the *asylum.* Today one can say conclusively that this project has failed. Since the 1950s and 1960s the psychiatric profession itself has accepted that the classic asylum can never become the genuinely medical environment it once aspired to be. But it has taken over a century for psychiatry to devise a formula for providing the infrastructure that can support a more plausible aspiration to a fully medical status, whilst being able at the same time to strengthen its social vocation. Viewed in this way the critiques of psychiatry in the nineteenth century represent a series of early attempts to devise an institutional, conceptual and legal framework for psychiatry, whose locus was not the asylum but the community. The decarceration of psychiatry has, however, proved to be as important and lengthy a process as the decarceration of the mental patient.

Critiques of psychiatry in the twentieth century

These share with the critiques of the nineteenth century an almost exclusive concern with its carceral apparatus, the asylum. From anti-psychiatry to mainstream psychiatry there have been attacks on various aspects of the asylum. Not all of these have sought its abolition. They have, nonetheless, provided support to a strategy that has been termed 'decarceration'.[15] In the worst examples of implementation of such a policy this has meant simply putting patients on the streets. This negative dimension of community mental health often means removing support. It can also mean changing the site of the asylum and reducing its size.[16] There is, however, another aspect to community mental health that is missed by those intent on attacking its shameful effects. This is the attempt to establish an institutional, administrative and therapeutic apparatus for psychiatry located within the 'community'. In the USA such a framework was established with the 1963 Community Mental Health Center and Retardation Act. In Britain the 1959 Mental Health Act provided for the possibility of such a move. The principal development following this legislation was, however, not the creation of a community mental-health apparatus but the integration of psychiatry into general hospitals. In France in 1960 the 'sectorization' of French psychiatry brought about a change towards the community as the locus for the deployment of psychiatric expertise.

My argument is that those critiques of psychiatry that take its institutional form as their explicit focus provide a key to understanding all the other critiques. It is in relation to psychiatry's institutional existence that the other aspects of its functioning are to be defined. Similarly, it is in relation to this institutional form that the other modes of critique can be viewed. One can divide the twentieth-century critiques levelled at the asylum into three broad groups. Whilst only approximate, this grouping has merits in that it allows us to identify the different strategies for the modernization of psychiatry to which they contribute.

The first of these lines of institutional critique can be termed *therapeutic*. This consists of a proposal to re-establish the therapeutic and curative ideals of the asylum, and to retain the asylum as their site of operation. It can be a powerful critique for all that. The eminent figure of Maxwell Jones represents one strand of this line of thought. He sought to retain the asylum, but to transform it into a genuinely therapeutic and curative establishment. This was a distinctive project to systematically utilize the positive possibilities of the institution and its administration for therapy.[17] A second strand sought to merely minimize the adverse effects of the asylum. This is represented by the work of Russell Barton.[18] 'Institutional neurosis' was the term Barton coined to designate a disease entity identifiable by apathy, lack of initiative, loss of interest in the outside world, submissiveness and resignation. However this did not lead Barton to recommend the abolition of the asylum. According to him the asylum should be retained, but attempts should also be made to rectify the negative consequences of institutional living.

The second line of critique of the asylum can be termed *political* in that its two principal dimensions concerned the power of the institution. The asylum was to be criticized for the power it gave society over certain categories of deviant individuals. It was also attacked for the power it conferred on the psychiatrist over the patient. Sometimes these two elements occur together, as in the writings of Franco Basaglia,[19] and sometimes separately.[20] For Basaglia the asylum was an institution of violence and oppression in which society exerted its power over the incomprehensibility of mental illness in the name of science. For his part, Goffman examined the processes through which the internal functioning of the asylum 'recruited' individuals into the moral careers characteristic of mental patients. As a 'total institution' the asylum exerted on behalf of society an absolute domination over the lives of those individuals who entered as patients.

The third line of critique of the asylum can be termed *reformist*. This is meant literally and not pejoratively. Under this heading can be placed a range of critiques, all of which have attempted reform of the asylum. The reform in question has a twofold character. First, it concerns the nature, size and functioning of the asylum. Second, it concerns the place of the asylum within the overall structure of what I have termed the psychiatric system. On the latter point the critique seeks to effect a redefinition of the role of the asylum, which should no longer be to provide the almost exclusive institutional framework for psychiatry, and which should be supplemented by a range of new institutions and practices.[21]

It is this third critique that has won ground in Britain. The asylum is criticized in the name of a restriction of its applicability, and of its insertion within a new institutional and administrative framework. The advantages of such a strategy are evident. It takes into account what I have termed the political critique of the asylum, yet insists on its retention on practical grounds, and also in the name of a comprehensive psychiatric service. And it provides a framework for a series of new professional alliances between psychiatry and professions such as social work.

It is, however, not just psychiatry's institutional arm that has been fiercely attacked in the twentieth century. As in the nineteenth century we see psychiatry's theoretical framework, its juridical basis, and its technological aspect all challenged also. The same four levels of critique occur, with the same prominence of the institutional critique. The critiques of its theoretical credentials have been varied and have concerned particular theoretical and diagnostic entities, an alleged excessively medical/somatic, as opposed to psychological, model for psychiatry, and also the very concept of mental illness. One category central to contemporary psychiatric practice, and which has been subjected to intense criticism for its weak diagnostic accuracy, uncertain aetiology and dustbin-like character, is that of schizophrenia. On the concept of schizophrenia, even the psychiatrist Anthony Clare has gone so far as to declare: 'Whether there is one condition, called schizophrenia, or several which are currently mixed up together under a common classificatory label is still an open question.

So too is the controversial problem of the cause.'[22] The critique of psychiatry's theoretical basis for being excessively medical-/somatic has come from two quarters. One of these is a modernizing group within psychiatry, or sometimes on its borders, that seeks to reform psychiatry by reducing the significance of the medical model and installing in its place a psychological model of disease and cure.The other is a more sociological mode of critique that equates medicalization with social control, one that depicts psychology in a positive light, as something good and to be promoted against the evils of medicalization.[23]

The critique of the very concept of mental illness is one that has come predominantly from within psychiatry itself, although not within mainstream psychiatry. The most famous example of this questioning of the notion of mental illness is the inversion in Laing's early work of the schizophrenic experience such that it came to be viewed as a rational and sane process. The implication is that there exists no more than a range of different ways of interpreting and experiencing the world – a primarily philosophical position.

A critique of the juridical basis of psychiatry has featured prominently in recent years in both Britain and the USA. The issues here concern patients' rights in general, the status of these rights in cases of internment and, in a broader sense, the question of the respective powers of the medical and legal professions over the mental patient. As psychiatry's carceral apparatus has been increasingly subjected to attack, its power over the process of entry to the asylum has also been called into question. The interchange or competition is between a strategy based on legal forms of argument and proof, on the one hand, and psychiatric modes of diagnosis, assessment and judgment, on the other. The rights argument might be viewed in this respect as the judicial equivalent of anti-psychiatry's valorization of subjectivity.

The final level of critique of psychiatry concerns the *technological* aspect of its operation. Despite the changes in psychiatry's mode of functioning over the past century, the issues here are strikingly similar to those that confronted psychiatry in the nineteenth century. Broadly speaking the issue that persists is this: how might we effect a salvage operation of the asylum, reinstating its aspiration to be a genuinely therapeutic environment, but doing so by restricting its sphere of operation and supplementing it by a range of mechanisms whereby it can operate on mental distress outside the walls of the asylum? A number of authors have offered support to the argument that since the early decades of this century, with the invention of the neuroses and the creation of such hygienic strategies as child-guidance clinics and clinics for the overhaul of entire families, an appropriate technology has been sought.[24] From being the last recourse in times of crisis and a proponent of exclusion and isolation, psychiatry's reformers would hope to place it as the first-line helper. Yet again, the issue here is the move away from the asylum towards non-carceral psychiatric interventions.

The therapeutic strategy for the modernization of psychiatry has little prospect of success today. Professional and public opinion is against the curative aspirations of a strategy based on reinstating the large isolated asylum as the almost exclusive locus of psychiatric activity. The objective of the political strategy is, by contrast, a complete dismantling of the asylum; it attacks the powers the asylum confers on psychiatrists over mentally distressed individuals. This has, however, also failed in Britain. Such a sweeping attack has always been regarded as naive by the psychiatric establishment, including the more progressive of its members. Its significance has, however, been its refusal to accept the separation of psychiatry and politics. This was helped by the redefinition of the conception of politics that occurred in the 1960s and that led to the inclusion of issues of personal liberation within the sphere of politics. As Castel has stated, this was a redefinition of the sphere of the political that allowed psychiatry to enter the realm of political critique.[25] The decline of such a conception of politics in the 1980s goes a long way towards explaining the decline of this strategy within a politics of psychiatry.

The reformist strategy is strongly critical of the asylum and of its non-curative and even iatrogenic effects. This is undertaken, however, in the name of *another* institutional, administrative and therapeutic apparatus – a new series of sites and practices within which the asylum has a place – albeit one of diminished importance. Such a strategy not only has the merits of 'realism', but of comprehensiveness in regard to the various critiques of psychiatry. It can incorporate within it the more popular radical critiques of the asylum as well as the more restrained calls for its modification. It offers a basis for the new professional alliances that will increasingly be needed as the policy of community mental health gradually installs itself. It offers a positive response to those critics of psychiatry who have sought to defend or establish the rights of mental patients. And it offers a great deal also to those who have argued that a greater role be attributed to psychological as opposed to medical models. The reformist strategy has emerged, one might say, as the 'natural' outgrowth of the varied critiques that have been mounted against psychiatry this century.

From anti-psychiatry to critical sociologies and historiographies of madness

Recent critiques of psychiatry based on the sociology and historiography of madness can be differentiated from earlier ones in two important respects. First, Anglo-American anti-psychiatry rose to prominence within a political culture in which notions of personal autonomy and subjectivity were accorded an increasingly central position. In this respect, much of anti-psychiatry's success can be attributed to its role within a more general process of cultural critique that extended beyond the boundaries of psychiatry. This accounts in large measure for anti-psychiatry's achievement in making psychiatry a public phenomenon.[26] Second, anti-psychiatry was primarily a critique of the more overtly repressive dimensions of psy- chiatry's practice – the asylum, electro-shock treatment, and the powers of the psychiatric profession. The critique here was primarily of the medicalization of deviance and of the powers society invested in psychiatry to ensure that this was seen to be carried out scientifically. Together these two features largely explain anti-psychiatry's success as well as its downfall. As the political culture within which it emerged declined, and as the attack on the medicalization of deviance proved increasingly wide of the mark, anti-psychiatry fell to the wayside. Or, rather, it changed track and was shunted into a sociological siding. It is there that it remains, changed a little by the years and supplemented by one or two new concepts and a modicum of historical evidence. In this form it can no longer be regarded a viable framework for the analysis or critique of psychiatry. Its inability to effectively engage with and challenge institutional psychiatry stems largely from its inability to grasp the nature of the contemporary psychiatric system. This system consists, as I have argued, of an ensemble of elements – theoretical accounts, institutional sites, legal codifications and therapeutic practices – that often compete and are related to specific strategies of social regulation. The asylum and medicalization are only two aspects of this system, not its entirety.

Anti-psychiatry and the more recent critical sociologies and historiographies of madness can be located along two dimensions – the diachronic and the synchronic. The diachronic entails a historical view of contemporary practices of psychiatry in terms of their continuation of a centuries-old practice of marginalization and confinement of deviance. From the witch-craze to the asylum the principle is considered to be the same – the confinement of those who are different and whom society refuses to tolerate. History here functions as a criterion for rendering intelligible the present. The synchronic looks at psychiatric practice at one particular moment in time, and entails a view of how psychiatry operates on specific behavioural characteristics of the individual, siphoning off its concerns from a vast pool of behaviours subjected to various distinct practices of social control (medicine, law, social work, etc.). Anti-psychiatry and current critical sociologies of madness obscure the analytical distinctiveness of these two aspects of psychiatric practice. The synchronic is collapsed into the diachronic, obliterating the novelty of the contemporary psychiatric system that has been establishing itself over the past half century, and reducing the explanatory framework to a number of rudimentary theoretical propositions centring on the notion of social control. One can forgive psychiatrists for experiencing a certain weariness in face of the monotony of the critique.

The attempt to explain contemporary psychiatry by its supposed origins five centuries ago is not just an academic exercise, it serves also to inform a politics of psychiatry. If psychiatry has failed to separate itself from its dubious origins then, the critique goes, history contains within itself a certain political logic. We can, on this assumption, have no truck with a practice that seeks to hide its overtly repressive actions with a cloak of scientific legitimacy. So, whilst psychiatry comforts itself with propagandist notions that it is developing and progressing towards sophisticated modes of treating mental distress, this critical sociology in turn comforts itself with the notion that what is emerging is an increasingly refined network of social control.

Anti-psychiatry is, of course, only a convenient label for grouping together a number of persons, writings and institutional practices. Of the former, the most prominent figures that appear under this heading are Goffman, Laing, Cooper and Szasz. The studies of Scheff and Rosenhan come into this category.[27] There have also been attempts to place the French philosopher and historian Michel Foucault under this heading, a categorization that is given apparent credence by the appearance of his *Madness and Civilization* in a series edited by Laing and introduced by David Cooper. I argue below, however, that to construe Foucault as an 'anti-psychiatrist' is mistaken. Anti-psychiatry is not just a matter of a number of names that can be counted on the fingers of one hand. It has been a phenomenon with the status of a wider cultural event. It found a cinematic form in films such as *One Flew over the Cuckoo's Nest*, *In Two Minds* and *Family Life*, and a literary version exemplified in the early days by Antonin Artaud and later on by Laing's literary writings.

The merit of anti-psychiatry has been to offer an interpretation of psychiatry that began with the personal and experiential dimension of the mental patient. Psychiatry's official practice and discourse was interrupted in this way by a view that draws attention to the deprivations and powerlessness of institutional existence (Goffman) and of becoming and being 'mad' (Laing) or labelled 'mad' (Scheff). Anti-psychiatry has also highlighted the processes through which the frontiers between the normal and the pathological are erected and, once erected, how difficult it is to move from the side of pathology to that of normality.

Anti-psychiatry currently has low status in the sociological literature. We should, however, remember that it was always a very uneven phenomenon, that it provided a salutary reminder that there was a view to be had from 'the other side', and that we should not simply attempt to obliterate this. But anti-psychiatry only achieved this by elevating the notion of subjectivity to such heights that it could provide the sole criterion for measuring the deficiencies of psychiatry's practice. Psychiatry was seen, in essence, as a domination. In the work of Goffman this took the form of a preoccupation with the degradations and profanations of the self that asylum psychiatry wrought. Laing's concern was with the existential experience of mental illness. And Szasz attacked institutional psychiatry for its harmful effects on the individual and its insufficiently contractual basis. In these different ways antipsychiatry was based on an *a priori* philosophical position that elevated to maximum importance the category of subjectivity. This does not, however, provide an adequate basis on which to develop a politics and critique of psychiatry. It entails a reduction of politics to a philosophical first principle, according to which power is evidenced by the suppression of subjectivity. This provides no means for evaluating the differing strategies within psychiatry, and their differing political trajectories. Also, it provides no means for understanding those forms of power that operate by seeking to invest the individual with subjectivity rather than to crush it.

A form of analysis and critique of institutional psychiatry that can be characterized by the notion of social control has supplanted anti-psychiatry since the late 1970s. As with antipsychiatry this is a mode of cultural analysis and critique that extends beyond psychiatry, which is merely one example (albeit a central one) of a practice that is seen to include the prison system and the judicial apparatus. This mode of analysis has recently subjected itself to a process of self-criticism in an attempt to refine and salvage the notion of social control.[28]

Social-control accounts of psychiatry can be identified schematically by a number of characteristics. First, psychiatry is viewed as a specialized, scientifically legitimated practice for the control of deviant groups in society. It is only one amongst many such practices that characterize all societies, although it assumes specific characteristics by virtue of the society in which it occurs. The notion of social control as a way of identifying such practices is not a neutral descriptive term but is condemnatory. Second, as one element within a more general social-control apparatus, psychiatry's emergence and transformation is often traced back to a causal principle located in the socio-economic production relations of capitalist society. As an institution of social control, psychiatry is seen to respond to specifically capitalist exigencies. Third, such practices of social control are related to the expansion of the activities of the state in capitalist societies. Psychiatry is one of the means by which the state extends its powers over conducts it had previously found difficult to regulate. Fourth, and finally, psychiatry is held to achieve this primarily through the medicalization of deviance. By medicalizing deviance psychiatry establishes a consensus that we should *do* something about such ill-health, and a legitimacy that centres on the claim that this is in the interests of the sick person and of society.

This account of psychiatry rose to prominence on a wave of 'revisionist' historiography that argued that history was not a matter of progress and reform.[29] British psychiatry received its revisionist honours rather late in Scull's narrative.[30] He identified the principal components of modern apparatuses of social control as threefold: first, the involvement of the state in the formation of a highly rationalized and centrally administered social-control apparatus; second, the treatment of deviance through segregation from the surrounding community; third, the careful differentiation of the various species of deviance and the assignment of different categories to different experts, which has as its corollary the emergence of the 'helping occupations'. Scull summarizes this in the following manner: 'From this perspective, the differentiation of the insane, the rise of a state-supported asylum system, and the emergence of the psychiatric profession can be seen to represent no more than a particular, though very important, example of this much more general series of changes in the social organization of deviance.'[31] Scull's study is an historically informed sociology. The details of this history of the growth of nineteenth-century British psychiatry are valuable, but the narrative labours under the weight of the sociological baggage it has to support. History becomes the linear accretion of the power of one particular group – the psychiatric profession – and the involvement of the state in this process. The culmination of this development is the totalization of such power in the 'therapeutic state'.[32]

One issue that has figured in social-control accounts of psychiatry is the way in which the psychiatric profession has achieved a dominant role within the mental-health industry in Britain.[83] An examination of this calls for attention to the social and political context in which the psychiatric profession has developed. The emerging political consensus on the question of mental illness in the early years of the twentieth century and the role of the Labour Party in particular in developing this consensus, is central here. Social-control accounts of such a process, however, have been weak in so far as they have tended to utilize a crude reductionist explanation in which developments in capitalism and the development of the Labour Party are linked together unproblematically to explain the emergence of a more generalized social-control apparatus.

The national specificity of what we might call a politics of health tends to be obliterated also in these accounts of psychiatry. So whilst George Rosen has supplied fascinating reports of the emergence of social medicine in continental Europe, what was specific to the countries he deals with – in particular the system of medical police – is lost in the reinterpretations of such studies.[34] What is required, instead of extrapolations from one specific country to a quite different context, is a demonstration of the ways in which a politics of health connects with specific governmental strategies. Virchow's astute comment that 'medicine is a social science and politics nothing but medicine on a grand scale' tells us little about the way in which a politics of health developed in Britain. Community care, for instance, cannot be viewed as simply involving more effective methods of social control. It needs to be related rather to a wide range of changes both in the internal structure of psychiatry itself as well as to the emergence of a variety of health strategies that seek to operate across the community rather than on the principle of separation, isolation and incarceration.

The attempt to locate the development of psychiatry in Britain in the twentieth century in relation to changes in the mode of intervention of the state in civil society is worthwhile. In this respect, the Labour Party as a major new political force would appear to have been an important factor in the shaping of a welfare politics that reinforced the power of the psychiatric profession and also helped to place psychiatry beyond the realm of the political. But to interpret this as mirroring the underlying conflicts of a class society that are resolved through an extension of the sick role obliterates the need for explanation. It is a type of sociological generalization that one can use for explaining all political events in relation to psychiatry in all societies and at all times. It obscures the heterogeneity of the psychiatric system today, the fact that psychiatry does not operate on deviance exclusively as something to be marginalized and segregated, put to one side of normal life, and also that it does not function solely through the state. In doing so it hides from view the current scope of the psychiatric system that incorporates not just psychiatrists and GPs but an entire army of petty functionaries whose concern is not with the deviant but with the normal mind.[35]

Psychiatry's political existence needs to be explained, but not by means of empty sociological generalizations of the medicalization of deviance through apparatuses of social control linked to the state. An understanding is required, rather, of psychiatry's social dimension, its reorganization in line with a more positive mode of government of the individual in advanced liberal societies. For government in a 'liberal' society no longer functions simply through repression and control, no longer operates via an external relation between the individual and the state, with its correlate the segregation of asocial behaviours. It entails, instead, that as far as possible individuals remain a part of society, become responsible for maximizing their potential contribution to society, and that when all else fails they be provided with just enough support to enable them to cope.[36] An account that depends entirely on the notion of social control and the suppression of deviance misses the fact that contemporary Western societies do not function according to the binary divisions of sane/mad, reason/unreason. Rather, they operate a continuum of differentiations that at one extreme entails segregation, and at the other operates on the normal mind in an attempt to optimize its functioning.

A reassessment of the notion of social control has emerged recently from certain of its former proponents.[37] The reassessment is itself confusing however, in that it entails a thorough demolition of the notion of social control as an explanatory concept, yet while still affirming its salutary value. Despite useful clarification of the concept, the lesson that surfaces is that the notion of social control will no longer suffice for sociohistorical analysis. A new and different explanatory framework is required.

One important point that emerges from this re-evaluation concerns the definition of social control. It has not always been a term used to express scorn: in the writings of Ross and George Herbert Mead it meant precisely the opposite.[38] Whilst the recent critical utilization of the concept has had a corrective value in relation to histories written according to the concept of reform, taken by itself the label 'social control' is often redundant. Moreover, when connected to the growth and development of capitalism it is often used as a way of avoiding explanation by simply dropping everything into the same bag. Without a much clearer definition of what social control is, what its pernicious effects are held to be, and what the mechanisms are through which it operates, we would do better without the concept. This last point raises a more general question of how we are to explain the relation between changes in social practices and ideas, and the structures that might be held to underly them. This way of putting the question follows from the view that reform of psychiatry should be explained in terms of changes in political, economic and social structures, and associated changes in the intellectual and cultural horizons of the dominant class.[39] Such a view has a certain appeal. It can be framed in a manner that largely avoids the charge of reductionism, whilst still enabling an explanation of reform that relates it to material interests. The difficulty, however, is that if one provides such an explanation in non-reductionist terms, it is not clear that it necessarily has any affiliation to an explanation of social control. Once the causal or determining links are weakened to a point where genuine historical interpretation is possible, the generalization of social control as an explanation for a vast range of phenomena becomes redundant.

A number of other issues concerning psychiatry as an institution of social control have been raised in recent discussions. One of these questions the notion that the state should remain the exclusive focus of debate and explanation. If we are concerned to retain the question of control as the focus, it is important to remind ourselves that the state does not have a monopoly of the punitive regulation of behaviour, and that its power and moral authority are not what binds society together. There is also the weakness of the functionalist assumption of social-control accounts. And there is a fundamental gap in social-control explanations. Whether or not psychiatrists act out of self-interest rather than to relieve suffering, we cannot leap from such an argument to the proposition that this necessarily leads them into activities that reinforce the social order. As has been perceptively remarked, there is little or no evidence that mental illness represents a threat to specifically *capitalist* social order.[40]

In so far as the notion of social control has featured prominently in discussions of psychiatry, its reassessment is of considerable significance. The problem, however, is more deep-
seated than some recent self-criticisms have suggested. It is
not a question of adjusting this or that dimension of the
explanation, giving a bit more emphasis here, lightening the
weight of causality there. What is at issue is the possibility of
opening up a new field of investigation with the aid of new
conceptual instruments. This is a process that has already been
commenced in the writings of Foucault and Castel as well as
others. We must emphasize that as a form of social and historical analysis this is not a more refined and non-reductionist
version of social-control accounts of psychiatry. Its concerns
have different starting points and are articulated through different concepts.

French historiographies of psychiatry

The tradition of historiography associated with the writings of
Michel Foucault, Robert Castel and others offers a theoretical
and historical interpretation of psychiatry that differs in a
number of important respects from the Anglo-American tradition. To identify this difference it may be helpful to begin
by sketching out the historical periodization they suggest as a
way of understanding psychiatry's emergence and transformation.[41]

A first period extends from the mid-seventeenth to the end
of the eighteenth century. This is the age Foucault refers to as
witnessing 'the great confinement'. His argument on this point
is that the mid-seventeenth century witnessed a dramatic shift
to widespread confinement of all classes of deviant and unproductive individuals. Madness was not differentiated systematically, provided with its own institution and status; insane
people were swept up along with beggars, the poor, the disabled and others. This was not the first time the poor and the
deviant had been interned. But it represented a qualitatively
new version of such a principle. This process of internment
had no medical ambitions but was simply a confinement. The
hôpital général through which this was accomplished in France
is explained by Foucault not in terms of a specific identity
accorded to madness, but in terms of a generalized concern of

order within the city, of 'police', a result of the imperative to labour, a new reaction to poverty, and one that was directly linked to monarchical power. This 'great internment' can be regarded as a failure, but Foucault argues that this 'failure' contributed to an ethical valorization of labour, an elevation of labour to the status of a moralizing and correcting activity regardless of the utility or profit that followed from it. The significance of this exclusion of madness along with a range of other unproductive groups was that madness came to be associated with questions of order, of moral regulation, of incapacity to labour, and of inability to integrate oneself with the group.

The great confinement of the mid-seventeenth century shut a variety of groups away together. But there was a significant element of individualization of madness within the world of confinement.[42] Foucault's critics generally seem to have missed this aspect of his account. This individualization of madness was limited, but it existed all the same. Changes occurred also across the Classical Age, a number of institutions opening in the middle of the eighteenth century reserved specifically for the insane.[43] Through such developments, and preceding the emergence of psychiatry in the nineteenth century, insane people achieved a degree of autonomy in relation to the other interned groups. Prior to its seizure by psychiatric *savoir*, and through changes within the world of confinement, madness became a singular object of perception. Multiple and varying figures of difference began to emerge.

It is important to remind ourselves that what Foucault provides in *Histoire de la folie* is not a history of psychiatry, but of its prehistory. Along with the much shorter *Mental Illness & Psychology*, which deserves to be better known, Foucault's researches have provided us with a study of the multiple transformations and sites of emergence that issued forth in the shape of psychiatry. The point of emergence of psychiatry with the figures of Tuke and Pinel is where Foucault's narrative ends. It is here that the beginning of the second stage of psychiatry's history can be located. This can be seen to extend from the late eighteeenth century to the early decades of the twentieth century. The best available analysis of this period, and one that shares much with Foucault's analysis, is contained in Robert Castel's still untranslated *L'Ordre psychiatrique*.[44]

The analysis of psychiatry's 'golden age' offered by Castel

takes over where *Histoire de la folie* ends. There is continuity in its concern to chart the social dimension of madness, and psychiatry's status as a political science. From 1790 and the abolition of the royal *lettres de cachet* to the law of 1838, which is still in force today in France, Castel charts the emergence of what he calls the 'modern problematic of madness'. The first element of this ensemble concerns the political context of the advent of legalism. Since the old basis of political legitimacy was removed by the Revolution, a new means of dealing with madness had to be found that was in accordance with the principles of a bourgeois 'contractual' society. The second element was the appearance of new agents, a reorganization of the relations between justice, local administrations and medicine, out of which the doctor emerged with a key position. The third element was the attribution to the insane person of the status of patient, madness coming increasingly to be viewed in medical terms and as differentiated from the control of criminals, beggars and vagabonds. The final element of the ensemble was the constitution of a new institutional structure, the 'special establishment', which provided psychiatry with its main site of operation for more than a century and a half.

The characterization of the nineteenth century as psychiatry's 'golden age' does not mean that across this period it ruled unchallenged. Castel demonstrates that this was far from being the case, and also that the nineteenth century was not homogeneous. As early as 1860, as I have noted above, profound criticisms were directed at psychiatry's institutional, theoretical, juridical and technological existence. One is, however, still entitled to talk of the nineteenth century as possessing a degree of coherence. The nineteenth century was a period during which psychiatry and the asylum were established across countries as diverse as France, Britain and the USA. And, despite constant criticism and attack, psychiatric expertise was not displaced from its position of absolute authority within the asylum, and from its status as being exclusively responsible for certain classes of extravagant behaviours.

The third period we can identify in psychiatry's history commences in the early years of the twentieth century, although as with the other divisions there is no clear-cut separation of one period from the next. Castel has analysed this modern age of psychiatry and the revolution it has brought about in psychiatry's mode of functioning in the USA.[45] The contours of the shift clearly vary from one national context to another. There are, however, remarkable parallels in psychiatry's development across the twentieth century. The inter-war years can be characterized as the beginning of psychiatric modernity. It was during this period that psychiatry, with the stimulus of psychoanalysis, moved outside the asylum and into the community. It was during this period that the neuroses were 'invented' and that child health and the family became objects for psychiatric intervention.[46] It was, however, not until the years around 1960 that institutional and administrative structures were to be provided that enabled psychiatry to function freely beyond the walls of the asylum. In the inter-war years psychiatry had its hands tied outside the asylum, and had to form alliances with social work, child psychology, and industrial hygienism. In 1960, however, there occurred the 'sectorization' of French psychiatry, in 1963 the Community Mental Health Center and Retardation Act was passed in the USA, and in 1959 the Mental Health Act in Britain was passed. In widely differing degrees these legislative changes provided an administrative framework for a psychiatry whose object would be the community and not exclusively the world of confinement.

If this schematic periodization has some value, the historiography of Foucault and Castel, further strengthened by that of Klaus Dörner[47] and discussed by Colin Gordon in chapter nine, offers considerable interpretive advantages over the Anglo-American tradition. We are not constrained by a view of psychiatry that reduces it to an agent of the state. Psychiatry can instead be studied in its functioning within the fabric of civil society itself. Nor are we limited to a view of psychiatry that reduces it to the asylum plus madness. An understanding of psychiatry is offered that grasps its emergence and transformations, and the modernizations that have led it to include within its sphere a whole range of 'normal' behaviours. We are free also from an explanation of the rise of psychiatry couched in terms of the medicalization of mental illness. The emergence of psychiatry is viewed rather as the rise of a carceral principle that individualizes madness, the subsequent attempt to medicalize this carceral apparatus, and the psychologization of the insane person. The twentieth century can be seen in this way to be fully in continuity with psychiatry's early development, in bringing about an increasing psychologization of social relations. It allows us also to provide an account of psychiatry's interrelation with specific strategies for the government and management of social life.

The distinctiveness of French historiography of psychiatry can be identified also in terms of its theoretical approach. There are four issues here that are important to note. A first defining feature of French historiography of psychiatry concerns its treatment of the state. Priority is accorded to the constitution in a number of sites throughout society of a specifically psychiatric concern with personal behaviours. The state is examined in so far as it contributes to this process, but it is not viewed as the sole or even principal locus of emergence of such a concern. This prioritization of psychiatry over the state contrasts with Anglo-American writings in which psychiatry functions more as a sub-plot to a history of the controlling power of the state than as an object of study in its own right. The concentration in French historiography on psychiatry itself and its constitution, conditions of emergence and transformation, leads to an analysis of the diverse sites of operation of psychiatric expertise and knowledge – the state asylums, the private asylums, private psychotherapy, GPs surgeries, etc. There is no *a priori* assumption that psychiatry is indissolubly an affair of state, although the state is, of course, a principal participant.

Just as the state is not used as an absolute datum for a history of psychiatry, neither is the phenomenon of madness. Rather than taking madness as the irreducible foundation of psychiatry, the focus is directed towards the different behavioural dimensions of personal life that have become objects of psychiatric knowledge and intervention. A principal advantage this offers is in the understanding of psychiatry in the twentieth century and its extension beyond unreason to the 'normal' population. Psychiatry viewed int his way becomes less a simple response to inexplicable and extravagant behaviours, and more a complex system of interrelated theoretical codes, therapeutic practices, institutional sites and legal codifications, traversed by and related to quite distinct socio-political strategies (incarceration, hygienic regulation of the community, self-care, etc.). As such it is not *an* institution that can be traced back to an originary strategist – the state, the economy, society's need for social control – rather, it operates within and through multiple and interlocking strategies of social regulation. One merit of this notion of a psychiatric *system* lies in its identification of the different levels of psychiatry's functioning, and the clarification it provides of the fundamental transformations or reorganizations of psychiatry's practice that occur from time to time.

A second defining feature of French historiography of psychiatry lies in the displacement it effects of the question of causality. Historiography has struggled too long under the weight of the demand to supply a causal explanation. The historiography of psychiatry is no exception. Too often an explanation is proposed as to the 'causes' of this or that change in psychatry's operation. Scull's proposed explanation of the phenemenon of decarceration is a case in point.[48] At a more general level, and beyond the specifics of psychiatry's history, when causality is absent profanation is declared to have occurred. The balance is now tipping the other way. Causal explanations are coming to be recognized as unsatisfactory on too many occasions. It is to be hoped that we shall soon be able to do without the notion of causality, and to then embark on the real work of untangling the complex of events that go to make up the operation of a practice such as psychiatry. One important direction in which such investigation should go is towards identifying the surfaces of emergence of psychiatric phenomena.[49] Instead of seeking to bridge the gap between 'mental illness' and the threat it is supoed to represent to capitalism, we should be looking at the specific sites where different forms of mental distress become constituted as psychiatric problems. How, where and through what processes do madness, depression and simple unhappiness become constituted as problems amenable to psychiatric treatment? Those sites that have already been shown to be of particular significance are the family, school, community, the judicial machine and industry.[50] It is these sites and their connections with changes in psychiatry that will repay closest investigation.

A third defining feature of French historiography of psychiatry follows from the view expressed by Foucault that power is not simply repressive, but also productive.[51] This thesis is often misunderstood to mean that all power is productive and, therefore, that repressive power no longer exists. The point to be stressed, however, is that Foucault in making this point was arguing for a fundamental reconceptualization of the notion of power, of its capacities, and its relationship to phenomena such as modes of personal existence, forms of interventions in the lives of individuals, discursive practices, and specific social categories such as the 'mad', the 'unhappy person', the 'neurotic'. Power is to be seen in relation to such phenomena as having a productive and constitutive role, not simply one that represses the individual's subjectivity. The latter comes instead to be viewed as something that is constituted in and through the operation of power relations. The notion that psychiatry can be understood in terms of its implication in the power relations that traverse Western societies means that it is in a significant respect constitutive of the social sphere itself.

A fourth and final characteristic of the French historiography of psychiatry is its philosophical dimension. The researches of Foucault and Castel on psychiatry and its emergence are permeated by a form of philosophical sensibility that is absent in Anglo-American writings and that is also profoundly misunderstood by certain British commentators.[51] There are two dimensions to the philosophical aspect of such studies. The first concerns the way in which psychiatry is located as an important component of modern technologies of the self.[52] As a relatively recent arrival on the scene, psychiatry is, from the outset, a mode of relating the insane person not just to the power of the doctor, but to the power of self-reflection and self-inspection. The notion of discipline applies here not just to the panopticon as a diagram of power that functions by means of spatial disposition and one's implication within a web of surveillance and observation.[53] Discipline operates most successfully through a process of auto-regulation of the person. From the moment psychiatry becomes a component integral to the individual's repertoire of self-evaluation and reflection, the personal tends increasingly to be redefined in terms of the psychiatric. The individual's interpretation of his/her conduct can be carried out in terms of psychiatric knowledge and principles. The varied dimensions of personal existence – fears, worries, happiness and unhappiness – can be understood according to the interpretive grid provided by psychiatry, enabling an instrumentalization of the personal according to psychiatric principles.

The second dimension of the philosophical approach of French historiography of psychiatry concerns psychiatry's implication in the constitution of the boundaries between reason and unreason, normality and pathology. Foucault has shown brilliantly how unreason becomes constituted as other, and as knowable only from the side of reason. From the moment that the truth of madness becomes something that can only be produced within the realm of reason, the mad person is deprived of the ability to pronounce on his/her condition. The twentieth century is not, however, a century of unreason. It is one in which reason and unreason no longer provide the means for effecting a division between normal and pathological mental states. Normality is no longer thought of in terms of reason, nor pathology in terms of its absence. The departure from the division of reason and unreason is of fundamental significance if we are to understand the nature of psychiatry today. The researches of Foucault and Castel have directed our attention to the division installed between reason and unreason, and the instrumentalization of this division according to the categories of the normal and the pathological. This serves as a useful reminder that as the distinction between the normal and the pathological is weakened across the twentieth century we need to develop an understanding of the nature of psychiatric interventions on the normal mind.

Conclusion

My concern in this essay has been with two distinct sets of issues. First, I have addressed the range of critiques that have been mounted against psychiatry since its inception. I have argued that these different critiques are a part of psychiatry's history and not simply external to it. They contribute to what I have referred to as different strategies for the modernization of psychiatry. Second, I have examined the more recent sociologically and historically based critiques. I have done so in terms of their contribution to the modernization of psychiatric practice, and in terms of the theoretical models they utilize for the understanding of psychiatry. My argument, based on identifying a number of themes in the writings of Foucault and Castel, has been that psychiatry cannot be understood exclusively in terms of madness, medicalization, the asylum and the state. We need, rather, to grasp the multiple sites of emergence and operation of psychiatric expertise, and their interdependence with specific strategies of social regulation. I have sought only to identify the general themes that might guide such enquiries. The rest of this volume looks at particular significant aspects of psychiatry's functioning.

My concern in identifying some of the theoretical issues at stake in the historiography of psychiatry has been with the analysis of the present. Historical analysis has much to contribute to the understanding of contemporary issues. It can do so, however, only on condition that it is not used as a basis for reducing the present to a past that has been superseded. This is what has happened in many socio-historical studies of psychiatry. I have argued that we need to understand psychiatric modernity in terms of a complex of practices that emerged in the inter-war years. Community psychiatry, or community mental health as many would prefer to have it called, needs to be seen in this light not as an alternative to psychiatry but as a modernization of its institutional and administrative matrix. Equally, we should be wary of celebrating psychological aproaches as alternatives to psychiatry. If psychiatry's history cannot be read simply as a medicalization of mental distress, then psychological approaches cannot be seen as unproblematic alternatives. As British psychiatry seeks to distance itself increasingly from the image and reality of the Victorian asylum, an evaluation of this modernization could usefully be undertaken in terms of a principle much older than psychiatry. Rather than adding the maintenance and optimization of his/her own mental health to the duties of the citizen, psychiatry should be judged according to its curative ability in the face of severe mental distress.

2

Psychiatry: the discipline of mental health

Nikolas Rose

Psychiatry seems an indispensable element of life in our modern society.[1] Its presence is not limited to those considerable numbers of people who receive medical treatment for severe mental disorders. Psychiatrists, mental hospitals, the mentally ill and the problems of mental health feature daily in political and social debates, in our newspapers, in television documentaries, exposés and soap operas. Psychiatric expertise has blossomed, and no phase of life is unknown to psychiatry and its ministrations: infertility, pregnancy, birth and the post-partum period; infancy; childhood at home and at school; sexual normality, perversion, impotence and pleasure; family life, marriage and divorce, employment and unemployment, mid-life crises and failures to achieve; old age, terminal illness and bereavement. When problems arise in our homes, on the streets, in factories, schools, hospitals, the army, courtroom or prison, psychiatry is on hand to provide its diagnoses and propose remedial action. Further, it is increasingly in psychiatric and psychological terms that we think and talk about our personal unhappiness. Psychiatry provides us with the very terms in which our problems are constituted, through its elaboration of the norms and images of healthy mental life, and its characterization of the features of pathology. These enable us to identify what is unhealthy, to classify and measure the problem, and to construe it as remediable. Mental life is now a domain that can be comprehended through, and may be managed by, scientific expertise.

How has our society come to be so traversed by psychiatry, by what means, in relation to what concerns, in what ways and to whose benefit? This essay will suggest that, in order to answer these questions, we need to free ourselves from the ways of thinking about psychiatry that have animated the critical literature for at least two decades. Despite their manifold differences, such sociological and political writings on psychiatry have established a set of themes that are commonly utilised in evaluating the social existence of psychiatry.[2] Many of these are examined elsewhere in this book. One central argument is that the power of psychiatry should be analysed in terms of the medicalization of social control – that psychiatry has been allocated its powers by the state in order to exercise and justify constraining individuals or groups who are deviant or troublesome. A key element in this scenario is the questioning of the claims of psychiatric medicine to have developed a scientific understanding of mental distress. Such claims are construed as mere means of legitimation of medical hegemony. Psychiatry, it appears, adheres almost exclusively to physical methods of treatment in order to back up its claims that mental distress has purely organic causes and hence that its treatment is analogous to that of physical illness. But, it is argued, drugs, electro-shock and psycho-surgery do not 'cure' mental distress but merely damp down or obliterate the capacity of the victim for those aspects of speech, thought and conduct that are considered socially threatening or undesirable; psychiatry nonetheless persists with its claims of scientificity and efficacy to back up its domination or exclusion of other forms of knowledge and types of treatment.

Such social and political analyses of psychiatry, explicitly or implicitly, suggest that these excluded or subordinate knowledges pose a radical challenge to the medicalization of madness. They reject the argument that mental distress is analogous to physical illness and hence can be treated in analogous ways. They draw attention to the social causes, conditions and judgments embodied in a diagnosis of mental illness. They deny the justification or the need for institutional confinement of the majority of mentally disordered people, not only if this is done under compulsion but also when entered into 'voluntarily'. Unlike psychiatric medicine, it is claimed, these alternatives recognize that so-called symptoms of mental illness are meaningful responses to interpersonal, familial or social circumstances. These symptoms need to be understood, and their causes recognized and transformed. Unlike psychiatry, it is suggested, these alternative techniques seek not merely to suppress socially undesirable conduct, but to restore mentally distressed individuals to a position where they have control over their own lives and can channel their resistance to circumstances into effective social action.

This approach thus bases its politics of psychiatry in the opposition to medical hegemony and campaigns to minimize compulsion in particular and institutionalization in general, in favour of care in the community. It seeks to promote the availability of social and psychotherapeutic techniques of treatment and tries to involve social workers, psychologists, psychotherapists, patients and ex-patients themselves in responses to mental distress. Its aim is to establish a service that does not merely react to 'mental illness' but that mobilizes social resources to promote mental health. But we should cease posing our analyses of the political functioning of psychiatry in terms of an opposition between a reactionary 'medical model' of madness that is supposedly blind to social factors in aetiology or in amelioration, and a progressive social theory whose explanations and remedies recognize the social conditions underlying mental distress. Such an analysis profoundly misunderstands contemporary psychiatry and the part it plays in the management of our economic, social and personal lives. In this essay, I shall examine the social role and vocation of psychiatry in order to disturb and fragment the assumptions that underpin much recent critical literature on psychiatry.[3] This will enable us to locate the political functioning of psychiatry in a new way and, perhaps, to make a different diagnosis of its ills and prescribe different antidotes.

The territory of psychiatry

In the early decades of the twentieth century, when 'organicism' in psychiatry was in its heyday, medicine was already establishing a social terrain for its operations. General medicine was concerned, at the beginning of the twentieth century, with a set of problems that were causing considerable political disquiet.[4] These concerned the size and quality of the population and its consequences for the success of military struggles abroad and for social and industrial efficiency at home. The political vocation of the old medicine of social hygiene was linked to large-scale schemes of environmental reform – sewage disposal, clean air and soil, pure water, uncontaminated food and satisfactory housing. But for the new hygienic medicine, the political health of the nation was dependent upon the physical health of the individual. The individual was no longer conceived of as merely a passive body awaiting infection from a contaminated environment. Through the details of their personal habits and lives, individuals were active elements in the spread of ill-health; hence reform of these habits could actively promote social well-being. Illness was to be minimized and health maximized by instruction of individuals in hygienic techniques for conducting personal and social lives. A complex apparatus of medical inspection, education in domestic hygiene, registration of births, infant-welfare clinics, health visitors, school milk and meals, health clinics and so forth were established to give reality to this new project of social hygiene. A profound shift had taken place in the objectives and techniques of government, a fundamental extension of political regulation of the habits of the population through detailed management of domestic life, not in the name of virtue or morality but in the name of individual health and social well-being. Individuals were to be obliged to conduct their personal lives in a hygienic manner; more importantly, they were to be encouraged to want to be healthy.[5]

In this period before the First World War, conventional psychopathology saw mental pathology in terms of a relation between an inherited constitution and the stresses to which it was subject in the life of the individual. The inherited nervous system might be insufficiently equipped with nerve cells, association fibres or otherwise organically incomplete. After conception, including during the *in utero* period, the nervous system might be damaged by stress. The brain might be injured, or harmed by toxins such as alcohol or by lack of nutrition or defects in the blood supply. In addition to such direct stress, the nervous system was also subject to the effects of indirect stress. Anxiety, inappropriate or over-demanding education, worries about employment or finance, intemperance or sexual excess, even religious fanaticism could adversely affect the nervous system, acting upon the brain through the production of impurities in the blood or through the exhaustion of nervous energy.[6]

But this organicism was not antithetical to a social role and vocation for psychiatry. A range of social ills were regarded as expressions of an inherited neuropathic constitution – epilepsy, alcoholism, mental defect, mania, melancholia could all be seen in this light. Not only might anti-social and immoral conduct result from such a predisposition, such behaviour might also provoke the onset of explicit pathology in those with such a predisposition and so could be criticized on medical as well as moral grounds. Careful management of infants was essential, not only from those children of families where previous pathology had manifested itself, to strengthen the constitution and build up habits that would minimize the risk of provoking onset, but also in all other families, since not even the strongest constitution was immune to damage. And, of course, the profligate breeding of those with severely tainted constitutions, lacking the morality or strength of character to restrain themselves, could lead to a swamping of the nation with neuropaths and a decline in national efficiency and the quality of the race. Hence the involvement of many key figures from the field of mental medicine in eugenic campaigns for the medical inspection of mental defectives, unemployables, criminals and others of the social problem group, and for their sterilization or permanent segregation.[7]

However, in the period following the end of the First World War, these negative and reactive tactics were gradually replaced by a positive strategy that redeployed the arguments of the new public health in a project of reducing the social ills caused by mental disturbance through the promotion of mental welfare and mental hygiene. Here the rationale of a new social psychiatry began to be formulated. This rationale found its first focus in the discovery of a new range of objects of administrative concern and psychiatric attention – the neuroses. These were mild mental disturbances that were sufficient to cause social inefficiency and personal unhappiness, although they did not disable the individual completely. If left untreated, these minor troubles would, very often, develop into more serious ills. And, as a corollary that demonstrated the point, it was claimed that many of those in our workhouses and prisons, our vagrants, criminals, delinquents and others who were socially or industrially inefficient, were so on account of mental pathology that had, very likely, begun in a small way in treatable neurosis. Hence the neuroses of childhood were of particular concern for they not only provided a fortunate early warning of troubles to come, but also, given the malleability of the child, could be successfully treated in the majority of cases.

The discovery of neuroses owed little to psychiatry; psychoanalysis, though more significant, was only indirectly responsible for the emergence of the category of neuroses as a way of construing and acting upon personal and social troubles.[8] The problem of the neuroses emerged outside both asylum and consulting room, in all those sites where individuals could be seen to fail in relation to institutional norms and expectations – the army, the factory, the school and the courts. Shell-shock accounted for 10 per cent of officer casualties in the 1914–18 war, and for 4 per cent of casualties from other ranks. More than 80,000 such cases were estimated to have occurred over the course of the war, and some 65,000 ex-servicemen were still receiving disability pensions in 1921 because of shell-shock. The more serious shell-shock cases were treated at special hospitals such as the Craiglockhart War Hospital for Neurasthenic Officers, and the similar establishments at Maghull, Nettley and Denmark Hill. Whilst senior military officers frequently regarded shell-shock as merely a disguise for cowardice, for which the appropriate treatment was improved morale, good officership and the threat of the firing squad, organicist physicians considered the condition to be a genuine one resulting from minute cerebral haemorrhages caused by the blast.[9]

The doctors in the shell-shock clinics were, however, unconvinced by such organic explanations, especially given the lack of independent evidence of the postulated lesions. Some publicity had been given in Britain in the pre-war period to the theories and techniques of Janet in Paris and of Freud in Vienna, and versions of their therapeutic methods were tried out on the shell-shocked with some considerable success. Shell-shock appeared to respond to a variety of approaches ranging from occupational training, through persuasion and a form of rational re-education, the use of suggestion, to a type of psychotherapy using hypnosis or free association. Their experience with this treatment converted many to a kind of dynamic theory of the will, one which conducted its analyses in terms such as instinct, repression and the intermixing of physical and mental symptoms. To understand the nature of neuroses such as shell-shock, it was indeed necessary to posit the existence of unconscious mental processes, elements repressed from consciousness as an attempt to resolve some intractable mental conflict. But in order to analyse and treat these conflicts one did not have to follow the psychoanalysts in their speculative and mistaken hypothesis of infantile sexuality – there were many instincts that could come into conflict, leading to the formation of a repressed complex that would produce illness through the misdirection of psychical energy. Such a theory of the dynamics of the psyche and the nature of the neuroses was to play a key role in the mental-hygiene movement, and it was within this movement that the conditions were laid for the new social psychiatry.

Soon after the end of the First World War, mental hygienists began to establish a connection between 'maladjusted' children who showed disorders of conduct at home or school – truanting, lying, quarrelling, night terrors, bedwetting, too much or too little emotion, too many or too few friends – and delinquent children who ended up before the courts. The juvenile courts, established in 1908, had brought together within a single forum neglected children, those in need of care, and those who had committed offences. Magistrates, probation officers and psychologists convinced themselves that no clear lines of demarcation could be drawn between them: in each case the problem lay in the home. The criminal act was just one of a range of possible symptoms of the emotional troubles of childhood. So the disturbed schoolchild would become the juvenile delinquent; the juvenile delinquent was, or had been, a disturbed schoolchild. Upon this connection would be built the child-guidance movement, with its key site – the child-guidance clinic – receiving children from home, school and court for evaluation, report and treatment.[10]

But the child-guidance movement was only one branch of the strategy of mental hygiene that was promoted by the Central Association for Mental Welfare, the Tavistock Square Clinic for the Treatment of Functional Nerve Disorders, by psychologists and penal reformers, and co-ordinated, from 1922, by the National Council for Mental Hygiene. This rationale underpinned the arguments made in a series of official reports, from that issued by the Board of Control after the First World War, through the Royal Commission on Lunacy and Mental Disorder that reported in 1926, to the Report of the Feversham Committee on Voluntary Mental Health Services published in 1939. Throughout this inter-war period, the new preventive medicine and social hygiene set the terms of debate. Poor mental hygiene was the cause of all sorts of social ills, and these were preventable by education in proper techniques for mental welfare and mental hygiene, by early detection of the signs of trouble and prompt and efficient treatment. Not only was poor mental hygiene a source of socially inefficient conduct, but the promotion of good mental hygiene was a feasible and valuable political objective. In the service of this strategy, obstacles to the promotion of mental welfare had to be identified and removed, and the appropriate facilities to enable its success had to be established.

The need for early and preventive treatment of mental disturbances was hampered by the stigma that surrounded lunacy, by the isolation of the asylum from other medical facilities, and by the legal procedures of 1890 that allowed asylums to take only patients who had been certified through a cumbersome process requiring the direct involvement of legal authorities. This discouraged individuals with mild problems from seeking help, and discouraged doctors from utilizing asylums, turning them into institutions for the incarceration of those considered beyond hope. Not only was this a counterproductive method of organizing services, it was also conceptually unwarranted. The separation of mental from physical illness was invalid – all illnesses involved both mental and physical components, and could be treated in similar institutions, through similar techniques, and by similar personnel. As the Royal Commission on Lunacy and Mental Disorder put it in 1926: 'insanity is, after all, only a disease like other diseases . . . a mind deranged can be ministered to no less effectively than a body deranged . . . The problem of insanity is essentially a public health problem to be dealt with on modern public health lines.'[11]

Treatment of insanity as a medical problem and on modern public-health lines entailed, first of all, a transformation in the form of institutional provision for the insane. As for physical illness, treatment should not require certification, compulsion or incarceration. Faciliites should be available in hospitals for out-patient and voluntary treatment to encourage easy access to help at an early stage of the disease. Prior to the First World War, the Lady Chichester Hospital at Hove had been the only special hospital for the treatment of neurotics.[12] Thus when Henry Maudsley made a gift of money to the London County Council in 1907, he stipulated that the hospital to be built should deal exclusively with early and acute cases, have an out-patients department, and carry out teaching and research on psychiatry in the context of medicine. Soon after the Maudsley Hospital was completed in 1915, and parliamentary sanction was obtained to allow it to take patients without certification, it was taken over by the military and used for the treatment of shell-shock cases until 1923.[13] When the Cassel Hospital opened, in Kent in 1919, its endowment was inspired by the wish to provide treatment similar to that used for 'shell-shocked' soldiers returning from the trenches for civilian patients with functional nerve disorders.[14]

The lessons of the mental-hygiene movement appeared to have been learned by the time of the Mental Treatment Act 1930, which renamed asylums 'mental hospitals' and stipulated that, in the majority of cases, lunatics should be termed simply 'persons of unsound mind'. Patients could now be received for in-patient treatment on their voluntary application, and local authorities were to make provision for the establishment of psychiatric out-patient clinics at general and mental hospitals. Some local authorities had already been utilizing voluntary associations to carry out early-care and after-care work, and the responsibilities of local authorities for lunacy and mental deficiency services were widened in those provisions of the Local Government Act of 1929 that followed the rec-ommendations of the Royal Commission on Lunacy and Mental Disorder.[15]

The principle of voluntary out-patient treatment for nervous disorders underpinned also the private psychiatric out-patient clinics such as the Medico-Psychological Clinic of London, which operated form 1913 to 1922, and the Tavistock Square Clinic, which opened its doors in 1920. It was the Children's Department of the Tavistock that provided the operational model for the child-guidance clinics, set up from the late twenties onward under the aegis of the Child Guidance Council, and funded by local authorities from the mid-thirties. These clinics, like the hospital out-patient departments, were to act as the hub for a comprehensive system of mental hygiene. Disturbed individuals could come to the clinics themselves, once they or others were educated in the signs of mental disturbance, and would now be free of the fears of stigma or incurability. Others were to be referred from school, court and elsewhere by statutory and voluntary agencies. In the clinics, assessment and treatment would be carried out, reports would be supplied to courts or schools, individuals would be referred to other institutions. But the clinics would also provide the base for a system of mental hygiene that could act more widely on the lives of patients, ex-patients and potential patients. Social workers, psychiatric social workers, probation officers, school-attendance officers and others would operate between the clinic and home, school or courtroom conveying information, advice and education. The new mental hygiene was to provide the basis of a project of general public education as to the habits likely to promote mental welfare. Mental health was to be a personal responsibility and a national objective.[16]

The very character of madness as a social phenomenon had thus changed: it was no longer some fundamental otherness of unreason that challenged the moral order. All those florid characters who had so liberally illustrated nineteenth-century textbooks were now below the level of social visibility, confined and rendered docile within the closed regime of the mental hospital, consigned to medical superintendence without limit of time. The paradigmatic subjects of the modernizing psychiatric apparatus posed a threat only in so far as they acted like grit in the institutional machinery of school, industry and elsewhere. They represented a source of social irritation, a loss of potential efficiency, and a future burden upon the state. Traces still lingered of the visions of degeneracy that had so structured the gaze of mental medicine in the late nineteenth century. Elements persisted of eugenic analyses, in which neurotics and the insane were allied with defectives, syphilitics, paupers, criminals, alchoholics and the unemployable, and proposals were made for attention to family history and for curbs upon the reproduction of this social problem group by sterilization or segregation. But such perceptions were already becoming anachronistic. Upon this new terrain of psychiatry, madness was construed merely as a problem of ill-health, personal unhappiness and social inefficiency. As a corollary, social inefficiency and personal unhappiness, as well as the symptoms of physical illness, became potential problems for psychiatric attention. In this transformation, not only were new psychiatric powers established, but a new field of social and personal life was rendered visible, calculable and governable.

The psychiatric community

The standard histories of psychiatric services look to developments in science and conscience to account for the move away from the asylum over the last quarter of a century in the USA, Britain and many other European countries, and towards the development of community psychiatric care.[17] The discovery, in the 1950s, of psychoactive drugs that had genuine ameliorative effects upon the symptoms of schizophrenia, manic depression, depression and anxiety, apparently enabled mental illness to be treated effectively and simultaneously did away with the necessity for long periods of institutional confinement. These discoveries confirmed that mental illness was an illness like any other, susceptible to treatment by the methods of clinical medicine. They also confirmed that the distinct categorization of mental illness enshrined both in law and in institutional provisions was unnecessary, and that custodial and segregationalist responses to mental illness were inappropriate and counterproductive. The segregation and isolation of those suffering from mental illness now had neither social nor medical justification.

In such accounts of psychiatric progress, it is suggested that further impetus was given to this move away from the asylum by the discovery of the poor conditions within mental institutions and the pathogenic effects of confinement itself. This concern may be traced back to 1921, when the account by Dr Montague Lomax of the conditions in Prestwich Hospital prompted the appointment of a committee of enquiry. This recommended that future hospitals be constructed on the villa system to enable separation of patients according to condition and home conditions and surroundings, and to keep new patients away from the asylum atmosphere. However, it is claimed, in the late 1950s, a number of publications gave further power and urgency to the shift away from confinement in mental hospital. Russell Barton diagnosed a condition he christened 'institutional neurosis' – a form of illness produced by the institution itself. Erving Goffman published his sociological account of the effects of the 'total institution' in stripping away the personality and identity of the inmate. These accounts were supported by the new group of social psychiatrists working outside the asylum system. Thus John Wing demonstrated that institutionalism – apathy, resignation, dependence, depersonalization and reliance on fantasy – was common to long-stay inmates of even well-run mental hospitals, and that reforms centering upon enriching the institutional environment were difficult to maintain in the face of institutional exigencies. It appeared that the pathogenic effects of the mental hospital were, themselves, intractable; the solution was not to reform the institution but to do away with it.[18]

Thus, it is suggested, medical and public attitudes changed towards the acceptance of the mentally ill back into the community and the ordinary medical services. Incarceration was not required for therapy – it was positively anti-therapeutic. Mental hospitals were custodial institutions that did little good, much harm and that consumed scarce resources that were better directed to the development of more effective forms of provision. Wherever possible hospitalization should be avoided, where necessary it should be in the ordinary medical system, the length of stay should be minimized, and individuals should be maintained in their communities where, rather than suffering the pathogenic consequences of institutionalization, they would be subject to the benign influences of normality. The enlightened era of community psychiatry had dawned.

Sociological critics of this account of psychiatric progress argue that the causal status attributed to the discovery of effective pharmacological treatments is misplaced.[19] They point to the repetitive history of enthusiastic claims for the efficacy of physical treatments of mental disorder followed by disillusionment occasioned by relapse, side-effects or other disappointments. This pattern can be discerned from the bleedings and purgings of the eighteenth century, through the use of sedatives such as chloral hydrate and bromides in the nineteenth century and barbiturates in the early twentieth century, thyroid extract or removal of tonsils, to the development of the 1930s. The inflated claims for insulin coma therapy of the thirties were followed in the forties by those for convulsion therapy, first using drugs and then electro-shock; a similar enthusiasm was shown, from the mid-thirties, for psycho-surgery. It is suggested that in each case, as for the modern drugs, major successes were claimed for the application of almost anything that serendipity or a leap of the medical imagination suggested might have a negative relationship with mental illness, without the carefully controlled trials that would show such claims to be ill-founded. Thus these critics cast doubt upon contemporary beliefs in the powers of the new drugs and point to their side-effects; they suggest that they have been adopted so widely not because of their curative capacity but because of the entrepreneurial skills of the drug companies and the professional interests of doctors seeking to found their claim for jurisdiction over mental disorder.

Not only do such critics dispute the efficacy of the post-war pharmacological developments, they also dispute their role in changing patterns of psychiatric services. They point to the lack of correlation between patterns of hospital bed-use and discharge rates and the use of such drugs in different areas and countries. They argue that the evidence suggests the early use of phenothiazine drugs in the 1950s was as much for control within the hospital as to facilitate discharge. Thus, it is claimed, the determinants of the move away from custodial responses to mental disorder must be found elsewhere. Similar scepticism is levelled at the role the standard histories accord to critiques of the damaging effects of incarceration. Such criticisms were made of the 'museums of madness' in the nineteenth century, but they did not have similar effects. Hence, it is argued, the determinants of the shifts in psychiatric policy cannot be either scientific or humanitarian.

On the contrary, the move away from the mental institution is understood in terms of the professional interests of psychiatrists and the economic interests of the state. At the professional level, it is claimed, what was at stake was not a desegregation of the mentally ill, but a desegregation of psychiatry, a desire of psychiatrists to end their isolation and gain access to the power, careers and status of other medical specialisms. The 'drug revolution' is thus regarded not as the origin of the move away from the mental hospital but as a pseudo-scientific legitimation for it.[20]

At the economic level, it is suggested, the shift away from institutional responses to mental disorder was part of a general shift in the rationale of welfare induced by a 'fiscal crisis of the state'. With the development of the apparatus of the welfare state, segregative modes of control become more costly and difficult to justify. In the nineteenth century the criticisms of the asylum could not be met, as 'outdoor relief' was regarded as an inducement to idleness, a subsidy to pauperism and an incitement to unemployment, undermining the necessity of entering into wage labour. But the welare state and social-insurance systems involve a change in the modality of social control that no longer requires confinement as the condition for state support. This combines with the increasing cost of incarceration, not only in terms of the maintenance and renewal of the fabric of the institution but also because of the increased levels of wages forced through by the unions representing the state employees running the system. At a time of fiscal crisis, where the state is finding it increasingly difficult to fund its welfare activities through the taxation system without unacceptable demands upon private profit, cheaper alternatives are sought to institutional care. The rhetoric of scientific progress and humanitarianism is utilized to mask and legitimate a move whose primary determinants are economic.[21]

It is clear that the cost of maintaining mental hospitals, which were largely built in the nineteenth century, has been a considerable factor in deliberations of national and local governments. But the economic arguments in themself are insufficient. The run-down of the mental hospital system began in the 1950s, during the post-war boom and before the economic 'crisis' of recent years. Cross-national comparisons show no correlation between moves away from incarceration and economic prosperity or crisis. And the financial savings have not been forthcoming, in the short or medium term.[22]

Further, it is true that changes in the organization of welfare provision have been important for the contemporary psychiatric system. Social insurance has made it possible for individuals without wage labour to be maintained without incarceration. Public housing facilities have provided the conditions for such persons to be physically sheltered outside the state institution, as have the development of private and charitable housing schemes. The foundation of a comprehensive system of primary medical care has enabled general practitioners to play a key role in the dispensing of the pharmaceutical treatments that would enable treatment to be maintained without custodial institutions. The consolidation of medical and psychiatric social work within the local authorities and the hospitals has enabled supervision of the patients outside hospitals. But such changes in the nature of welfare have not been merely external conditions making possible a shift in the organisation of psychiatry; the changes in psychiatry have been an intrinsic element in the new rationale of welfare. The post-war modernization of psychiatry was a positive strategy, not a mere rationalization for financial savings. What was at stake was a new way of thinking about mental distress, a new way of linking it to social ills, and a new way of practicing in relation to it.

The shaping of psychiatry by war

Official discussions of psychiatry in the post-war period appear merely to reiterate and extend the themes already established before the Second World War. The recommendations of the Feversham Committee, to set up a National Council for Mental Health to co-ordinate voluntary societies and statutory authorities, were published in 1939 and acted upon soon after the outbreak of war. When Dr Carlos Blacker published his report on *Neurosis and the National Health Services*, in 1946, he drew attention to the problems hampering early treatment, their consequences and their solutions in familiar terms. *The Future Organization of the Psychiatric Services*, published in 1945 after discussions between representatives of the Royal Medico-Psychological Association, the Psychological Medicine Section of the British Medical Association and the Royal College of Physicians, stressed the similarities and interdependencies between mental and physical ills both clinically and organizationally; it was this that underpinned its arguments for treating psychiatry like other branches of medicine, and fully integrating its administrative structure, resources and facilities within the comprehensive health service established in the National Health Service Act, 1946. Similarly in 1953 the Report of the Third Expert Committee of the World Health Organization argued for a move from the 'classical' system, in which the mental hospital dominates, to the 'modern' system, in which in-patient, out-patient, day care, domiciliary care, hostels and so forth operate as 'tools' in the hands of the 'community' and a 'medico-social' team. And the Royal Commission on Mental Illness and Mental Deficiency, which was set up in 1954 and reported in 1957, posed the issues in a similar way, as did the Mental Health Act 1959 that followed on from its recommendations. As the Minister put it, what was involved was a 're-orientation of mental health services away from institutional care towards care in the community'. Hence the Act extended the open-door policy, established informal admissions as the norm, extended local authority powers, encouraged liason between health and social services, and so forth.[23]

Thus, while it is true that the Mental Health Act of 1959 allocated considerable discretionary powers to doctors in respect of involuntary admission to mental hospital and the administration of treatment without the patient's consent, it would be a mistake to view it as a further medicalization of social control. It was neither an extension of the coercive powers of the authorities nor a triumph of organicist medicine over other theories of the origin of mental disorder or other professional claims for a role in a mental-health system. On the contrary, the strategy sought to minimize the role of incarceration in the social responses to mental distress, to establish links, relays and alliances between medicine and other social agencies, to facilitate the movement of individuals amongst and between the different branches of the mental health system, to encourage each of us to take responsibility for the preservation and promotion of mental health.

But the apparent continuity between the official pronouncements after the Second World War and the programmes of mental hygiene in the pre-war period is misleading. The pre-war psychiatric population was split between the neurotics – maladjusted and delinquent children, inefficient workers and shell-shocked soldiers and the like – and the psychotics. These latter were those certified under the various sections of the Act, segregated from the sufferers of physical illness, and confined in the large, isolated, custodial mental hospitals. The psychiatric complex dreamt of by the epigones of mental hygiene had obtained only a limited purchase on reality: the provision of out-patient clinics was confined to a few geographical areas; only a small number of the more recently built asylums had established separate facilities for new acute patients; very few beds for in-patient treatment were provided in wards of general hospitals; some, but not all, municipal hospitals had set up 'observation wards' where mental patients could be confined under short sections for limited periods for assessment and diagnosis before being discharged or committed to a mental hospital.

In the 1930s, mental hospitals had an average population of around 1,200 but some contained up to 3,000 patients. The majority of patients were there for long periods – if not permanently – and active therapeutic intervention was spasmodic. It was accepted that most patients were suffering from psychoses that were often hereditary in origin and, by and large, incurable. The old ideals of moral treatment had largely been discarded; the asylums were communities where the better patients 'lived a life of contented servitude, working as orderlies, storemen, or domestic servants in a cosier world than that outside'. With the melancholic, paraphrenic or deluded, certain attachments formed between staff and patients; for others the regime varied from neglect, through surveillance and containment, to degradation and brutality.[24]

However questionable their claims to efficacy, the new physical treatments that developed in the 1930s did rupture the stasis of these hospitals, by offering doctors an image of themselves as healers of the sick and not merely superintendents of the institution. Waves of enthusiasm for these treatments swept through the hospitals. Physical treatments were selected and applied according to the latest reports in the medical literature or the predilections of the medics – removal of tonsils, administration of thyroid extract, insulin coma-therapy, convulsion therapy and, in some cases, psycho-surgery – sometimes leading to dramatic recoveries. Nonetheless, the asylum was an unsatisfactory locale for the encouragement of these curative aspirations. The principal task of asylum doctors remained the containment of chronic patients, it often required the use of coercion, and offered few prospects for innovation other than more efficient administration.

A fissuring was occurring within mental medicine. A certain hostility was growing between the long established sector of asylum superintendents, defenders of the need for separate and distinct institutions for the treatment of the mentally ill, who dominated the Board of Control, and the physicians who sought the integration of the practice, training and facilities of psychiatry with those of the general hospital. The events that presaged a brighter future for psychiatry were largely taking place outside the asylums, or at any rate outside their mainstream. They were happening in the insulin units of the mental hospitals, in the development of new physical treatments in the general hospitals, in out-patient clinics, in private practice, in psychotherapy and psychoanalysis. The Second World War was to decisively shift the balance between these two wings of psychiatry.[25]

Psychiatric involvement in the First World War had initially been marginal, consisting in the rejection by medical officers of recruits with gross nervous disorders – certified insane or with epilepsy.[26] But the experience of that war had shown the military cost of this concentration upon the numerically minor problem of psychosis to the exclusion of the much larger problem of neurosis. Numerous casualties had apparently resulted from the admission and deployment of men ill-suited to the strains of military service, whether by temperament or the present or past condition of their nervous or mental health. In 1938 a memorandum of the Royal Medico-Psychological Association predicted the prospect of three to four million acute psychiatric cases occuring within six months of the outbreak of hostilities. But, while the British Army had been slow to learn the lessons of the First World War in the twenties and thirties, the same had not been true of our allies or, more significantly, of our enemy. Indeed, whatever the loathsome objectives of the German war machine, their efficiency in the maximization of the potential of their manpower through organizational means was much admired.

Perhaps it was because of his intermediate position – based neither in hospital psychiatry nor in the camp of psychoanalysis – that John Rawlings Rees, Director of the Tavistock Clinic, was appointed consulting psychiatrist to the British Army. Or perhaps it was because the problems at issue in wartime were precisely those of functional nerve disorder over which the Tavistock had established its jurisdiction. In any event, the consequence was that the new tasks of psychiatry were to be thought from within the rationale of mental hygiene. These tasks of the war were fivefold: selection; prophylaxis by training and man management; the maintenance of morale;

the treatment of psychiatric casualties; the rehabilitation of returning prisoners of war.

In the task of selection, psychiatry could act on mental health by administrative means. The objectives were both negative and positive: negative in that, by careful selection and allocation of individuals to task and role according to psychiatric criteria, disciplinary problems, neurotic breakdowns and military inefficiency could be minimized; positive because, simultaneously, personal contentment, group morale and organizational efficiency could be maximized. Something like 15 per cent of recruits were referred to psychiatrists by the recruitment boards for assessment, with a view to selecting out potential problem cases. These were of two main types. There were the dullards who were unsuitable because they could not learn to carry arms, use them efficiently or obey orders. And there were the unstable who were liable to break down in active service at the front. The size of this task was a considerable stimulus to the development of methods of intelligence assessment that could be carried out in groups, and to the invention of practical devices for personality assessment.

Of course these techniques were just as important in the selection of officers. The early years of the war showed a high rate of psychiatric breakdown of officers, partly thought to be due to the commissioning from the ranks of men with a history of psychopathy – maladjustment or neurotic disorders. Encouraging results were obtained by psychiatric interviews and assessment with intelligence tests and projective and other tests of personality. Selection boards for all candidates were restructured to include psychologists and psychiatrists, and they rapidly assumed the key role. Later Bion's leaderless group principle enriched the armoury of assessment devices. Here a group of candidates without an appointed leader were given a problem to solve; much could be learned by psychiatric observation of the roles individuals took within the group. After the war, this test was displaced by the new psychological technology of personality testing. But whilst the group had only a limited life as a technique of personality assessment, it was to have powerful consequences: in an inverted form it provided the first sketch for a psychodynamic group therapy.

A new domain of social reality had become thinkable, calculable and manageable; psychiatrists and psychologists col-
laborated in the expanding project of managing the human
factor in group life. The processes of selection accomplished
this through fitting individuals to their particular niche in the
light of their mental qualities. But one could also transform
these mental qualities by training. Psychiatry enabled the
adjustment of training techniques in order to enhance the fit
between the mental and the organizational, thus enhancing
contentment, mental health and morale. One could, for example, use the psychiatric principle of 'battle inocculation' by
which men were adjusted to battle conditions through exposure
to gradually increasing doses of explosion. Similarly, morale
could be maximized by methods of man-management that
would promote solidarity through acting on the psychiatrically
important aspects of group life. Men were not to be welded
into efficient fighting units by instilling artificial hatred of the
enemy, but by producing a sense of aim and purpose, of
individual competence and value within the group. These techniques could also be applied to the maximization of the operation of the industrial machine that supported the war effort,
to make the most out of the human factor in production. These
were the beginnings of the methods developed after the war
at the Tavistock Institute of Social Relations, which used a
kind of psychoanalysis of industry to analyse and cure the
unconscious conflicts within the enterprise that were hampering
productivity.[27]

Psychiatrists appointed by the army saw almost a quarter of
a million cases during the Second World War, even discounting
those referred from army intakes, those seen in selection testing and patients seen in psychiatric hospitals.[28] Whilst only
about 8,000 of these were diagnosed as psychotics, some
130,000 were considered to be neurotics. The invaliding rate
for psychiatric disabilities was over 30 per cent of that for
discharge for all medical causes. Whilst military neurosis centres did manage to return about 80 per cent of their cases to
duty, the results of treatment overall were poor. This certainly
emphasized the need for new treatment techniques. More
fundamentally for post-war developments, it confirmed that
psychiatry should not focus upon the confinement of the small
number of psychotically deranged persons. To fulfil the task
that society required, it needed to shift its attention to the

detection and treatment of those large numbers of the population who were now known to be liable to neurotic breakdown, maladjustment, inefficiency and unemployability on the grounds of poor mental health. The lessons of the war displaced asylum medicine from centre stage; issues of public health, mental hygiene and social efficiency were now at the heart of the programme for the reorganization of state-funded psychiatric services.[29]

Developments in professional sectors outside psychiatric medicine made it possible for this new psychiatric programme to establish itself. Prior to the war, psychology had aspired to become an autonomous clinical instance alongside medicine, having under its jurisdiction all those maladjustments of conduct from delinquency to industrial inefficiency.[30] But these aspirations were hampered by the limitations of their technological repertoire and were largely thwarted. A limited psychologization of industry had occurred, both at the level of the enterprise and at the level of the labour market. This was promoted by the Health of Munitions Workers Committee, the Industrial Fatigue Research Board and the National Institute of Industrial Psychology. Within the enterprise it used the measurement techniques traditional in psychophysiology – measures of sensation, discrimination, attention and co-ordination – to advise on the technical organization of the production process, and its effects upon efficiency, fatigue and accidents. In selection for employment and vocational guidance, the problem of the lack of appropriate technical means of assessment was severe. Psychological assessments operated by trying to establish an individual's position in relation to the norms of functioning, and distribution of scores, in the population as a whole. During the 1920s, the intellect had been made calculable in this way, and intelligence tests had been constructed and standardized on the basis of assumptions concerning the statistical distribution of mental powers in the population as a whole and its correlation with estimates of social or educational adaptation. But a measure of intelligence was insufficient for the allocation of individuals to industrial roles. Devices were needed that would quantify and rank personality and aptitudes in a way amenable to managerial judgments. These devices needed to use an easily administered assessment schedule completable in a short time. Whilst many such schemes had been invented in the inter-war years in the

USA, none of them had firmly established itself on the toolbag of practical psychologists in Britain.[31] They eschewed the dynamic diagnostic systems like the Rorschach and the Thematic Apperception Test (TAT), which had been developed for clinical use. Their enterprise was grounded upon the rationale of psychometrics, which conceptualized the psyche in terms of distinct traits or dimensions, largely heritable, distributed according to the normal curve, and quantifiable by standardized measures of adjustment. For them, psychology had been formed in the image of the standardized test and this defined the limits of their conceptual universe and practical contributions.

The war changed things on a number of fronts. The concern of the military with efficient utilization of manpower led to the promotion of research on techniques for assessment of personality and aptitude that would be useful in screening for pathologies and allocation to tasks. This not only overcame resistance to the use of available techniques, it also led to the development of new devices that would enable the expertise of the psyche to extend its remit to the personality in a big way. The British War Office Selection Boards and the US Office of Strategic Services engaged in a heroic struggle to construct systems of psychological assessment that would accurately predict performance in real-life situations. If selection could become an activity governed by scientific expertise, it would not only minimize rates of failure. It would also eliminate the suspicion that class bias was influencing decisions as to recruitment and promotion. This was damaging to morale and discouraged applications for commissions from the ranks.[32] Large populations were now available for psychological investigation and measurement, funding was plentiful, and advanced statistical techniques such as factor analysis could now be applied to these problems. The fruits of this wartime labour included the Minnesota Multiphasic Personality Inventory (MMPI), enabling assessment of hysterical, neurotic, schizoid and other attributes, and Cattell's Sixteen Factor Personality Questionnaire. The factorization of the personality enabled it simultaneously to be represented in thought and utilized in reality.

The experience of wartime not only produced the psychological technology of the personality, it also shifted the relations between psychologists and psychiatrists, laying the

basis for an enhancement of the role and responsibilities \
accorded to psychological expertise. Whilst clinical psychology
would continually bemoan its inferior position within the psychiatric system, and claim to be more than merely a technology
of testing, at least it now had a more convincing repertoire of
activities to occupy it, and a domain of vocational guidance,
and industrial psychology in which it could substantiate its
claims as an independent body of expertise. Upon this basis it
was to promote its clinical status through the claims made for
the normalizing techniques of behaviour therapy.[33]

The development of the post-war apparatus of the welfare
state also enabled the extension of psychiatric social work from
the child-guidance clinics and mental hospitals into the heart
of social casework.[34] Psychiatric social workers were employed
not only in the prison and Borsal services, in care committees
and so forth, but also in the extensive work of rehabilitation
of ex-service men and women, working in the mental health
advisory services set up for this purpose under the National
Health Service Act of 1946. And, further, psychiatrically
trained social workers were now operating as Children's Officers under the Children Act of 1948. Pretty soon, the aspirations
of the founders of psychiatric social work in the inter-war years
were to be realized: all social work would have to attend, to
a greater or lesser extent, to the psychological investments and
conflicts that underpinned even those presenting problems that
were apparently entirely practical.

Thus the transformations of the psychiatric system in the
1950s and 1960s do indeed mark a significant shift in the social
dispensation of psychiatry. It is true that the criticisms of the
asylum were not new, and neither were the claims made for
the curative potential of drug treatments. But in the context
of the new rationale for psychiatry as a part of public health,
what they represented was an extension of the process of
modernization to those sectors of the psychiatric system that
had previously been recalcitrant. The closed asylums with their
populations of chronic and psychotic patients were not only
sucking in social resources that were more usefully deployed
in the other sectors of the system, but were also actively
damaging in their effects. And the new pharmacological technologies of treatment, whether or not they worked as claimed,
provided the conditions for *conceiving* of the management of
the severely deranged or psychiatrically disabled upon the new

psychiatric terrain. The medical complex of general practitioners, out-patients departments, and ordinary general hospitals could administer the drug-based therapeutics without the segregative institution. Social insurance and social workers could service the ill person without confinement. And madness – as merely illness, unhappiness and inefficiency – no longer constituted a fundamental threat to reason and order that required incarceration. The asylum had become unnecessary.

The policy landmarks of the new configuration are clear enough.[35] Enoch Powell, Minister of Health, in his 1961 speech to the National Association of Mental Health, announced the objective of halving the number of places in hospitals for mental illness over the next fifteen years, and the closure of the majority of the existing mental hospitals. The Ministry circular following this speech confirmed the decline in bed spaces, urged planning for closure of 'large, isolated and unsatisfactory buildings', and laid out the four kinds of accommodation to be provided in the new system: acute units for short-stay patients, usually in general hospitals; units for medium-stay patients; units for long-stay patients, often in hostels or annexes of general hospitals; and secure units provided on a regional basis. In 1962 the Hospital Plan for the next fifteen years envisaged the phasing out of all specialist hospitals, such as those for the mentally ill and the chronically sick, and their incorporation into District General Hospitals. In 1963 *Health and Welfare: the Development of Community Care* urged the desirability of 'community care', but did not specify what this entailed. In 1971 *Hospital Services for the Mentally Ill* proposed the complete abolition of the mental-hospital system, with all in-patient, day-patient and out-patient services provided by departments of District General Hospitals, linked in to services provided by the local authority social services, general practitioners and in consultation with the Department of Employment.

This policy was continued throughout the 1970s, irrespective, it appears, of the political complexion of the government or minister of the day. The lines of argument were similar in *Better Services for the Mentally Ill*, produced by Barbara Castle's Labour ministry in 1975, and in *Care in Action* and *Care in the Community* produced in 1981 under the aegis of the monetarist conservatism represented by Patrick Jenkin.

Now the strategy was posed in terms of the creation of a comprehensive psychiatric service, a continuum of care, a community psychiatric system: prevention through education and the encouragement of practices to promote mental health; early treatment entailing the removal of stigma, ease of access, minimization of legal formalism and the education of professionals so that they may pick up the early signs of mental disorder; out-patient treatment in clinics, sheltered housing, through domiciliary service and with social-work support; in-patient treatment to be minimized, for as short a period as possible and within the district general hospital; after-care on discharge provided by the out-patient services. And, despite the controversies over the passage of the 1982 Mental Health (Amendment) Act, we can see that its emphasis on care in the community, on the minimization of hospitalization and compulsory detention and so forth, is actually consonant with the direction of psychiatric modernization.

The community, in the debates over community psychiatry, has a reality which is neither geographical nor that of a network of informal social relationships. It is a social sector, a sector brought into being and marked out by the strategies and practices of social management. In this community of psychiatry, elements previously dispersed can be brought into a functioning relationship with one another. The disputes over forms of treatment, professional rivalries and institutional hostilities do not undermine the establishment of this territory, quite the reverse. The emergence of a variety of theories of mental distress, competing professional groupings and technologies of treatment other than those favoured by the medical orthodoxy, enable alliances to be struck up, and an expanding psychiatric population to be distributed across a proliferating field. The paramedical sectors that made their own claims over and against those of medicine – community and group therapies, nursing models, clinical psychology, quasi-professional voluntary groupings – in fact operate through a series of overt or tacit alliances with 'official psychiatry', in which they are allocated certain categories of patient – the chronics, psychopaths, hysterics, phobics, and the old, and so forth – in order to free the modernized psychiatric institution for the most promising material, to enable it to support its claims for effectiveness and to free it from the taint of custodialism. Opposition to the psychiatric institution and the dominance of medicine in the name of community mental health for all is not only pushing at an open door; it has also been intrinsic to the process whereby all issues of personal unhappiness have been translated into problems of mental health, problems that may be ameliorated with the assistance of one of the many brands of professional technicians of the psyche.

Technologies of the self

Critical accounts of the state of psychiatry tend to suggest that the 'official' psychiatric apparatus is hegemonized by physical and pharmacological responses to mental distress. It is claimed that psychiatry is antithetical to, and has marginalized, psychodynamic and social models of aetiology and techniques of treatment. And it is suggested that a radical politics of mental health should seek to support these techniques against those deployed within psychiatric medicine.[36] However such analyses obscure the rather more complex links between treatment technologies, the political conditions of their emergence and utilization, their objectives and consequences.

At the outbreak of the Second World War, the techniques available in the psychiatric armoury were somewhat limited: continuous narcosis, insulin coma-therapy, sedation with barbiturates, occasional use of individual psychotherapy, some experimental use of hypnosis or pentathol for abreaction. But in the post-war period a range of new techniques became available, many invented in response to the exigencies of wartime. These were to play a key role in the realignment of the psychiatric system in the 1950s and beyond. We can roughly distinguish five lines of development: physical and pharmacological treatments; social therapies; psychoanalysis; behaviour therapy; and therapies of normality. Physical and pharmacological treatments have been much discussed and much derided in the critical literature on psychiatry. As far as physical interventions like psycho-surgery and electro-convulsive therapy are concerned, the criticisms have focused upon the coercive and intrusive nature of such techniques, their damaging effects, unknown mechanisms and unproven efficacy. More pertinent for our present purposes, such treatments are viewed as paradigms of those offered by psychiatric medicine as a whole, and a general critique of psychiatric treatment is, as it were, extrapolated from these physical interventions. But to understand the power of contemporary psychiatry we need to approach the spectrum of treatment from the other end, and to ask instead what has been made possible by those technologies for the management of selves which are, apparently, more benign.

Pharmacological treatments

From the early 1950s psychiatric pharmacology was a growth industry. New drugs proliferated, making claims for specific modes of action and efficacy in the treatment of particular conditions: phenothiazine-type drugs for the treatment of schizophrenia; lithium-based therapies for manic depression; tricyclic, tetracyclic and monoamine oxidase inhibitors for depression; the benzodiazapines used as tranquillizers, sleeping-pills, anti-depressants, and much else. By 1977, such psychoactive drugs accounted for 25 per cent by number, and 17 per cent by cost, of all National Health Service prescriptions. But these drugs were not merely deployed in the hospitals or to counter major mental disorders. A massive psychiatrization of everyday worries appears to have taken place. By 1984, 23 per cent of the adult population of Britain – nearly 10 million people – had taken tranquillizers; around 3.5 million people for more than four months; with 1.5 per cent of the adult population taking them on a long-term basis and close to a quarter of a million people having taken them for seven years or more.[37] These minor tranquillizers, principally prescribed by general practitioners, were deployed for ills ranging from broken homes, through poor digestion, insomnia, divorce, nerves, changes of employment, unemployment, high blood pressure and all the other minor troubles of life, often as a matter of routine.

Such a proliferation of drugs is frequently criticized for merely suppressing inevitable symptoms of social, racial, sexual and economic injustice. It is also criticized because it fails to suppress such symptoms – for the restricted efficacy of the drugs and their harmful side-effects. There is, no doubt, much truth in the criticism that these interventions leave the causes of problems unaltered, merely attempting to maintain individuals as subjects who can cope with their social roles. But it would be a mistake to assume a fundamental opposition between drug therapies and other modalities of treatment. This is not simply because drugs are frequently utilized in combination with other treatment modes, despite their apparent discrepancy at the level of explanatory codes and therapeutic rationales. It is, more importantly, because the more 'benign' forms of treatment often share very similar normalizing objectives.

Social therapies

Wilfred Bion is credited with the first recognition of the principle underlying the social therapies;[38] Maxwell Jones came to regard it as fundamental: 'social environmental influences are themselves capable of effectively changing individual and group patterns of behaviour.'[39] With John Rickman, Bion was drafted into Northfield Military Hospital near Birmingham in 1943 to deal with unruly conditions that had developed in its Training Wing. Whilst Rickman engaged in group discussion, Bion sought to act upon the conduct of the men through manipulating authority relations in the Wing. The neurosis was first made visible by relaxing the authoritarian framework that had provided both the framework of community life and the structure for resistances to it. When the men themselves had to take responsibility for organizing tasks, and for defining and disciplining miscreants, they would learn that the disruption was not grounded *in* authority but in their psychological relations *to* authority. When the group realized the psychological origins of its distress, it could release its full energies in self-cure. The object was thus to promote group solidarity through the management of psychological relations.

Although this experiment ended after six weeks, it was followed by a second 'Northfield experiment'. In this, Thomas Main sought to produce what he referred to as a 'therapeutic community' in which the hospital was to be used[40]

> not as an organization run by doctors in the interests of their own greater technical efficiency, but as a community with the immediate aim of full participation of all its members in its daily life and the eventual aim of the resocialisation of the neurotic individual for life in ordinary society . . . a spontaneous and emotionally structured (rather than medically dictated) organization in which all staff and patients engage.

For such a reformatory technology, the institutional regime is construed as a system of relations that are more emotional than technical.There is also a shift in relations of expertise. The role of the doctor is no longer direction but interpretation. All those around the sick person – patients, domestics, nurses – are drawn into the field of the illness and its cure. The social relations of group life are now conceived not only as a means of treatment of neurosis, but also the field where neurosis is manifested and may be exacerbated: the origin of neurosis itself is to be found in problems of social relations.[41]

At the same time, a parallel experiment was developing an analagous technology.[42] In 1942 a cardiologist (Pat Wood) and a psychiatrist (Maxwell Jones) became joint directors of a 100-bed unit for the treatment of 'effort syndrome'. The Mill Hill Neurosis Unit was one of two establishments for the treatment of war neuroses run by the Ministry of Health, with staff drawn from the Maudsley Hospital. Whilst the other unit utilized short-term treatments like modified insulin, ether abreaction, continuous narcosis and narco-analysis, at Mill Hill the emphasis was on the application of sociological and psychological conceptions of treatment. The investigators concluded, after detailed cardiological examination, that effort syndrome – breathlessness, palpitations, left-chest pain, postural giddiness, occasional fainting attacks and fatigue – was not related to heart disease. On the contrary, it was deemed a psychosomatic complaint. A discussion procedure involving nurses was developed to explain to the patients the physiological mechanisms that produced their symptoms, seeking to allay the anxiety that exacerbated the problem and to change patients' attitudes to their symptoms.

These discussion groups soon expanded, beginning to deal with problems raised in life on the ward and elsewhere, and taking the form of group discussion and, often, dramatization of the problems. It gradually appeared that the whole of hospital life could affect the illness, provoking deterioration in the condition or participation in therapy. Further, the patient's reactions to the hospital community mirrored his or her reactions to the community outside, hence the latter could be affected by working upon the former. This entailed social interpenetration between doctors, nurses and patients, made easier by the fact that doctors were, in the main, from outside the mental hospital system, that nurses were drawn from educated, mature women with some status, and that patients were principally from the armed services.

When the war ended, the Ministry of Labour embarked upon a massive enterprise of labour resettlement. Twenty civilian resettlement units were established, with the aim of rehabilitating ex-prisoners of war for civilian life. The techniques deployed in these 'transitional communities' for 'social reconnection' were those that had been developed in the community treatment of neurotic soldiers.[43] Jones was made responsible for the unit set up at Southern Hospital, Dartford, in Kent, and re-used the procedures developed at Mill Hill, additionally seeking to connect up the 'transitional community' with the local community that surrounded it. Where rehabilitation had previously been a mere adjunct to therapy conducted by other means – mediating between life under the dominance of medicine and life as a private matter – it now became continuous with, indeed the essence of, the therapeutic intervention itself. The patient was one who had lost his or her capacity to function as an adjusted social individual; treatment was to reinvest the malfunctioning individual with the rights, privileges, capacities, moralities and responsibilities of personhood.

Jones' major achievement was the realization that these techniques could be applied to any other socially maladjusted individual.[44] The problems of disabled labourers prompted the establishment of an elaborate social apparatus in the immediate post-war period. The Disabled Persons (Employment) Act had been passed in 1944; at the beginning of 1950 just under one million persons were registered disabled, there were 366 full-time and 1,450 part-time Disablement Resettlement Officers, and twelve Industrial Rehabilitation Units located in the big cities, containing workshops with factory-like conditions. As far as the National Advisory Council on the Employment of the Disabled was concerned, the most troublesome aspect of the problem was the hard core of chronic unemployed. Whilst only around 50,000 registered disabled persons were classed as psychiatric, for this hard core, whatever their diagnostic label, unemployment had led to the development of anti-social attitudes. Hence their problem had become a psychiatric one – a problem of maladjustment requiring rehabilitation. The Roffey Park Rehabilitation Centre had utilized community treatment for maladjusted industrial workers with some success;[45] shortly after, in 1947, the Industrial Neurosis Unit at Belmont Hospital was set up to investigate methods of treatment and resettlement of this hard core to feed back into general planning for rehabilitation of inefficient or maladjusted workers. The population of chronic unemployed neurotics it received from all over the country included inadequate and aggressive psychopaths, schizoid personalities, early schizophrenics, various drug addictions, sexual perversions and chronic psychoneurotics. To this unpromising and heterogeneous population, unified only by their social inefficiency and maladjustment, were applied all the community techniques for restoring the neurotic to adjustment to his environment in order to maintain functional efficiency. Thus there were large discussion groups for abreaction and the socializing influence of group approval, with doctors supplying episodic psychodynamic interpretations of group processes. There were small groups to encourge participation, lead the patient to develop a sense of acceptance and belonging, foster the development of responsibility for fellow group members, allow social pressures to modify personality, and provide the opportunity for occasional judicious interpretations by group leaders. And there was psychodrama, which was therapeutic in that it promoted group formation, allowed the abreaction of individual patients, and showed that there could be social acceptance of previously hidden intimate problems.

Therapeutic communities were not inspired by a simple humanitarian impulse; all aspects of the regime sought to manage the individual from a pathology conceived of as social maladjustment to a normality construed in terms of functional efficiency. Each of the four themes of this ideology of the therapeutic community can be understood in this light.[46] Democratization certainly refers to the belief that each member of the community – staff and patients – should share equally in the exercise of power in decisions over both administrative and therapeutic aspects of community affair, but the object here is not simply a moral commitment to ending hierarchy, or even the utilization of the latent skills and potential of patients. It is to remove the reality basis for the stereotyped use of authorities as loci of hate or blame, hence allowing such phenomena to be interpreted and analysed in terms of transference, with a view to transforming attitudes to authority. Permissiveness, the toleration of a wide range of distressing or deviant behaviour, facilitates the expression of inhibited materials, allowing them to come to the patient's awareness, and be analysed and worked through. Communalism, the establishment of tight-knit inter-communicative relationships seeks not only to enforce participation upon the isolate, but also to counter the affectionlessness produced in patients by early pathological family situations. Reality confrontation, the continuous presentation of interpretations of behaviour to patients, seeks to show the maladjusted how their behaviour affects others, reveal its disruptive consequences, and counteract the denial, distortion, withdrawal and other mechanisms that interfere with the capacity to relate to others in the normal world. A benign innovation perhaps, but the adoption of these techniques was not motivated by a simple humanism but as part of a profound strategy of normalization of maladjusted selves. Through these devices, sexual, criminal, industrial or social deviants, whose behaviour was now construed as a manifestation of an underlying personality disorder, were to be managed back to a state of adjustment in which they could function smoothly within the institutional regimes they had previously disrupted.

It required but a simple shift of perspective to see that the traditional mental hospital violated all these therapeutic maxims. Hence in the 1950s a two-pronged attack on such institutions was mounted under the banner of the therapeutic community. On the one hand, a series of research studies of psychiatric institutions, principally American but rapidly imported into Britain, confirmed the pathogenic features of their organization and management.[47] On the other hand, a series of 'adventures in psychiatry' were undertaken, which sought to reorganize the mental hospital more or less according to the new rationale. Thomas Main at the Cassel, David Martin at Claybury and David Clark at Fulbourn sought to incorporate some or all of the new techniques of administrative therapy into their institutions, supplemented by accentuation of distinct aspects of analysis or practice, and sometimes in combination with chemotherapy or individual therapy.[48] It is sometimes thought that these developments were isolated and short-lived; that psychiatrists seeking to promote the merger with general medicine scandalized about the goings-on in such hospitals, criticised the therapeutic efficacy of these attempts to use the institution as a positive element in the production of the cure, and simultaneously utilized the arguments about the negative effects of mental hospital life in order to further their cause. But we need also to recognize what these new techniques of normalization added to the psychiatric system.

First, there was a widespread adoption of a policy of 'opening the doors' throughout the 1950s, a policy confirmed and promoted by the legislative reform of 1959. 'Opening the doors' stood for two responses to the critiques of the debilitating effects of the hospital environment. On the one hand, there was administrative reform of the asylum, whose emblem was the unlocking of wards but which also entailed a general reduction in the regimentation of bodies in time and space; on the other, there was the adoption of a policy of accelerated discharge. Unlocked wards were certainly not new, but now they rapidly became the norm. T.P. Rees at Warlingham Park Hospital opened the doors of 21 out of his 23 wards in the early fifties; by 1956 22 out of 37 wards of Netherne Hospital were opened and 60 per cent of patients were allowed out on parole within the boundaries of the estate; MacMillan opened the doors at Mapperly Hospital Nottingham in 1954, Stern did likewise at the Central Hospital Warwick in 1957 as did Mandelbrote at Coney Hill, Gloucester.[49]

Simultaneously, the new therapeutic dimensions made practicable by the rationale of the therapeutic community were exploited and professionalized. Of course, nurses had gained a new significance within the drug-based rationale for community psychiatry: they were perfectly capable of dispensing the therapeutic agents and could ensure regular medication through domiciliary visits, thus extending medical scrutiny beyond the hospital and into the home. Their voice, however muted, was beginning to be heard amongst the rival claims to status in the new psychiatric community. But the new techniques of administrative therapy provided a more secure base for claims to scientific expertise and professional status. Doctors could not claim special skills in the manipulation of the dynamic relations between members of the institutional community; yet these were now to be systematically utilized in the construction of a normal identity for the patient. Put crudely, nurses could now claim jurisdiction over the twenty three hours a day (at least) when the patient was not seeing the doctor. In the psychiatric wards of old mental hospitals and new psychiatric units, and in the day hospitals and half-way houses that began to proliferate, new techniques of nursing were developed and deployed; psychiatric nursing linked up with a shift within general nursing. The nurse's gaze was restructured; the patient was no longer to be seen as a series of tasks, but as a person to be actively engaged in the process of recovery.[50]

Alongside these developments within nursing, one sees the emergence of schemes of occupational therapy and industrial therapy – the former having as its rationale the increase of muscular co-ordination, and hence of self-confidence; the latter encouraging the development of the habits of labour through routine assembly work stressing task orientation and industrial efficiency. As mental disorder began to be seen, at least in part, as inhering in the inability to adjust efficiently to the exigencies of employment, work itself began to be seen as a vital element in the treatment of mental disorder.[51]

Programmes of hospital closure did not interrupt this expanding trade in lunacy, but allowed it to develop in new institutional contexts – in day hospitals run by the hospital service, day centres run by local authorities, half-way houses, hostels, group homes and a variety of other residential and non-residential institutions. The transformation of madness into a problem of maladjustment, and of treatment into a technique of rehabilitation, made custodialism and segregation as redundant as did drugs, and similarly facilitated the extension of psychiatry beyond the asylum into the new institutions of the psychiatric community.

A place was also to be found for the authentic therapeutic communities.[52] The community at Belmont continued, now known as Henderson Hospital, and catering for much the same sections of the psychiatric population. Maxwell Jones himself both spread the gospel in the USA, and deployed and developed his methods at Dingleton Hospital in Scotland. The Cassel Hospital continued under the directorship of Thomas Main. And mini-therapeutic communities have been attached to many psychiatric units in general hospitals, despite the apparent incompatibility of their rationales. Outside hospitals, the colours of the therapeutic community movement are worn by specialized rehabilitative institutions in the prison system, by many provisions for maladjusted, delinquent and criminal youths, by houses for drug-users and alchoholics – often run by ex-patients – by the houses of the Richmond Fellowship, and in many other residential establishments in the public, grant-aided, charitable and private sectors.

The proliferation of such communities demonstrates clearly the differentiation of the psychiatric population and the specialization of social responses to it. Therapeutic communities should not be seen as a threat to orthodox psychiatry. Rather, they provide a therapeutic rationale for the containment of those sectors who are, in one way or another, resistant to its techniques of normalization – the young neurotics and the personality disordered, the persistently self-damaging, the repetitively suicidal, the ostentatiously anti-social, those who continually act out and those who are continually manipulated by others. For those whose illness consists only in a disruptive failure of social adjustment, treatment can be seen as co-extensive with, and exhausted by, a systematic programme of resocialization: the re-constitution of the patient as a person.

Psychoanalysis

These social therapies clearly have an ambiguous border with a third technology of treatment – psychoanalysis. Despite the boost given to individual psychoanalysis after the Second World War, with the influx of European analysts into Britain, individual analytic work never gained much of a place in the hospital system or in other state-funded sectors. Dynamically inspired therapies were sometimes deployed in state clinics for children, and state agencies would sometimes refer children to the private sector. Individual therapies loosely drawing upon psychoanalysis were available on a contractual basis to those with money to pay, time to give, and a psyche to realign; we shall return to these later. What psychoanalysis principally contributed to the psychiatric system was a new way for non-psychiatric professions to conceptualize and actualize a specialized expertise, and an extension of the scope of psychiatric normalization to the 'private' domain of familial relations.

We have already seen how, in the social therapies, psycho-analysis was amongst those inventions that made a whole new field of group realities surrounding illness and cure thinkable and practicable. Similarly, psychoanalysis provided the conceptual and practical rationale for much of the expanded profession of social work in the fifties and sixties, underpinning much of the pressure towards a generic family service.[53] This centred on dangerous and endangered children, extending the early rationale of the child-guidance movement into a general programme for the production of healthy personalities by acting upon the emotional interchanges of family life. Nerves, maladjustment and delinquency were not evil tendencies or bad habits but symptoms of a psychologically malfunctioning family. The subjectivity of the child was a kind of internal representation of the psychodynamic relations between varied and sometimes incompatible family roles – husbands and wives, mothers and fathers, parents and children, sons and daughters, brothers and sisters. Social workers were thus uniquely placed to link up the problems of any one individual with the problems of them all, to interpret the family disturbance and reveal the hidden and unconscious conflicts playing across the inter-subjective field of the family, to bring insight to family members and thus to rectify the problem at its root – in the family itself. Such a psychoanalytically inspired social work thus brought love and guilt, jealousy and dependency, phantasy and desire within the ambit of government; it was now possible for the production of subjectivity to be socially managed by professional expertise.

Behaviour therapy

In the 1950s, the technological inventions made in pharmacology, social therapies and psychoanalysis were joined by a new mode of thinking about, and acting upon, psychological maladjustment: behaviour therapy.[54] As psychology began to consolidate the conceptual and technical hold it had obtained over the domain of personality during the Second World War, it simultaneously began to stake a claim for a slice of the therapy market. In order to do this it had to fight on two fronts. First, it needed to establish a working relationship with psychiatry. Second, it had to legitimate itself over and against psychoanalysis, with whom it competed at the level of its theoretical codes, diagnostic techniques and treatment modalities. At the technical level, it sought to discredit the reliability and validity of the dynamically inspired tests of personality. At the level of theoretical codes, it claimed that what was good in psychoanalysis was incorporated within learning theory – especially the recognition of the motivating role of anxiety – whilst what was not incorporated was the speculative and unestablished notions concerning the depths of the psyche which were, in any event, not amenable to scientific specification. And, at the level of therapy, it sought to use the language of scientific psychology and its repertoire of systematic research techniques to demonstrate that the claims of psychoanalysis to therapeutic efficacy were ill-founded.

Behaviour therapy linked up four elements. First, a psychological conception of the personality as consisting of a combination of a small number of measurable traits or dimensions, in which individuals varied – this had been the basis of the most successful wartime tests of character and temperament. Second, a theory of the development of personality through the cumulation of responses learned through the effects of conditioning upon the inherent susceptibilities of the individual. Third, a theory of neurotic symptoms as patterns of behaviour learned in the normal way but, for some reason or other, unadaptive. And, fourth, a normalizing technique based upon the principle that the processes of conditioning and deconditioning could be systematically exploited to resocialize behaviour into patterns deemed adaptive. Here was a mechanism that did not require us to refer to underlying disorders or complexes in the psyche, but remained at the level of the problem itself: the discrepancy between behaviour produced and behaviour desired. But, further, here was a technique that did not require reference to organic malfunctions, for we were not dealing with an illness but with the contingent mis-shaping of a psychology that was not sick, by means of processes that were themselves normal. Hence, psychologists could make a claim to a clinical expertise that was neither a threat to medicine, nor subordinate to it. Behaviour therapy required, in its pristine form, not the techniques of the consulting room and the bedside but those of the laboratory and the research project. Psychologists could thus claim this particular corner of the market in psychopathology without challenging the jurisdiction of the psychiatrist over the medical care of the patient.

Indeed, such an alliance proved rather fruitful. Beneath the surface of the fratricidal strife that obtained between psychologists and psychiatrists, a practical division of labour was established within the psychiatric units, hospitals and clinics. Psychiatric diagnosis was initially necessary to rule out underlying organic causes of the condition. One must certainly avoid the temptation to reduce all mental disorders to mere psychological malformations of personality. But within these constraints, under medical guidance, given a tightly specified problem and a desired end-state, clinical psychology was let loose upon specific targets: alchoholics, anorexics, bullemics, phobics, obsessives and the anxious could now have their behaviour managed back to normality through a programme employing the systematic use of sanctions and rewards. This programme could be undertaken on an out-patient basis as, say, in the case of specific phobias, or through a kind of merger with the social therapies of rehabilitation, in day hospitals and specialized in-patient units. In the latter, all aspects of ward life could be incorporated into a systematic programme for the reshaping of behaviour, suitably adjusted to utilize the individual desires and dislikes of the patient.

There has been a tendency to criticize behaviour therapy on the grounds of its harshness – as in the production of unpleasant states through drugs or shock in aversion therapy for alchoholics or homosexuals – and on the basis that it is imposed coercively upon those whose only illness is to resist socially approved norms of behaviour. But to take exception merely to this 'hard' end of behavioural techniques would be to rather miss the point. The techniques of behaviour therapy have spread far beyond the hospital scene, far ouside the control of medical psychiatry, and far wider than aversion therapies. In education and special education, in social work and nursing, in the prison and in management consultancy, in every area where human action is to be shaped up in the service of individual or social goals, behavioural techniques may be deployed. From giving up smoking to management of anxiety, from sex therapy to assertion training, from cognitive restructuring to change values to reformatory techniques for the kleptomaniac, these techniques can be employed. Behavioural techniques can be used to reconceptualize all situations in which the human factor is to be utilized at its most efficient in relation to any set of objectives.

Therapies of normality

Behavioural techniques are thus an essential constituent of the new 'therapies of normality' that have blossomed since the 1960s. These new techniques are not deployed in attempts to cure gross intellectual, emotional or volitional incapacities. Rather, they use psychiatric expertise to reshape subjectivity in desired directions, with the claim that they can produce certain functional capacities or psychological attributes.[55] The new technologies of subjectivity have not been applied coercively by state functionaries in order to constrain or eliminate deviant behaviours. They have grown up in the private sector, or have been promoted by voluntary organizations and philanthropists of the psyche. On the one hand, the apostles of these new techniques have held up images of what we could become; on the other, individuals have sought them out to help them fulfil the dream of realigning what they are with what they want to be.

Prior to the Second World War, psychoanalysis was virtually the only form of psychiatric expertise available in the private sector. In the last quarter of a century a host of new professions and techniques have come to operate upon the territory of psychiatry. Their services are available to all of us, for they promise succour to anyone who experiences a discrepancy between the reality of their lives and their desires. Hence these techniques are not limited to the problems previously covered by the category of neurosis. The new techniques certainly apply themselves to these neuroses, but they also radically extend the aspects of personal and social life that can be construed as remediable through psychiatric expertise. They work by instrumentalizing and elaborating our phantasies of happiness, pleasure and achievement, promoting an ideal of what we might be and working in the space that is thus opened between our wishes and our lives. With their assistance we can realise that infertility is not just a medical condition but a potentially damaging psychological problem, we can make all our children happy and exceptional, we could all achieve sexual pleasure, we can turn our marriages from ethical obligations into personal fulfilments, we can overcome the blocks that prevent us realizing our potential, we can even free ourselves from the awe we feel at the prospect of our finitude – death has become a manageable psychological problem.

These therapies of normality transpose the difficulties inherent in living on to a psychological register; they become not intractable features of desire and frustration but malfunctions of the psychological apparatus that are remediable through the operation of particular techniques. The self is thus

opened up, a new continent for exploitation by the entre-
preneurs of the psyche, who both offer us an image of a
life of maximized intellectual, commercial, sexual or personal
fulfillment and assure us that we can achieve it with the assistance of the technicians of subjectivity.

The discipline of mental health

This examination of some aspects of the genealogy of our
modernized psychiatric system disrupts many of the beliefs
upon which much contemporary 'radical' criticism of psychiatry
has been based. The psychiatric system that has taken shape
in Britian – and in Europe and the USA – over the last fifty
years has not been characterized primarily by coercion and
segregation, delineated by the mental hospital, hegemonized
by the medical profession or dominated by a narrow organicism
at the level of theory and treatment. At the programmatic
level, psychiatry would constitute a 'continuum of care' that
would run from custodial measures for those with major mental
derangements, through voluntary treatment for minor mental
troubles, to prophylactic work by propaganda, advice and the
reform of personal life in the interests of mental health. The
hospital retains a key role in this system; not now the isolated,
segregative and custodial institution, but the psychiatric wing
or ward of the district general hospital. The psychiatric population is highly differentiated and distributed across a range of
specialized sites: secure units, local-authority group homes,
specialized units for children, alchoholics, anorexics, drug-
users, and so forth. And relations have been established
between such institutions and other sites where psychiatric
expertise is deployed: the child-guidance clinic, the courtroom,
the counselling centre, the prison and the classroom.

   This ensemble is not hegemonized at the level of its theoretical codes or therapeutic practices by a socially blind organicism. Psychiatrists have long allowed a key role for 'social
factors' in the precipitation and prevention of mental distress,
have sought a prophylactic role by injecting psychiatric considerations into debates over social policies, and have solicited
collaboration between medical treatment in hospital and the
aid of other social agencies. In the contemporary psychiatric
system, key roles are played by non-medical professions –

nursing, social work, probation, psychology, education – and increasingly by quasi-professional 'voluntary' or self-help organizations. Whilst the 'eclecticism' of psychiatry is sometimes criticized, it is precisely this eclecticism that allows the system to function, enabling the coexistence of therapeutic ideologies and techniques that appear fundamentally opposed: from individual psychotherapy to co-counselling, from dynamic group therapy to behaviour modification, from drug treatment to primal screaming. Hospitals using psychotropic medications, therapeutic communities, feminist self-help groups, social-work group homes, community nurses and many other strange bedfellows have combined to chart the domain of mental health and develop technologies for its management.

The critiques of the custodial and segregative project of the asylum, far from standing outside psychiatry, have actually contributed to the reorganization of psychiatry and the formation of this new complex of powers over mental health. The move away from the asylum has extended the range of social ills seen to be flowing from psychiatric disturbance and has, simultaneously, psychiatrized new populations – children, delinquents, criminals, vagrants and the work-shy, the aged, unhappy marital and sexual partners – all become possible objects for explanation and treatment in terms of mental disturbance. In the majority of cases, such treatment is not imposed coercively upon unwilling subjects but sought out by those who have come to identify their own distress in psychiatric terms, believe that psychiatric expertise will help them, and are thankful for the attention they receive.

Some guidelines can thus be suggested for investigating the power of contemporary psychiatry. Rather than seeking to explain a process of de-institutionalization, we need to account for *the proliferation of sites for the practice of psychiatry*. There has not been an extension of social control but rather *the psychiatrization of new problems and the differentiation of the psychiatric population*. Nor has there been an illegitimate extension of the mandate of medicine, instead what has taken place is *a new distribution of professional powers*. Indeed, there has been no simple medical monopolization of mental distress, but rather the development of a *free market in expertise*. Thus we cannot base our analysis of the power of psychiatry upon an opposition to the medicalization of madness, but need to evaluate the consequences of *a multiplicity of techniques of normalization*. The modern dispensation of psychiatry, far from being merely repressive or negative, has constituted a new *discipline of mental health*. Hence, rather than basing a politics upon the demand for mental health for all, perhaps we should examine the implications of the construction of subjectivity as a site of self-examination and technical remediation, and question the desirability of conceiving of our personal fulfilment in terms of mental health.

3

Psychiatry and the construction of the feminine

Hilary Allen

A cursory examination of mental health statistics suggests that women are mentally sicker than men. More women then men are admitted to psychiatric units every year; once discharged they have more frequent readmissions, and more women receive treatment for psychological disorders from GPs and out-patient clinics. This relative excess of women occurs across almost all the diagnostic categories of psychiatry, with the exception of alcoholism and personality disorder, but is most marked in relation to depression and the psycho-neuroses. Of all patients receiving any form of psychiatric treatment, by far the largest group is that of women receiving psychotropic drugs, normally tranquillizers and anti-depressants, through their general practitioners.[1]

In this sense, the inclusion in a book such as this of a single chapter addressing the 'special' issues of psychiatry's approach to the female, as if in some way analogous to its 'special' approach to racial minorities, is curious and misleading. The female is not the 'special' but the *normal* form of the psychiatric patient – throughout, when this book refers to patients,, it is predominantly referring to women. The same is, of course, true of the standard texts in psychiatry, even though there, as elsewhere, the convention is maintained of uniformly referring to the patient as male.

Psychiatry itself has given little direct attention to the sexual discrepancy in psychiatric epidemiology. Sexual variations in epidemiology are a matter of interest but not on the whole of perturbation to the medical profession, and the understanding that women suffer more mental morbidity than men is so well established and so congruent with stereotypical views about women generally – as unstable, irrational and changeable – that its statistical confirmation evokes little surprise or reflection. For a polemical feminism, on the other hand, whose interest in the matter is political rather than clinical, this apparent female morbidity is a matter of mixed discomfort and concern. To the extent that the figures appear to confirm an unwelcome stereotype of women, they are embarrassing to feminism, and there is every reason to deny their validity. On the other hand, to the extent that they attest to the ubiquity of women's suffering, they are a matter of concern for feminism, and there is every motivation to propose a reading of this suffering that will unite it with all the other troubles of women, as a function of women's social oppression.

Embarrassment tending towards denial and compassion tending towards indignation: out of these two tendencies there has emerged a feminist analysis of psychiatry whose main thrust has been towards the demonstration of a patriarchal complicity in the apparent mental morbidity of women, and whose main conceptual schema comprises an elaborate interlinking of women's mental troubles with the social imposition of a debilitating norm of femininity. This form of analysis, first developed in Phylis Chesler's *Women & Madness*,[2] and subsequently indissolubly linked with her name, has for more than a decade coloured almost every feminist dicussion of psychiatry and female psychopathology.

The body of feminist work that has since been produced is stylistically diverse, and includes both popular polemics aimed at a general feminist audience,[3] and more scholarly contributions in the academic and professional literature.[4] These works have added little, however, to the basic theoretical analysis that Chesler's study establishes and, more importantly, they adopt without question the same unspoken assumptions about the kind of issue upon which a feminist analysis of psychiatry must be grounded. Rather misleadingly, the British edition of Chesler's book is subtitled: 'When is a woman mad and who is it who decides?'. But the interrogation around which the analysis is actually organized might more aptly be summarized as 'Why is it *women* who are mad and who is to blame?' Although much of the later literature is less aggressively inquisitorial in its tone, there remains the assumption that the primary task of feminist intervention in the field is to account for the high incidence of diagnosed female pathology, and to do so in terms that securely demonstrate its social aetiology in women's oppression. Thus for example Al-Issa's lengthy volume, which is intended largely as a resource for university courses in psychology, sociology and women's studies, summarizes the major problematics of the field in the following questions: 'Why are women in the Western World labelled 'crazy' more often than men? Is it that women are more vulnerable to mental illness, or have they fallen victim to social and psychological pressures inherent in our society? Are they discriminated against by the mental health profession? And how do the causes, effects and treatments of mental disorders differ between the sexes?'[5] In answering these questions Al-Issa marshals all the conventional machinery of academic research, citation and argument in order to reproduce and elaborate the same basic theses that are proposed more polemically by Chesler.

This essay locates itself in direct tension with Chesler's analysis and with the work that has followed from it. It shares with this body of work a central concern with psychiatric patients as *women*, and a conviction that a feminist politics in the field of psychiatry is legitimate and necessary. There is every reason to break the long silence over the unspoken 'she' of psychiatry and expose to feminist attention the wards and waiting rooms full of women who lurk behind the bland 'he' of the psychiatric textbooks. But beyond this shared and central concern with *women*, my argument parts company with Chesler and those who follow her. I examine the questions that are prioritized in their approach, argue that the answers provided are unsustainable, and also challenge the centrality of the questions themselves. I suggest that the prioritization of these questions, and the seeming imperative to answer them in particular ways (at whatever cost to the credibility of the argument) derives from certain unnecessary and unhelpful preconceptions about the theoretical requirements of a feminist politics of psychiatry. In arguing these points I shall refer repeatedly to Chesler's original development of the analysis. Her text remains the most systematic and explicit formulation of the position that later works have either taken for granted or sought to elaborate; it is thus exemplary of the preoccupations of the field as a whole.

I regard Chesler's analysis as unhelpful for a feminist politics of psychiatry not only because its arguments seem ultimately unconvincing, but also because in practical terms it tends both to obscure many areas where a feminist intervention might be pertinent and categorically to foreclose certain others. In the second part of this essay I consider the question of practical feminist intervention in more detail. I begin by briefly looking at feminist therapy, which I take as an example of the kinds of practical intervention Chesler's approach *does* allow, but also as illustrating some of the limitations of involvement that this approach implies. I therefore turn to the possibility of developing additional and alternative approaches, and suggest some less constricting grounds upon which a feminist politics of psychiatry might be based. These are not dependent on either the denial of women's mental illnesses, or the demonstration of an exclusive patriarchal blame for them, and they involve a major shift in what is to be understood as a feminist politics of psychiatry. In the concluding pages I seek to illustrate the implications of such a shift, by specifying some of the areas that it might open up for feminist examination and intervention, and identifying some of the gains and losses that might be entailed.

Chesler: a feminine complaint

The existing feminist analysis forms itself in the gap that is left by the deletion of an inadmissible argument – the argument that women are 'really' and 'naturally' madder than men, as a function of their inherent feminine condition. In describing the argument as 'deleted', I am not suggesting that it is not allowed to appear *at all*: on the contrary, it is commonplace in feminist discussions of psychiatry to find a painstaking reconstruction of the argument, using judicious quotation from historical and other texts, to demonstrate the existence within psychiatry of a conception of female psychopathology as arising from an inherent emotional, intellectual or moral deficiency of the feminine subject. Seidenberg and De Crow, for example, quote the following excerpts from nineteenth-century texts, as illustrating the attribution of female psychopathology to the failings of female biology: 'Woman has a sum total of nervous force equivalent to a man's, but this force is distributed over a greater multiplicity of organs . . . The nervous force is therefore weakened in each organ . . . it is more sensitive, more liable to derangement.' 'With women it is but a step from extreme nervous susceptibility to downright hysteria, and from that to overt insanity.'[6] Other writers, such as Howell,[7] and Chesler herself, concentrate upon a selective reading of Freud and later psychoanalytic writers, quoting such passages as the following to demonstrate the attribution of female psychopathology to the inherent vicissitudes of femininity: 'A woman . . . often frightens us by her psychical rigidity and unchangeability . . . There are no paths open to further development; it is as though the whole process had already run its course and remains thence forward insusceptible to influence – as though, indeed, the difficult development to femininity has exhausted the possibilities of the person concerned.'[8]

Such theoretical positions are not expunged absolutely from feminist discussions, but they are presented in a purely inquisitorial fashion: the detection and exposure of such heretical tendencies in the works of psychiatry's notional forebears is taken as evidence of a fundamental bad faith at the core of psychiatric ideology. They are deployed in the feminist texts as simultaneously discredited and discreditable. They are depictions of female vulnerability that can be taken as already discarded, and their quotation is thus used – by an unspecified extension or association – to imply that *any* suggestion of female vulnerability must be both preposterous and disingenuous.

Yet despite the fact that such arguments seem to be placed beneath the threshold of serious debate, there is a sense in which they insist, implicitly, as the critical threat around which the feminist battle lines are drawn. The analysis appears to assume, unreflectively, that to even to countenance the possibility of an inherent female vulnerability to mental illness would in principle be devastating for any feminist position. Beyond the general pillorying of such explanations, an alternative must therefore be proposed – an explanation that will safely pre-empt the territory of female psychopathology and leave no space into which notions of any inherent feminine weakness could be inserted. The parameters of the argument thus come to be defined somewhat defensively; unsurprisingly perhaps, the alternative that is provided takes up the explanation of women's psychopathology in almost precisely the same terms and by quite the same *form* of argument as that which it seeks to preclude. It does not in any sense challenge the notion that the preponderance of women within psychiatry must be theorizable by reference to some universal, homogeneous and deleterious condition to which all women are subject – let us call it 'femininity' – but instead merely redefines the origin of this condition. The central thrust of the feminist analysis depends upon the demonstration that this deleterious and sickening femininity is not an inherent, essential condition of women as such, but something external, imposed upon women through some direct or indirect oppression. The rebuttal of the inadmissible challenge thus takes the form: yes, women's femininity makes them sick, but this femininity is not an essential condition of women (so there is possibility of change) and furthermore it has been coercively imposed upon women (so it is men and not women who are to blame).

At this point three central conditions of the analysis can already be identified. Each reflects a certain preconception about the necessary theoretical conditions of a feminist politics of psychiatry. First, there is the refusal of any appeal to an inherent vulnerability of women in the explanation of women's psychiatric morbidity – without which it is assumed the analysis could not constitute itself as *feminist*. Second, there is the explanation of women's psychopathology in terms of uniform and overarching conditions to which in principle all women are assumed to be subject – without which it is assumed the analysis could not be *theoretically* adequate. Third, there is the attribution of patriarchal blame – without which it is assumed that the analysis could not be *political*. I shall suggest that none of these assumptions are necessary, and that the development of a feminist politics of psychiatry does not require that these analytic conditions are fulfilled. First, however, let us briefly examine how the existing analysis brings these three components together.

There are two prongs to the analysis. The first of these makes women's mental illnesses a more or less direct product of the oppressive feminine role, a role imposed by a patriarchal order of society. In its weak form, in which women's mental breakdowns are conceived as the objective result of insufferable stresses to which women are characteristically exposed – economic dependence, social isolation, domestic violence, lack of satisfactory status or occupation, and so on – the argument claims empirical support from a variety of well-documented studies from within the mainstream of academic and medical research. Brown and Harris,[9] for example, find the development of depression in women to be strongly correlated with certain social circumstances that are in some degree typical of the conditions of young working-class mothers – social isolation, responsibility for children at home, lack of employment. And there are also a number of epidemiological studies that indicate that women's mental ill-health is concentrated amongst women cohabiting with men – in women without men the rate of mental illness is low.[10] In men, however, the relationship is reversed – the inference being that in conventional cohabitation women's domestic responsibilities place insufferable strains on their mental health, whereas men do rather nicely from the arrangement.

In this weak form, the argument is not fundamentally an argument about femininity as such, but about the deleterious impact of the stresses to which women in our society are characteristically exposed. The objective conditions under which many women live are depressing/sickening/maddening, and women's psychopathology is merely the mark that is left upon women by these material circumstances. Certainly the argument concerns female subjects, but it neither relates to *all* female subjects, simply in their capacity as female, nor in principle *requires* female subjects. In so far as the approach could be seen as predicting anything about men, it would predict that under these same objective conditions men would also develop mental illness: only if it were discovered that they did *not* respond in this way might it be necessary to introduce a variable such as 'femininity' to account for the differential response of women.

But there is a stronger and more radical form of the argument, in which a relationship between mental disorder and a unifying femininity is more significantly posed. Here the 'patriarchal social order' is assumed to determine not only the objective conditions under which women will typically live but also – through some mechanism of ideology – the kinds of subjects they can be, the ways in which they can respond to stresses, the terms in which they can experience reality. It is this system of *internalized* constraints upon women, operating ideologically across *all* women, regardless of their specific material circumstances, that constitutes the feminine condition and that is construed as mentally crippling to women, and the origin of their propensity to mental ill-health. Thus femininity re-enters the argument as that which will once again explain women's psychopathology. Indeed, women's most typical expressions of mental ill-health are construed as little more than femininity 'writ large' – women's depression, hysteria, anorexia, attempted suicide, anxiety states, etc. – are theorized as simply the perversely self-destructive exaggeration of all those debilitating traits in which femininity is seen to inhere: dependency, self-effacement, emotionality, triviality, timidity, passivity and so forth. Joanna Ryan gives a typical example of this reasoning in her discussion of depression:

> We . . . have to consider what it is about depression that is specific to femininity, especially since for many women depression does not seem to be related to identifiable losses or events, but is much more something that comes and goes in their lives. What does depression express about being a woman in our society? Firstly, being depressed is a very typically female form of distress in the sense that it is a passive and socially inoffensive mode of being. Depression is containing, exhausting, and stupefying. It exudes powerlessness and is the antithesis of activity and control. In all these ways it is simply an exaggeration of what women are all too often seen as. Secondly depression involves an enormous amount of self-blame and self-hatred and collapse of self-confidence . . . Here again it is only an intensification of the ways in which so many women feel about themselves anyhow.[11]

This form of analysis paints a bleak picture for women. Women are externally disadvantaged, internally crippled, driven to sickness and then exposed to psychiatry. And, since the logic of the argument is framed in terms of patriarchal structures in which psychiatry is clearly implicated, it is not surprising that psychiatry is not credited in these arguments with any wish or power to improve the situation. On the contrary, psychiatry is presented as not merely complicit with the patriarchal system within which these troubles are produced, but as its key henchman: the 'treatment' of the psychiatric patient is construed as the further enforcement of that debilitating femininity – that passive dependence, self-effacement, and so on – that initially occasioned the psychatric intervention. Small comfort for women that Chesler's analysis denies any 'essential' mental pathology of women, born of any 'essential' femininity: the socially engendered pathology, born of a socially engendered femininity, seems almost equally ineluctable. All that seems to have shifted is the locus of responsibility for this unfortunate state of affairs from an inescapable 'nature' to an inescapable 'patriarchy'.

To make the picture even bleaker, Chesler provides a second prong to the argument, on which to impale any woman who attempts to shake off the crippling shackles of femininity. Here women's struggles to *refuse* or *reject* this femininity are also portrayed as grounds for a psychiatric diagnosis: those conditions, such as schizophrenia or psychopathy, which cannot easily be characterized as a desperate exaggeration of femininity are here characterized as the equally desperate refusal of it. Women will equally be labelled as mad (or may actually be *driven* mad – it is never theoretically clear whether this madness is to be construed as merely an oppressive label or a real condition of these women) if they somehow escape the full internal debilitation of the feminine role and react to their social oppression with an appropriate rage, hostility and rebellion.

In its content this argument draws upon both a series of casual observations about mental illness and a series of specific empirical findings. Casually, it makes allowance for the observation that many psychiatrically diagnosed women show seemingly masculine traits (violence and assertiveness for example) that cannot easily be fitted into the model of an exaggerated femininity, and that historically many unruly, independent and 'masculine' women have been incarcerated as mad.[12] More specifically, the argument draws upon certain research findings, particularly concerning schizophrenic women. Chesler thus cites the work of Cheek,[13] and of McLelland and Watt,[14] as finding that schizophrenic women showed more masculine and fewer feminine traits than 'normal' female controls. What is argued on this basis is that the aberrations from the norm that are here detected are not merely 'symptoms' of a disorder but its constitutive condition: the role rejection is what the so-called pathology is all about.

Whilst the content of the argument is specific, its general form rests firmly in the tradition of anti-psychiatry, and operates the same central inversion: it is not the patient but society that is pathological. The patient's symptoms are that she refuses society's pathology, and acts reasonably, even if powerlessly and thus self-destructively, in an unreasonable situation. What is added to this now familiar line is a specifically sexual theory of the originary alienation, in terms of femininity, and the attribution of a specifically patriarchal role for psychiatry. In the terms of this theorization, psychiatry provides the final coercive instance against women who fall radically out of line with femininity – policing, punishing, and silencing them.

In Chesler's analysis, these two prongs of argument are deftly incorporated into a single encyclopaedic explanation of women's apparent propensity to mental illness:

> *What we consider 'madness' whether it appears in women or in men is either the acting-out of the devalued female role or the total or partial rejection of one's sex-role stereotype.* Women who fully act out the conditioned female role are clinically viewed as 'neurotic' or 'psychotic'. When and if they are hospitalised it is for predominantly female behaviours such as 'depression', 'suicide attempts', 'anxiety neuroses', 'paranoia' or 'promiscuity'. Women who reject or are ambivalent about the female role frighten themselves and society, so much so that their ostracism and self-destructiveness probably begin very early. Such women are also assured of a psychiatric label and, if they are hospitalised, it is for less 'female' behaviours, such as 'schizophrenia', 'lesbianism' or 'promiscuity'.[15]

Many criticisms may be levelled against the details of Chesler's presentation, and from many different angles. It is an unashamedly polemical text and its kaleidoscope of statistical, empirical, historical, mythological and anecdotal data is deployed with a singlemindedness that disallows any contrary argument or conclusions. It is not, however, the particular eccentricities of the text that concern me here, but a much more fundamental problem with the general thesis it proposes: this is the empirical difficulty of substantiating the basic claim on which her case rests. Chesler claims that psychiatry, as a privileged intermediary between women and the patriarchy, is centrally organized around a complex maintenance and policing of gender roles, and that its categories of pathology are ultimately reducible to categorizations of the expression or the rejection of a devalued femininity. Psychiatry, I suggest, simply does not operate like that; its categories are not organized in that way.

Before going on to substantiate my objection with some specific observations about the treatment of gender within psychiatry, it is necessary to identify the particular device whereby Chesler seeks to establish the inferences she claims: the refusal to make any differentiations between what is constitutive of psychiatry and what is contingent to it. Properly speaking, her argument can only hold if the psychiatric sexism with which she concerns herself is *constitutive* of psychiatry and its categories. By this I mean that her argument claims to relate to the underlying structure, objectives and conditions of possibility of psychiatry, exposing the maintenance of gender roles as its fundamental project – as that without which psychiatry would simply cease to exist. Let us be clear, she is not simply claiming that psychiatry is 'as it happens' full of sexism, or that psychiatric categories are 'in practice' operated asymmetrically, or that in the name of psychiatry much violence has 'in fact' been done to women. All of this can be true of psychiatry but, nonetheless, be merely contingent to it. And if all this psychiatric sexism *is* merely contingent to psychiatry, so that it could in principle be eliminated without implying the fundamental evacuation of psychiatry or the dissolution of its categories, then Chesler's argument disintegrates: psychiatry cannot then be seen as organized around gender-role maintenance and the categories of women's mental pathologies are not simply tokens of an oppressed femininity.

It is not difficult to demonstrate that psychiatry is contingently sexist, normative, and guilty of many abuses against women. Indeed, given the general conditions of society *outside* of psychiatry, it would indeed be curious if one could not find such features inside psychiatry as well. Many feminist texts, including Chesler's, have documented outrageous abuses of women by psychiatry and its agents.[16] And of perhaps more general significance, Broverman et al.'s much quoted study of the stereotypical attitudes of psychiatric personnel demonstrates vividly that those working in the field operate a double standard of expectation of men and women, attributing to 'normal healthy women' relatively few of the positive traits that they associate either with 'normal healthy men' or even 'normal healthy adults'.[17] The scales are already unbalanced at the moment of expectation: psychiatrists approach women with assumptions about female mentality that may condition what they 'see' and influence how they respond. Certainly, psychiatrists' normative expectations concerning mental health in a woman are bound to influence what attributes they perceive as abnormal and what objectives they seek to achieve in treatment. Almost as certainly, these normative expectations will often operate, from a feminist perspective, to the detriment of women patients: at best doing no more than maintaining them in conditions of stereotypical disadvantage and, at worse, compounding their burdens – as happens, for example, when the unhappy housewife has tranquillizer addiction added to her catalogue of troubles.

There is every reason for a feminist politics of psychiatry to take seriously the pervasiveness of psychiatric sexism ; this is not in dispute. What I am arguing, however, is that it is entirely illegitimate – and ultimately entirely unhelpful – to claim from this evidence that this sexism is itself constitutive of psychiatry, that the maintenance of this sexism is a central project of psychiatry, or that without this, psychiatry (and by implication women's mental illness) would cease to exist. I am arguing that none of the evidence that Chesler brings to bear can legitimately be taken as substantiating such a claim. What kind of evidence then *would* one need to adduce in order to support such a conclusion?

Two possibilities seem obvious. The first would be to demonstrate that psychiatric discourse is organized, overtly or otherwise, around a uniform division of gender, with different categories of pathology for men and for women, and with categories of female pathology whose symptomatology is reducible to the various functions and dysfunctions of femininity. The second would be to demonstrate that irrespective of the external form of this discourse (which might be no more than an ideological mystification), what actually occasions psychiatric intervention and determines its direction is uniformly related to the fulfilment or non-fulfilment of gender roles.

There is no evidence that psychiatry operates uniformly in

either of these ways. Indeed, what may be characterized as the 'psychiatric system' is so radically heterogeneous in its objects and theories that it is far from clear how it could be expected to operate in *any* way uniformly. Certainly, if there is anything uniform about the way issues of gender are taken up within the various branches of psychiatry it is an entirely negative uniformity: a uniformity in a general marginalization of issues of gender, in whatever terms they are posed, as more-or-less extraneous to the psychiatric project. There is not space here to look in detail at the way issues of gender are taken up across the whole (wide and fragmented) field of psychiatry. For the sake of economy it will here suffice to make some general points about what might be regarded as the 'solid middle ground' of psychiatric theory and practice, and to high-light a few rather specific examples of the direct discrepancy between the actual operation of psychiatry and that which would be predicted on the basis of Chesler's analysis.

One way to conceptualize this solid middle ground is in terms of the standard psychiatric classifications of disorders, illnesses, symptoms, etc. that structure psychiatric diagnosis and provide the central organizing categories of formal psychiatric discourse. Here we find a conceptual framework that, to a large extent, serves to obviate the need for any specific attention to gender. With very few exceptions the modern psychiatric categories are defined and described in sexually neutral terms, delineated by the presence of symptoms and signs that might in principle be identified as pathological in whatever subject they appeared. The approach objectifies the symptoms and the disorders, making the subject of psychiatry merely the bearer of pathologies which are themselves, in their notionally pure form, delineated in some non-subjective space. Conceived thus, the subject of psychiatry is only tangentially a gendered subject. Of course, since there *are* no others, the subjects in whom mental illnesses appear must 'in fact' be gendered subjects, just as they must be subjects of a particular age, race, height, education and so on, and these personal characteristics may be acknowledged as conditioning the particular mani-festations of these illnesses. The persecutory voices of a female schizophrenic may have characteristically different things to say from those of a male, but it is the presence of the voice that comprises the symptom; women and men may have

characteristically different ways of 'expressing' their symptomatology, or dealing with it or disguising it, but these differences are regarded within psychiatric discourse as no more
than a kind of background 'noise', as much distorting as revealing the pure – and sexually undifferentiated – form of the
medical pathology.

There are only two major exceptions to this: that of personality disorder, which includes hysteria and sexual deviation;
and that of the various psychological disturbances seen as
arising from the female reproductive cycle. What is interesting,
however, in both these cases, is their progressive *marginalization* from the field of psychiatry.[18] Chesler suggests that
women who reject their sex-role stereotype are liable to be
categorized as psychopathic or personality disordered (the two
diagnoses are for most purposes interchangeable). To some
extent this would indeed seem to be the case: sexual deviance
in women, violence towards self or others, or inability to
maintain the close family or domestic relationships expected
of women are all identified as symptoms of personality
disorder, and may lead to this psychiatric diagnosis. And there
is undoubtedly a widespread assumption that such women are
mad: many of them do come into the hands of psychiatrists,
through GPs and general hospitals, through social-work agencies and the courts, and through self-referral. The demand is
constantly made that psychiatry should take charge of them,
to intervene in their troubled lives and their troublesome
departures from 'normality'. What is striking, however, is that
psychiatry increasingly refuses responsibility for doing so.
Where gender-role deviance is the primary complaint, psychiatry uses the labels 'personality disorder' and 'psychopathy'
not as a legitimation for intervention but as a ground for
declining to intervene; it defines these diagnostic categories as
outside the domain of psychiatric disorder. Deviations of gender role are defined not as mental illnesses but as abnormalities
of personality, and the domain of personality variation is then
defined as outside that of psychiatry. Psychiatry notes and
identifies these deviations as pathological, indeed claims an
exclusive competence to do so but, nonetheless, refuses to
police the territory that it thus marks out. These patients are
labelled as pathological, but the pathology is marginalized from
the sphere of psychiatric attention or intervention.

A comparable marginalization is operated in relation to

disorders conceived as arising primarily from a disturbance of female biology. These might easily be seen, within Chesler's framework, as exemplary cases of the excessive acting out of the female role – the exaggerated emotionality of the premenstrual syndrome,[19] the weepiness or excessive excitement of postnatal psychosis,[20] the frustration and distraction of menopausal depression.[21] What is more, their exclusive applicability to women patients, and their distinct theorization in terms of the female condition would appear to make them ripe examples for an analysis of the kind that Chesler proposes. But, in fact, to the extent that they are conceptualized in terms of femininity, psychiatry again tends to marginalize them, or flatly refuse jurisdiction. Where they are theorized as arising primarily from a disturbed female biology – as in the case of premenstrual psychopathology – they are routinely referred or transferred to specialists in endocrinology or gynaecology rather than psychiatry, as not 'properly' psychiatric disorders at all. On the other hand, where they are conceived as merely the exaggeration of a 'normal' feminine response, as in much of the less florid puerperal disturbance, they have increasingly been treated as requiring social-work intervention more than psychiatric treatment. Where there is clear psychiatric symptomatology, on the other hand, as in severe depressive or psychotic reactions, the tendency has increasingly been to minimize the dimension of sexual specificity, by treating the biological factors as no more than non-specific 'precipitating factors', triggering a depressive or schizophrenic illness. The effect is to assimilate these disorders to the standard (sexually non-specific) categories of mental disorder, with their sexually non-specific criteria of diagnosis and treatment; indeed, it is now common in psychiatry to deny the specificity of such disorders altogether.

It may be misleading, however, to rely wholly on the formal discourse of psychiatric textbooks and standard classifications as indicative of the mainstream of psychiatric practice. These texts mark out a domain of theory and practice that properly belongs to a hospital-based psychiatry, operating within the same kind of institutional and conceptual frameworks as physical medicine. Its fundamental unit is the healthy or unhealthy person, and its concept of health or ill-health is that of an abstract attribute inhering within the bounds of the person (and thus clinically accessible to observation or intervention in whatever environment the person happens to be).

But along with the growth of community psychiatry and the sprawling extension of the 'psychiatric system' out of the hospital, the mainstream orthodoxy of the textbooks and the classificatory systems has been somewhat supplanted. This development does not consist simply in the relative decline of the hospital as the privileged site of psychiatric activity, nor even in the independent and absolute growth of psychiatric activity elsewhere. It also comprises a more fundamental shift, from an abstract ideal of 'mental health' to a pragmatic, economic and functional norm of 'coping in the community'.[22] An increasing proportion of psychiatric activity and resources are focusing upon the psychiatric 'support' – largely through the prescription of tranquillizers in general practice – of individuals afflicted with sub-acute disturbances and troubles, of indeterminate nature and indefinite scope. Much of this development has occurred beneath the threshold of theoretical visibility for psychiatry. It is a massive expansion of psychiatric practice within the residual spaces of standard psychiatric orthodoxy: the 'psychosocial disorders', the mild chronic and largely undifferentiated 'troubles of coping', the 'other and unspecified' categories of the standard classifications. It is a domain in which diagnostic classification and illness-specific treatments are given relatively little weight, and where the general medical model of the treatment of disease entities is superseded by a more modest, social model of 'supportive' therapy, 'maintenance' in the community, and intermittent 'crisis' intervention.

It is hardly necessary to point out that in practice this psychiatry of 'coping' is very largely a psychiatry of women, and that the particular forms of sub-critical survival that it tends to foster consist, very often, of the maintenance of a minimal and conventional status quo – a line of least resistance that offers little hope of radical improvement for many women. In terms of the operation of psychiatric sexism it is perhaps here, rather than in the more dramatic domain of acute mental derangement, that the field is most depressing. But despite this, the shift from a medical model of ill-health within the person to a functional model of 'social coping' tends if anything to reduce any constitutive psychiatric investment in maintaining norms of 'healthy' role adjustment. The criteria of social coping are modest, and in principle do not require of the individual anything as elaborate as a successful adjustment to gender role; indeed, where a specific *departure* from the normative gender role seems liable to foster 'coping' this may even be encouraged. There have been a number of attempts, for example, to deploy Seligman's thesis of 'learned helplessness' in relation to the treatment of chronic depression in women.[23] An analogy is here drawn between the state of learned helplessness and the internalization of a 'feminine' role consisting of passivity, dependence and self-effacement. Treatment then consists of a series of interventions aimed explicitly at *disrupting* this feminine position, and encouraging the women concerned to adopt such 'non' feminine behaviours as assertion, independence, and the expression of anger and self-confidence. These approaches undoubtedly do cut across common assumptions of members of the psychiatric profession – particularly the assumption of a general coincidence between a feminine role adjustment and women's health – and are in that sense novel and atypical within psychiatry. But to the extent that they are deployed, more or less successfully, to foster the general objectives of standard psychiatry, they are in no constitutive sense alien to the psychiatric project, and can be assimilated by psychiatry without any radical disruption of its terms.

Feminist therapy: subversion or diversion?

I have sought in these arguments to demonstrate the inadequacy of the existing feminist analysis of psychiatry, as a patriarchal institution that is fundamentally and necessarily oppressive to women. Given that I am quite willing to concede that despite all these arguments, psychiatry is in fact shot through and through with sexism, the distinction that I have been labouring may seem academic. But I have stressed it precisely because it has fundamental implications for the terms in which a feminist politics of psychiatry could be organized. If psychiatry is conceived as inherently and fundamentally an instrument of 'the patriarchy', there is clearly no space for a feminist intervention 'within' it. Taking this conception to its logical conclusion, it demands that any feminist project that concerns itself with mental health must, in principle, be a project *against* psychiatry; at the very least it must organize itself in the context of a more or less radical secession from psychiatry.

The possibility of developing feminist mental-health strategies *outside* the existing institutional frameworks seems of itself unexceptionable. Regardless of whether one views the existing psychiatric services as inherently oppressive to women, it is clear that they neither exhaust the possibilities for intervention in mental health nor deal effectively with many of the problems women currently bring to psychiatry. Certainly, as is illustrated by feminist therapy, there may be gains for feminism in seeking to establish alternative and independent strategies for dealing with women's psychological troubles. Since the development of feminist therapy has been both the most conspicuous of feminism's practical achievements in the field of mental health, and an achievement predicated upon very much the kind of analysis that I have been discussing here, it may at this point be relevant to use it to illustrate some of the implications of this kind of analysis for the development of practical strategies in the field. The object of this discussion is in no sense to provide an introductory account of the aims, methods and achievements of feminist therapy; these are discussed in detail in a number of widely available texts.[24] Nor is it to disclaim or undermine the usefulness of feminist therapy within the parameters that it sets for itself. Rather I wish to make certain points about the *limits* of this approach, and to argue that these are limits which the shortcomings of the existing feminist analysis make inevitable.

Feminist therapy, as represented, *inter alia*, by the Women's Therapy Centre in London,[25] directs itself to the treatment of women's psychological problems through a range of psychotherapeutic measures. In no way does it see itself as a branch of the existing psychiatric system, which it depicts (flatly, and with explicit deference to Chesler) as an 'institution of patriarchal power', that feminist practice must 'turn upside down'. It claims to offer a 'radically new psychological theory of women, based upon feminist principles'.[26] The psychological theory that is proposed draws heavily upon the psychoanalytic tradition, but modifies this approach in a number of critical ways.[27] The central characteristics of feminist therapy are here outlined by Joanna Ryan:

It seems to me that what is specific to feminist therapy is its concern to understand internal and external reality together. It does this in a way that recognises how external reality forms and oppresses women, at the same time as understanding the autonomy and powerfulness of internal reality. It relates inner and outer reality within a total perspective as well as keeping them separate and distinct. Feminist therapy has also provided the means by which women may free and heal themselves from some of the more damaging and internalised effects of their lives, without their social reality or political beliefs being invalidated, and with an understanding of women's liberation as well as women's oppression.[28]

The understanding of women's psychological distress as arising from an oppression that operates in the interplay of women's internal and external reality is the hallmark of feminist therapy. As indicated in this passage, women's external reality is understood in terms of women's patriarchal oppression, and in this sense an overtly sociological and political component is added to the more exclusively psychological concerns of traditional psychoanalysis: what is important is not simply the internal organization of the psyche but also the external matrix within which the psyche is formed and operates. The 'internal reality' of women's lives is theorized in terms that more closely approximate to those of conventional psychoanalysis, with the emphasis being placed upon the early mother-child relationship, the complex path to gendered adulthood, and the vicissitudes and failings of the resulting experience of self.[29] As in conventional psychoanalysis, the achievement of a gendered identity is conceived as the culminating stage of the developmental trajectory, and as conditioning the later psychological experiences of the adult. But even at this level a fundamental link is established, which is absent from conventional psychoanalytic theory, between the psychical and the social: the particular trajectory of development seen as constitutive of the female psychology is theorized as culturally determined by the particular social relations of patriarchy. As is stated baldly by Eichenbaum and Orbach: 'It is out of our experience in society that an understanding of women's psychology must be sought; not, as is usually taught, the other way round.'[30]

It is in this context that feminist therapists have gone on to delineate and theorize a series of central problems that are seen as underlying the psychical distress to which women are prone. It is important to understand that these central problems (which are concerned, amongst other things, with issues of dependency, neediness, anger, the body, control and guilt) are not conceived simply as problems to which women are prone, but as problems to which they are prone *as women*. In outlining an approach for feminist therapists' own assessment of their female patients, Eichenbaum and Orbach thus propose: 'We suggest that therapists ask themselves the following questions: How do they understand the woman's distress? What does this distress have to do with the experience of being a woman? How is her gender central to what she is experiencing? How does the presenting problem or distress relate to her struggle to be an adult woman?'[31]

Out of these preoccupations has been developed an approach that is finely tuned to the analysis and treatment of a variety of women's psychological troubles. At the same time as recognzing this achievement, however, I suggest that it is imperative to recognize the limitations of this approach. I wish to argue that however valuable a contribution may be made by feminist therapy to the advancement of women's mental well-being, this can only be viewed as in some way *extending* the existing field of the psychiatric system, and not as subverting or supplanting it. Further, I would argue that any attempt to treat feminist therapy (either as it exists now or as it could be developed within its existing theoretical parameters) as providing a paradigm for a feminist politics of psychiatry, will be severely limiting and unhelpful. Certainly, there is a degree of overlap in the problems and the persons dealt with by conventional psychiatry and by feminist therapy. However, any privileging of feminist therapy as the paradigm for feminist intervention in the field of mental health generally is liable to obscure the much larger area in which feminist therapy and psychiatry *diverge*. And here I would assert two points. First, the problems with which psychiatry deals but feminist therapy does not are real problems worthy of feminist attention. Second, the fact that these are problems with which feminist therapy does not deal should be recognized not simply as an omission 'in fact', but as a limitation *in principle*, imposed by the fundamental terms in which feminist therapy is conceived and organized.

Like Chesler's analysis, feminist therapy is locked in the

space between three founding assumptions about what a feminist politics of psychiatry must be. On one side is the requirement that such a politics be able to rebuff any charge of an inherent mental instability of women; on another, the requirement that such female psychopathology that may arise be theorized as the direct and culpable responsibility of the patriarchy; on the third, the requirement for a unifying analysis of women's mental troubles in terms of femininity. Like Chesler's analysis, feminist therapy assumes an existing field of patriarchal psychiatry, organized around an oppressive psychiatrization of the feminine and, in antithesis to this, structures itself as an anti-patriarchal therapy organized around a liberating anti-psychiatry of the feminine. In feminist therapy we thus *can* find a psychotherapeutic practice organized constitutively around questions of gender. Here women's mental troubles are theorized and treated as arising from the vicissitudes of their fundamental condition as women, and here we find the insistent conception of women as a homogeneous class, unified by the commonality of 'women's experience'. Through this unification we find resurrected the conception of a fundamental and sexually specific psychopathology, in which all women are, to a greater or lesser extent, implicated. Typically, and perhaps ironically, this psychopathology of women is depicted as located in the familiar and 'feminine' territory of disturbed emotional and domestic relationships, conceived as expressive of an internal disruption of the feminine psyche and resolvable through individual therapy.

I suggested earlier that Chesler's analysis could be seen as an attack on a somewhat imaginary enemy: modern psychiatry simply does not exist as she depicts it, and it is no coincidence that in order to find exemplary instances of the psychiatry she does depict – a psychiatry engrossed with questions of gender – she has to look to the statements of early psychoanalysis rather than modern mainstream psychiatry. In a somewhat parallel way, I suggest that it is no coincidence that it is not mainstream psychiatry but psychoanalysis that provides the critical reference point towards and against which feminist therapy orientates itself. It is the theoretical preoccupation of psychoanalysis with gender – and not the operation of gender categories within psychiatry itself – that feminist therapy takes up, interrogates, challenges, reformulates and ultimately reproduces. And, whilst it challenges the historical deployment of psychoanalysis for the patriarchal regulation of daughters and wives, it offers, concretely, the same form of material services, through the same kinds of institutional structures and practices. This reproduction of the theoretical preoccupations and practical arrangements of psychoanalysis destine feminist therapy to operate over much the same clinical territory as psychoanalysis and to compete over much the same clientele: women judged coherent and articulate enough to participate in the talk of therapy, young enough to justify its deferred rewards for effort, usually rich enough to consider private treatment, sufficiently conforming from the outset to desire and accept the proffered version of mental health and to co-operate with treatment, and suffering from disorders of apparently non-organic origin, which neither are so debilitating as to require institutional care nor engender such dangerous behaviour as to require institutional custody. Certainly, for this group of patients, feminist therapy may be able to offer a recuperated psychoanalysis which in feminist terms has many advantages over either traditional analytic therapies or the out-patient or general practitioner treatment which might otherwise be offered. To the extent that this population does include many women who might otherwise get absorbed into the nondescript and unproductive fringes of the psychiatric system, feminist therapy can indeed be seen as providing a valuable strategy of intervention within a politics of psychiatry. But, at the same time, it is important to note that the central core of psychiatry's female patients are absent from this population, and to them – the senile, the mad, the disorganized, the deluded, the 'insightless', the impoverished, the dangerous and the inarticulate – feminist therapy has little or nothing to say.

I am not suggesting here that feminist therapy has in some way failed by not addressing the needs of these groups, or that it could or should extend its sphere to encompass the field of psychiatric involvement more fully. I am not rehearsing yet again the old complaint that feminism spends too much time with privileged middle-class women to the detriment of the more urgent problems of working-class sisters, or claiming that feminist therapy might be better employed in some other area of endeavour. On the contrary, I am suggesting that the current limits of feminist therapy are limits in principle, imposed by the absolute limits of its theoretical horizons. It is not simply that it does not, or does not yet provide a general model for feminist intervention in the field of mental health: it cannot do so. What it seeks to oppose and rebuild has little relationship to modern psychiatry, and the problems that it seeks thereby to remedy are not on the whole those with which psychiatry is required to contend.

Towards the complex and the specific

So far the movement of this essay has been predominantly critical, attempting to show the weakness of certain feminist approaches to psychiatry that seem ill-founded, constricting, and unnecessary. I have done so, however, with the objective of opening up rather than foreclosing the field. In this final section I should, therefore, like to draw out, on the basis of the arguments I have raised, certain points concerning the direction that a feminist politics of psychiatry might now take.

Any attempt to provide a unified and unifying theory of psychiatry is thwarted by the actual heterogeneity of the field, not only in terms of its theoretical and practical approaches but also in the range of disparate problems and conditions that it seeks to treat. I suggest that the recognition of this heterogeneity is as important in the context of the development of feminist strategies as it is elsewhere, and that there will be little gain for feminism in any attempt to unify the field of political analysis or political intervention in psychiatry. A dispersed, fragmented politics, addressing specific troubles and specific practices is likely to be more productive – even if less elegant.

In this context, it may be helpful to acknowledge that women's apparent over-representation within psychiatry may have multiple origins and need not in principle be susceptible to any grand and unifying explanation. It is not necessary to assume that psychiatry appropriates all its female subjects uniformly, or that it appropriates them 'as a class'. There is no need for an overarching analysis in terms of some uniform condition of all women: a feminist politics does not have to be a politics of femininity. One may note, for example, the association between depression and the conditions of many young working-class mothers, and draw important political conclusions from this, without inferring that these political conclusions relate to all women, to all depressed women, or even to all depressed working-class mothers. Equally well, the development of a feminist politics of psychiatry does not have to rest upon the establishment of a universal patriarchal responsibility for women's extensive psychiatric morbidity. One may note, for example, that thyroid dysfunction and its associated psychiatric symptomatology occur very much more frequently in women than in men, without either assuming that this is in some way the product of patriarchal relations or excluding the suffering and the treatment of these women from the domain of a feminist politics of psychiatry.

In this context I suggest it is necessary to rethink what might be meant by a feminist politics of psychiatry, and to remap, perhaps more broadly than before, the ground of such a politics. Most psychiatric patients, of either sex, are amongst the most vulnerable, disvalued, and economically disadvantaged members of society; the fact that the majority of them are also women is liable both to compound the real disadvantages that they suffer as individuals and reduce further their social power as a group. Obviously, these observations do not exhaust the grounds of feminist concern with psychiatry, but I suggest that they are, nonetheless, *sufficient* grounds for such feminist concern, and that psychiatry may thus be constituted as a proper site for feminist involvement, quite independently of any commitment to the founding assumptions of Chesler's analysis.

First, there is space for a feminist politics *whether or not* women are inherently more vulnerable to mental disorder than men. Certainly it would be *sad* for feminism if this were the case, just as it is sad for feminism that women are in many ways more physically vulnerable than men. But, as with women's physical vulnerability, such a possibility is anything but devastating for a feminist analysis: clearly it would have implications for the development of feminist strategies but would surely not undercut the need for them. Second, there is space for a feminist politics *whether or not* women's psychopathology can be theorized as arising from the material or ideological oppressions of women. It is already clear that certain forms of distress amongst women *can* be theorized in this way, but the privilege that such forms of explanation have been given has served to distort the field of feminist attention. Not only has it resulted in a more-or-less overt resistance to evidence of alternative causal or contributory factors in

women's psychopathology (such as the embarrassingly per-
suasive mass of evidence for a genetic component in schizophrenia), but also, and more importantly, has led to a near
total inattention to those areas of psychiatry such as senile
dementia, where social and psychodynamic explanations of the
pathology have little grip. I suggest that there are feminist
concerns to be canvassed in these areas too, and that they in
no sense need to be predicated upon a political analysis of the
aetiology of these disorders. Third, there is space for a feminist
politics *whether or not* 'the patriarchy is to blame'. Again, as
I have already discussed, there is ample evidence of a pervasive
psychiatric sexism, in addition to the general sexism that exists
everywhere, and there is every reason for feminists to expose
and challenge this sexism, and to analyse the ways in which it
contributes to female psychopathology or impedes its proper
treatment. But there are feminist battles to be fought that do
not depend upon any such attribution of patriarchal blame,
and many that might best be fought by taking psychiatry as an
ally rather than an enemy. In sum, the separation of feminist
politics of psychiatry from a commitment to the assumptions
of the earlier feminist analyses frees such a politics from the
limitations imposed by these assumptions, without precluding
attention to the issues they reflect. On the contrary, rather
than taking them as founding principles to be indiscriminately
asserted and defended at any cost, in opens them up as *real*
issues, requiring a serious feminist attention in the context of
the particular and disparate cases in which they arise.

The case of senile dementia provides an illustration both of
the complexity of the field that is thus opened to feminist
involvement and of the simplicity of the concern that grounds
this involvement. Senile dementia is an irreversible degener-
ative condition arising primarily from the organic deterioration
of the ageing brain, and women are grossly over-represented
amongst those who are hospitalized as a result of it. There are
many reasons for this. The most important is biological: more
women than men survive to the age of greatest risk – in men
other organs tend to fail earlier, before mental deterioration
becomes a problem. But there are also social factors affecting
the rate of hospitalization: many senile old men are nursed at
home by their (younger and more domestically competent)
wives; by the time women develop the condition, by contrast,
many will be widows and those husbands that survive may be

unwilling or unable to take on the (feminine) role of nurse. The aetiology of senile dementia probably lies well outside the domain of politics, but what happens to those afflicted with it clearly does not, as the recent closing of psychogeriatric units in parts of London has made clear. The question of what care, priority and rights should be accorded to these armies of redundant and deranged women – many of whom will have spent their lives in unpaid service and be economically impoverished as a result – is surely of feminist concern.

Posed at this level, in relation to specific problems, groups of patients and approaches to treatment, the terms of a feminist analysis and intervention would become both more complex and less programmatic. The kinds of questions that would have to be asked in relation to senile dementia, for example, would be very different from those connected to the access of women patients to their children, and different again from those concerning the prescription of tranquillizers as a means of blunting the suffering that so many women report to their GPs. And the kinds of answers that might be reached would of necessity be specific, localized and, in all likelihood, compromising. The refusal of an overarching theory of all women and their madness allows neither the questions nor the answers to be simply 'read off' from an established credo, but it does allow more of the problems to become visible, and to be articulated as of feminist concern.

At the same time, this approach allows the *treatment* of women's complicated troubles to be taken seriously, and not merely drowned in a howl of polemical outrage. Many of the psychological troubles for which women curently seek treatment might well disappear if social relations were different, and there is every reason to work towards such changes; but other troubles of women may very well persist. Either way, women's suffering is, in the meantime, very insistent and cannot easily be expected to wait for treatment until the patriarchy finally goes away. In this extended 'meantime', there are real problems for those seeking to provide treatment. Much of women's depression, for example, may quite easily be interpreted as the result of intolerable social circumstances, which neither the women concerned nor the doctors to whom they turn for relief can materially transform. Everyone knows that medicine does not have the 'answer' to the problem – but does this mean that such limited and equivocal relief as medicine can provide should in principle be refused? By analogy, everyone knows that medicine does not hold the answer to the environmental pollutants to which industrial workers are often exposed; the answer is in the environment and in the social system and no amount of medicine will cure it. But should we assume from this that doctors are wrong to offer such limited relief as they can for those suffering from lung cancer or emphysema? The adoption of compromising approaches by medicine may signify bad faith but it does not have to do so.

Finally, the arguments that I have raised have implications for the feminist approach to the deeply ingrained sexism that doubtless characterizes much psychiatric practice. The radical analysis that makes this sexism a constitutive feature of psychiatry and presents the psychiatric establishment as the ultimate bulwark of the patriarchy renders pointless any attempt to 'clean up' psychiatry: one might as well try scrubbing the dirt off the walls of a mud hut. But, by the same token, this radical analysis offers a certain cause for optimism, at least for the combative and the utopian; it offers psychiatry as a site *par excellence* for feminist attack – the overthrow of psychiatry would itself be revolutionary. The approach I am suggesting is more modest and less exciting. To regard the sexism of psychiatry as no more than the mindless reproduction of a sexism that is everywhere pervasive certainly blunts the edge of any singular political thrust. Political intervention in psychiatry is robbed of any widespread – let alone apocalyptic – significance, and even local gains are liable to constant erosion from without. But, at the same time, this approach implies that within the limitations of these constraints, a feminist politics is not necessarily bound to fail: it suggests that there may be real and achievable gains through seeking to raise the consciousness of the mental-health professions to feminist issues, and through seeking to develop and propagate methods of treatment that counteract rather than compound the disadvantages of women patients. It opens the door for constructive feminist work within rather than against psychiatry, with all the mixed and compromised blessings that such a reformist politics implies.

4

Racism and transcultural psychiatry

Kobena Mercer

In recent years the subject of black peoples' mental health and illness has become an issue. It has attracted increasing attention from psychiatrists, doctors, social workers and other professionals in 'welfare' services and has become a focal point of interest and activity in the Afro-Caribbean, Asian and other communities. What are the key questions of concern around this issue? What are the terms of debate and who are the main protagonists? This essay aims to stand back from current debates in order to situate questions of race and mental health and illness within a political framework.

Currently the agenda for debate on these issues is defined by the discourse of 'transcultural psychiatry', which has posed questions and analyses concerning the encounter between black people and the psychiatric system. A certain concept of 'culture' is central to the way in which this prevailing agenda perceives, examines and understands the issues. This essay argues that the transcultural framework, though it has yielded many insights, also limits our understanding of how black people encounter the institutional working of the psychiatric services. It explores, first, the ways in which the concepts of 'culture' and 'ethnicity' function in transcultural psychiatry, by looking at their deployment around race and the diagnosis of schizophrenia. It then compares contemporary transculturalism with earlier research literature and suggests that the concept of 'culture' plays an integral role within new strategies of regulation and government of black people's lives, through interventions based on professional norms of mental health. The essay concludes with some tentative outlines for an alternative approach to the questions raised by transcultural psychiatry.

The major areas of concern that feature regularly in contemporary discussion on race and psychiatry are, first, the numbers of black people in mental hospitals in Britain; second, how they got there, in particular the relations between law and psychiatry in admissions to mental hospitals; and, third, diagnosis, which defines the nature of black peoples' encounter with psychiatry as a medical practice.

The concern over the numbers of black people in the care of psychiatry centres on evidence that 'race' appears to be associated with different rates of admission to mental hospitals. According to research conducted in the early 1970s on the distribution of mental illness in migrant communities settled in Britain, West Indians had a rate of admission of 539 psychiatric patients per 100,000 population compared with the national British average rate of 494 per 100,000. Indians and Pakistanis had a comparably lower rate of 403 and 336 admissions per 100,000 population, respectively.[1] In official language, Britain's black populations constitute an 'ethnic minority' in that, demographically, black people account for something like only 3–4 per cent of the British population. What is disturbing about the picture of 'race' in psychiatric institutions is that in some areas it is suspected that black people are *over-represented* among psychiatric patients.

Since Odergaard's research on high rates of mental hospitalization of Norwegian migrants to the USA in the 1930s,[2] evidence of higher rates of mental illness among migrant groups has often been explained within psychiatry as a consequence of the traumatic experience of uprooting and resettling in a country with different social and cultural values. This explanation may have had some plausibility in the 1960s but black people in Britain are no longer 'immigrants'. Yet recent studies based on mental hospital admissions in the London area in the mid-1970s also indicate a significantly higher rate of admission for black people.[3] The concern over this issue has centred upon how black people are identified, referred and then admitted to psychiatric hospital. Of particular significance here is the role of compulsory admissions in bringing large numbers of black people to the attention of the psychiatric services.

There are two basic routes through which people enter psychiatric hospitals: admissions are either voluntary or involuntary. In the latter case the decision to admit is made without the consent of the prospective patient. Various sections of mental-health legislation, embodied in the Mental Health Act of 1959 and its successor of 1983, make provision for bringing potential mental patients to the attention of psychiatry without their consent. Various institutions and agents have legally defined roles and responsibilities, ranging from relatives and members of the patient's family, to doctors in general practice, social workers, police officers, court magistrates, probation officers and prison medical staff. Since the fundamental changes in psychiatric provision brought about by the integration of services into the National Health Service in the 1950s, compulsory admissions have accounted for fewer and fewer overall admissions and voluntary ones have become the 'norm'.[4] This contrasts starkly with the picture before the 1930s when all admissions to mental institutions involved legal certification, a procedure itself introduced to safeguard the potential patient against medical discretion. The dividing line between law and medicine has shifted significantly.

But, despite this shift, while voluntary admission is the 'norm' for white patients, black people are more likely to enter the psychiatric system under compulsion. Section 136 of the 1959 Mental Health Act, and now Section 136 of the 1983 Mental Health Act, empower police officers to detain someone for up to three days in a 'place of safety' if that person is seen in a public place and regarded to be a danger to him- or herself and others. This section of mental-health law has attracted attention and concern, for evidence suggests that black people are more likely than white to be 'caught' by its use. Littlewood and Lipsedge have suggested that blacks eventually diagnosed as psychotic were *twice as likely* as their white counterparts (in terms of age, gender and social class) to be detained under Section 136 and be referred to mental hospital in this way.[5] Further research has shown that of a sample of patients born either in the New Commonwealth or elsewhere outside Britain, black people were *three to four times more likely* than their white counterparts to have been admitted through these forms of compulsion.[6] Not surprisingly, this aspect of mental-health law has focused the concerns of the black communities and has earned itself the nickname of the 'mental-health sus law'.[7]

Other aspects of the relations between law and psychiatry and black peoples' encounter with their coercive dimensions can be seen in the linkages between policing, the prisons and psychiatry.[8]

The third issue of concern in current debates on race and psychiatry is the process of diagnosis and, in particular, the diagnostic category of schizophrenia. From as early as the mid-1960s, research on black settlers hospitalized under the category of schizophrenia began to call into question the validity of this diagnosis. By comparing the symptoms of black patients with conventional descriptions of schizophrenia, it was found that only a small percentage conformed to the model symptomatology of this major 'psychotic' mental illness.[9] The epidemiological survey research of the early 1970s showed higher rates of admission under the category of schizophrenia as opposed to 'neurotic' mental illnesses such as depression or mania. Cochrane's study found that while 87 per 100,000 British-born men were hospitalized as schizophrenic, the figure for West-Indian-born men was over three times as high, at 290 per 100,000. Also, against an identical figure of 87 per 100,000 population for British-born women, the figure for West-Indian-born women was 323 per 100,000.[10]

The overall thrust of contemporary research on this key issue of race, schizophrenia and the diagnostic process suggests that the regularity of the use of this diagnostic label is an indication of a deeper 'problem'. Research supports the view that the medical validity of this diagnosis of mental distress in black people is questionable, and that what is at issue is *misdiagnosis*. Two leading exponents of contemporary transcultural psychiatry, Maurice Lipsedge and Roland Littlewood, have devoted much of their extensive research to this problematic area of diagnosis. They argue that British psychiatrists, trained in the conventional manner, fail to correctly recognize the true medical significance of black patients' symptoms because they lack an adequate knowledge of the black person's culture and how it influences the manifestation of mental illness. Without such a 'cultural' knowledge the white psychiatrist is liable to misinterpret black peoples' expressions of emotions such as grief, distress and anger as signs of schizophrenia.

One of the most disturbing implications of evidence of misdiagnosis is that mistreatment is one of its consequences. Black people who may be experiencing temporary breakdowns and who are just unable to 'cope' with stress may find themselves being regarded and treated as chronic psychotic patients because of a mistaken and inappropriate diagnosis that prescribes powerful chemotherapy and electro-convulsive therapy (ECT). Evidence suggests that in this area of psychiatric treatment black people are less likely than their white counterparts to be offered non-physical types of treatment such as psychotherapy, and that differentiated responses from psychiatrists and certain forms of discriminatory practice have become more-or-less institutionalized in mainstream psychiatric provision.[11] The issue of misdiagnosis is crucially important because the process of identifying and classifying symptoms is the point at which the 'scientific' medical knowledge of the practioner is applied. Like the legal act of a verdict, the act of diagnosis decides whether someone is 'really' ill or not and, if so, what kind of treatment will be prescribed to solve the problem. Questioning the validity of the diagnosis of schizophrenia in black people therefore also questions the medical and scientific claims on which the psychiatric profession is based. For this reason, the issue of race and diagnosis is of particular concern to psychiatric professionals. By considering this issue in some detail we will be able to examine the strengths and limitations of contemporary transcultural psychiatry.

Schizophrenia, race and misdiagnosis

'Transcultural psychiatry' is neither a movement, an ideology nor the result of an institutional or policy initiative. Rather, it consists of a particular vocabulary, a specific set of terms of reference and a distinct grouping of a range of concerns all addressed to the subject of 'race' in the context of psychiatric theory and practice.

As a discourse, transcultural psychiatry depends on a concept of 'culture' derived from its roots in the discourse of medical anthropology that emerged in the colonial social formations of Africa, India and South East Asia in the 1920s and 1930s.[12] However, the considerable body of research literature that has been built up around the subject of black people living in Britain since the 1950s also borrows concepts from other disciplines, such as social psychology and sociology. Contemporary transcultural psychiatry can be summarily defined as an intellectual response to the black presence in Britain's mentally ill populations. This intellectual response began in the early 1960s with studies on 'psychotic' illnesses among Caribbean migrants. In the work of Gordon, Tewfik and Okasha, and Kiev the concern is with the issue of schizophrenia, diagnosis and the role of cultural values, practices and beliefs in shaping patterns of mental illness among Afro-Caribbeans.[13] In the research from this period there is also a concern with the incidence and prevalence of rates of mental illness in migrant groups distinguished by biological attributes. This concern with the distribution of psychiatric morbidity across racial groups in Britain comes to the foreground in the research of Bagley, Cochrane and others, produced in the late 1960s and early 1970s.[14] From the mid-1970s onwards, contemporary transcultural psychiatry has shifted the focus of concern again on to the clinical encounter between the white doctor and the black patient, while retaining many themes and preoccupations from the earlier periods of psychiatric research on the black presence in Britain.

Contemporary transculturalism is by no means a homogeneous phenomenon. Phillip Rack is one leading contemporary figure who occupies a 'centrist' position in debates. Rack helped establish the Transcultural Psychiatry Unit at Lynfield Mount hospital in Bradford after a survey, initiated in the early seventies, prompted changes in service provision with regard to take-up by the local Pakistani community.[15] Rack is concerned specifically with 'ethnic' groups from the Indian subcontinent and the focus of his work, shared by other figures such as John Cox,[16] is on pragmatic issues arising from the encounter between Asian patients and the psychiatric services. By contrast, two other leading figures, Littlewood and Lipsedge, specialize their concern with 'race' and psychiatry around Caribbean groups. Where Rack's main text, *Race, Culture and Mental Disorder* presents itself as a manual oriented towards practical issues, Littlewood and Lipsedge's *Aliens and Alienists* avows, 'This is not a handbook'[17]. Their text is the culmination of extensive clinical research filtered through a wide-ranging theoretical framework that draws on concepts from anthropology, sociology, psychoanalysis and even semiology. Their sophisticated mode of analysis has

articulated a critique of institutional psychiatry for its depersonalization and stigmatization of black patients and, in this
respect, they occupy a position to the 'left' of figures like Rack.

There are also other positions. Julien Leff's work, although
concerned with both clinical and epidemiological aspects of
'race' in psychiatric practice, is rooted in an international cross-
cultural comparative approach similar to that pioneered by
Murphy and the Leightons in the 1950s.[18] Leff occupies a
more conservative position and is not a major protagonist in
contemporary transcultural discourse. Occupying a more radical position than Littlewood and Lipsedge is Aggrey Burke,
whose work on patterns of mental distress in Caribbean patients in Britain and the West Indies emphasizes the role of
social conditions in psychic disturbance.[19]

As the major protagonists in the discourse of transcultrual
psychiatry, figures such as Rack, Littlewood and Lipsedge and
Burke have all been centrally involved in the Transcultural
Psychiatry Society (TCPS) in Britain, a forum for researchers
and practitioners established with Rack as its first chairperson
in 1976. The TCPS is important because its agenda on race
and psychiatry has taken the lead in offering a framework for
discussing issues to do with black people and psychiatry.

The initial aims and objectives of the TCPS show how central
the concept of 'culture' is to its 'way of seeing':

> The aims of the society are to initiate and sustain interest in
> transcultural psychiatry; to increase awareness and understanding
> of the effects of culture upon health and illness; and to encourage
> practitioners to develop sensitivity to the cultural values, skills and
> systems of thought by which people organise their lives, including
> in particular, the factors which are most relevant to mental illness.[20]

The concept of 'culture' provides a set of terms for the analysis
of 'problem-areas' concerning the black presence within mental
illness institutions. It provides a discourse organized by professionals with a special interest in 'race', addressed on the
whole to other psychiatric and welfare professionals. At this
level it has similarities with other discourses on 'race' in social
policy, such as the discourse of 'multicultural education': its
agenda for debate is geared towards the interests of professionals as opposed to non-professionals, and its central
notion of 'culture' acts as a code-word or euphemism for race.

Let us look at how the concept of 'culture' functions as an analytic tool in transcultural discourse on the issue of race and the diagnosis of schizophrenia.

The issue of the validity of the diagnosis of schizophrenia is not new. It was first registered as an issue for research in the early 1960s and since then a considerable body of research literature has evolved around it. It has been around the area of diagnosis that transcultural discourse has questioned medical knowledge of 'race' through its culturalist framework: the issue of diagnosis pinpoints the concerns of psychiatric professionals whose ethical codes are based on claims to scientific knowledge. While available evidence suggests that both Asian and Afro-Caribbean people are equally more likely than their white counterparts to be diagnosed as schizophrenic, I have chosen to concentrate on the latter for two reasons. The first is that, over the years, a number of crude diagnostic pseudo-categories such as 'West Indian psychosis' and 'Caribbean psychosis' have come into operation and lead a semi-official life within the psychiatric system. These categories have not been coined as a result of theory and there is no research to legitimate their practical use. Instead they have arisen as handy, descriptive labels referring in an empirical, common-sense way to the Caribbean presence in Britain's mentally ill populations. 'West Indian psychosis' is a psychiatric stereotype. Its existence provides a clue to the manifestation of racism within the psychiatric system. The term implies that Afro-Caribbean patients have syndromes and symptoms that are so different that they do not 'fit in' with any of the existing codes and classifications of psychiatric knowledge, that a special term had to be invented to designate this difference. The birth of the medical stereotype 'West Indian psychosis' reveals the diagnostic process as a 'problem-area'.

The second reason for concentrating on the Afro-Caribbean encounter is that within transcultural psychiatry authors tend to concentrate on either of these two main constituencies of the black population. Littlewood and Lipsedge have devoted their work to Afro-Caribbean patients and have focused on the 'problem-area' of race, diagnosis and schizophrenia through their extensive work on 'acute psychotic reaction' among Afro-Caribbean patients. Their work is important because it seeks to produce a conceptually rigorous analysis.

Furthermore, it carries an implicit critique of ethnocentrism in mainstream psychiatric provision at the point of diagnosis. Littlewood and Lipsedge argue that 'the increase in the diagnosis of schizophrenia in the West Indian born may be due in part to the occurrence of acute psychotic reactions which are diagnosed as schizophrenia.'[21] It is on this basis that they argue that a process of misdiagnosis is taking place. Their use of this new clinical term, 'acute psychotic reaction', and their alternative approach to the issues allows them to argue that, 'it appear(s) likely that the elevated rates of classical schizophrenia reported among the West Indian born are exaggerted.[22] The essence of their analysis is that psychiatrists who are trained in the conventions of psychiatric education fail to recognize what is in fact a temporary breakdown caused by social stress, because such practitioners lack the relevant knowledge of the patient's culture and how it shapes the way symptoms are presented.

The starting point for Littlewood and Lipsedge's research was evidence that black patients were much more likely than white to have their diagnosis changed during the course of hospitalization. They suggest that this indicates a high degree of uncertainty on the part of the psychiatrist and imply that ethnocentric medical perception may be responsible for the misdiagnosis of schizophrenia among black, Afro-Caribbean, patients.

Their clinical study began with a sample of African and Afro-Caribbean women admitted to mental hospital in the London area and initially diagnosed as schizophrenic. The method sought to explore possible correlations between the change in 'official' diagnosis and the religious life of the patient, as it was posited that these cultural expressions were misinterpreted by the psychiatrist as signs of a psychotic illness. The profile of the black women that emerged was of patients who had experienced stressful events such as the threat of eviction, marital conflict, arguments with growing adolescents or quarrels with neighbours. Such events precipitated a breakdown characterized by dramatic delusions and hallucinations bearing themes of persecution, religious prophecy and exhortation, often coupled with accusations of malevolent witchcraft or appeals to magical and supernatural entities. As this tended to occur in a public place and to be accompanied by excited

and agitated actions that could be seen as potentially aggressive, most cases were admitted under compulsory procedures
involving the police. After initial sedation on admission the
mood of the patient alternated between elation and
withdrawal, but within a matter of days (and under routine
chemotherapy treatment for schizophrenia) the patients
became more stable in their behaviour; they were discharged
after a period of about four weeks. Littlewood and Lipsedge
add that over a period of years and under similar personal and
social circumstances the episodes were repeated, but that self-
referral became more common and the official diagnosis of
schizophrenia tended to become less likely and was replaced
by categories such as 'affective psychosis' or 'abnormal personality'.[23]

There are striking similarities between this profile of 'acute
psychotic reaction' and the description of 'West Indian psychosis':

> It [West Indian psychosis] is characterised by the sudden onset of
> apparently bizarre, often violent behaviour, with florid (i.e. –
> dramatic) delusions and hallucinations. Such patients can only be
> handled with extreme difficulty in the community and are usually
> admitted to hospital. They invariably recover rapidly and spon-
> taneously. The outcome of this condition is good and patients
> rarely fail to return to a state comparable to that prior to the onset
> of their illness.[24]

This account suggests that the medical stereotype has arisen
in response to the unusual features of the change in symptoms
over a short period of time. It implies that this may be the
locus of diagnostic confusion and uncertainty. Littlewood and
Lipsedge's interpretation takes up the notion that the condition
is a 'catastrophic reaction to stress'.[25] By introducing a new set
of clinical, social, psychological and cultural terms, they theorize the connections between 'stress' and 'symptom'. There
are three basic elements to their interpretation; let us look at
each in turn and then at how they are interrelated.

Medical perception

Littlewood and Lipsedge point out that religious, magical and
supernatural beliefs provide the references for the symptoms of

delusion and hallucination, but do not in themselves constitute evidence of classical schizophrenia. They are concerned to show that the Caribbean-born patients' beliefs in Old Testament prophecies, the Will of God, and witchcraft, are not 'crazy ideas' produced by individual psychopathology, but are elements of 'normal' belief systems that are collective and social in nature. They question the way in which psychiatrists readily identify such normal cultural expressions with schizophrenia. Their intervention implies that the medical perception of thought and belief is ethnocentric. Without a knowledge of other cultures, the Western-trained psychiatrist is liable to misinterpret the black patient's words and actions and to identify what appears to be unusual, unfamiliar and unintelligible conduct with evidence of an underlying mental illness of the psychotic type. By introducing a knowledge of systems of religious and supernatural belief in Caribbean societies, such as Obeah, Pentecostalism and Rasta, Littlewood and Lipsedge aim to correct this distorted ethnocentric perception and argue that the apparently bizarre nature of the symptoms are 'intelligible in terms of the patient's life-situation and culture'.[26] Transcultural psychiatry seeks to elucidate the specific cultural determinations that shape the way symptoms appear in the psychiatric encounter.

Aetiological explanation

By separating what is normal, social and cultural from evidence of individual mental illness, a new form of explanation of the origins and causes of the condition is offered. The two salient features of alternation between excitation and withdrawal, and the rapid recovery in a short period of time are regarded as traits that make the 'acute psychotic reaction' atypical. According to Littlewood and Lipsedge, it would be expected that such a condition would progressively develop into a recognizable psychotic syndrome. But, after evaluating the features of their sample against a range of such categories, they conclude that there is something atypical and unique to the Afro-Caribbean women in Britain:

> Each episode of acute psychosis, on resolution of the disturbed florid presentation, *revealed depressive features* . . . It would be unwise to classify the reactions as depressive, but it might be fruitful to consider them . . . as equivalents or alternatives to depression,

particularly in view of the fact that over time they become less frequent and tend to be 'replaced' by more typical reactive depression.[27]

Littlewood and Lipsedge suggest that the cause of the 'acute psychotic reaction' is social in nature: the breakdown is precipitated by stress. Although examples of stress are given, such as eviction, family conflicts, unwanted pregnancies, it is not defined as such: rather the associated term 'coping' comes into play and the mental illness experienced by the women in the sample is seen as a crisis of coping with stress.[28]

According to David Armstrong the concept of 'coping' developed with the emergence of 'social psychiatry' after the Second World War and was used to focus on 'neurotic' illnesses seen as consequences of traumatic and stressful experiences (see also the discussion in chapter 2).[29] Transcultural psychiatry effects a similar shift in medical perception, although it is applied to the interpretive framework through which the symptoms are viewed. These are redefined as indicating not a psychosis but a neurosis, and are seen to be caused by external social factors.

Culture plays an important role here as it mediates the expression of coping with stressful social and interpersonal conditions. Religion in its widest and most general sense is viewed as a cultural institution created for the release of stress and frustration and is held to play a psychological role in satisfying basic needs for security, belonging and group solidarity. Caribbean religion is thus seen to have an over-determined importance as a psychological 'coping' mechanism. While the women in the sample had been involved in worship and church attendance for most of their lives, their declining involvement is seen as a response to the inadequacy of religion and the church to provide such a means of 'coping'. The Pentecostal churches which some of the women used to attend, 'did not appear to offer the social integration and satisfactions expected'.[30] The 'acute psychotic reaction' is, therefore, seen as an expression of personal distress that takes the symbols of religion to structure its manifestation. Littlewood and Lipsedge argue that, whilst this indicates a failure of previous modes of coping with social stress (the church), the religious symbols and beliefs through which personal distress is expressed are retained. The cultural institution of religion therefore mediates the expression of individual distress. This process of mediation gives rise to the symptoms that are clinically decoded as signs of schizophrenia, but the long-term profile of the condition reveals them to be the outward manifestation of what is essentially a neurotic condition, a crisis of 'coping'.

Psychotherapy

Having clarified the role of culture in the production of symptoms, Littlewood and Lipsedge advance claims for the use of psychotherapy with black patients misdiagnosed as schizophrenic: 'If the psychosis is not primarily of an endogenous nature, it might be useful to pay attention to the precipitating factors and concentrate on a psychotherapeutic approach to enable patients to use more successful ways of dealing with their problems.'[31] This is a bold claim as elsewhere the denial of access to such non-physical treatment options for black patients has been pointed to as an aspect of discriminatory practices within psychiatric services.[32] The claim is based on the theoretical argument that the black patient's symptoms are 'symbols' and that the illness is a communication that has to be interpreted. Although the case study of 'Beatrice Jackson' acts as a model of cross-cultural interpretation it is not clear what kinds of 'more successful ways of dealing with problems' it has given rise to.[33] The salient theme running through Littlewood and Lipsedge's arguments for ethnic psychotherapy, however, is that black patients should have the opportunity of equal access to such non-physical forms of treatment. They criticize the way that psychiatric provision 'de-Caribbeanises [sic] and de-authenticates' the black patient,[34] and from this point of view their arguments for psychotherapy amount to a call for the 'humanization' of the treatment of black, Afro-Caribbean, patients.

Indeed this theme of perceiving the black patient not as a problem but as a 'person with a problem' features in the work of other transcultural psychiatrists, such as Rack.[35] Transcultural psychiatry seeks here to promote a personalized relationship of empathy and identification 'across' the cultural differences between the white doctor and the black patient. The practitioner not only requires a cognitive 'knowledge' of the black patient's culture in order to make more accurate diagnoses, but he or she also needs a personal capacity to identify with the predicament of the black patient in order to provide a more individualized treatment. Although Littlewood and Lipsedge are isolated in stating the case for psychotherapy with black patients, the argument is based on a radicalization of a central transcultural concern with the individual personality or subjectivity of the black patient.

The value of Littlewood and Lipsedge's work is twofold. Firstly, by suggesting that black patients are misdiagnosed and possibly mistreated as a result, they point to ethnocentrism operating within the psychiatric encounter with the black person. This is important because it gestures towards an analysis of the way that institutional racism manifests itself within the psychiatric system. They suggest that Afro-Caribbeans in particular are objects of a kind of medical stereotyping, one that identifies them as 'psychotics' within the diagnostic process. Similarly, the option of psychotherapy is denied to Afro-Caribbean patients because psychiatrists, 'regard black patients as incapable of verbal self-expression with a tendency to physical expression of emotional difficulties'.[36] At the point of treatment it could be said that discriminatory practices within the psychiatric service are rationalized by white, Eurocentric, stereotypes of black, Caribbean, people.

Littlewood and Lipsedge, along with transcultural psychiatry as a whole, do not propose a comprehensive political critique of racism within the psychiatric system. The implicit critique of ethnocentric assumptions, attitudes and expectations is accompanied by a commitment to cultural relativism applied to the clinical context. Such a critique has limitations in that it is based primarily on *moral* arguments and positions and proceeds as if a 'knowledge' of culture is a sufficient condition for changing discriminatory practices in diagnosis and treatment. Littlewood and Lipsedge's views are, however, important because, by introducing a knowledge of culturally mediated expressions in the analysis of misdiagnosis, they point to the primary role of social (as opposed to biological) conditions in constructing mental illness. This shifts the ground of the 'medical model', rejects a search for 'diseases of the psyche', and points towards a social definition of mental illness as a crisis of coping with stressful social circumstances.

Elsewhere, Littlewood and Lipsedge attempt to test out such an explanatory approach, looking for causal links between 'social conditions and mental illness'.[37] Their account highlights the unequal racial distribution of health-chances and stressful life-events that may render racially oppressed social groups more vulnerable to forms of mental distress. Whilst not conclusive, this offers a point of departure for a more explicit attempt to analyse the ways in which racism functions in the social production of mental illness as well as in its institutional regulation and management.

In summary, Littlewood and Lipsedge's extensive research on 'acute psychotic reaction' is important because it represents one of the most sophisticated and radical sets of analyses and arguments offered from within transcultural psychiatry. The overall thrust of their work is to bring a knowledge of the 'culture' of the black – Afro-Caribbean in this case – psychiatric patient to bear on the psychiatrist's perception and treatment of the individual patient, in order to displace ethnocentric stereotypes such as 'West Indian psychosis'. While certain themes and preoccupations with issues of aetiology and psychotherapy are specific to them, Littlewood and Lipsedge's mode of assessment and analytic intervention in the 'problem-area' of misdiagnosis is of common concern to the discourse of transculturalism as a whole.

Culture, knowledge and communication: the transcultural problematic

At the centre of transcultural psychiatry's perspective on diagnosis is a concern with the pracititioner's knowledge of the 'ethnic' patient's culture. Without an adequate knowledge of how different cultures mediate the presentation of mental illness, the practitioner is unable to effectively communicate with the black patient and may misinterpret the medical significance of the symptoms. For Littlewood and Lipsedge the starting point for the diagnosis of schizophrenia was the practitioner's inability to clearly distinguish between normal forms of cultural expression and signs of potential mental illness. The normal/abnormal distincton was to be 'relativized' by emphasizing the role of 'culture' in the mediation of a response to stress. Other exponents of transculturalism also share this approach. For Rack, 'culture' is also a means of clarifying what is perceived in the black patient's symptoms to be a culturally mediated response to stress: 'An English person under unmanagable stress may respond with anxiety, depression, hysteria or other neurotic symptoms: but he is unlikely to develop delusions, hallucinations, confusion, thought disorder and other signs of schizophrenia. Among Asians, Africans and West Indians however, such reactions are not uncommon. The presentation is indistinguishable from schizophrenia but the consequences are different.'[38] Against the absence of a comparative knowledge of different cultures and the limitations of Eurocentric assumptions, transculturalism offers a 'new' knowledge that seeks to correct, adjust and realign the axiomatic distinctions between normal and pathological, psychoses and neuroses, in order that more effective clinical communication between white doctor and black patient can take place.

In certain respects the thrust of cultural relativism, fundamental to transcultural psychiatry, is not new. The theme of an implicit critique of Eurocentrism in psychiatric perception and treatment of non-European patients was present in earlier research literature: 'The British doctor will have been trained to recognise a classical picture of disease which has arisen in European culture and has therefore been described in European terms. It is too often assumed that this is the normal pattern for other people from other lands. This assumption is far from correct.'[39] Contemporary transcultural psychiatry is also concerned with the points raised here. It questions the implicit Eurocentric bias to the medical education of the psychiatrist, which informs his or her abilities to perceive, recognize and classify (diagnose) symptoms of mental illness. And it is concerned with re-establishing the distinction between the normal and the abnormal, relative to a plurality of different cultures.

Common to past and present discourses on race and psychiatry is a relativism that seeks to loosen the static, fixed and Eurocentric assumptions of the white practitioner in the encounter with the black, 'ethnic' so-called, patient. However, what appears to distinguish contemporary cross-culturalism from earlier analyses of race and mental illness is that its 'culturalism' is echoed in practices such as education, social work, community work and the youth service. Unlike the research on black people and psychiatry in the 1960s, contemporary transcultural psychiatry articulates its concerns with 'culture' in terms that have become established in mainstream social policy. This wide range of discourses on 'race' is framed by an over-arching concept of culture as learned or acquired human conduct; common to it is the notion of 'ethnicity'. In the discourse of multicultural education, for example, the encounter between the black child and the schooling system is analysed and understood in terms of the 'culture' of the former: specific 'problem-areas' such as underachievement in Afro-Caribbean pupils are conceptualized in terms of the 'problem' of cultural identity of the black child.[40] The specificity of trans-culturalism lies in its utilization of cultural pluralism in the medical context of psychiatric services – its particular concern with the normal and the abnormal is anchored on to the highly specific area of diagnosis. But, in so far as transculturalism utilizes the 'ethnicity' paradigm for the representation of a plurality of cultural differences, it shares less with previous concerns of race and psychiatry than with the policies of cultural pluralism that have become institutionalized within the practices of the contemporary welfare state.

Across these different institutional settings the encounter with 'race' is problematized in terms of communication. In psychiatry, an anthropological framework that defines culture as learned human behaviours enables the representation of a diversity of 'cultural factors' deemed relevant to the practitioner's competence. The term 'culture' acts as a portmanteau capable of carrying a wide range of multiple references. It facilitates psychiatric discourse on a diversity of aspects of the black person's way of life: from migration and settlement, family, household and kinship structures, gender roles and relations to child-rearing, dietary habits and preferences, magical, supernatural and religious beliefs and folk-conceptions of health and illness. 'Culture' acts as the organizing term for a mobile system of representation that opens on to a plurality of referential objects. These 'objects' are aspects of the personal and social relations in which the black person lives. The inherent vagueness of the concept of culture provides the means whereby a wider range of social relations are brought into the psychiatrists' view in the process of diagnosis. Anchored by the two major concerns with symptoms and stress and the normal/abnormal distinction, 'culture' is used to construct a knowledge on the part of the psychiatrist that will facilitate more effective communication in the clinical encounter with the black subject. Around the problem of the practitioner's lack of knowledge of culture in the diagnostic process, the transcultural problematic locates its object of intervention in the space of the doctor-patient relationship. It is at this point that transculturalism joins the more pervasive culturalist logic of the 'ethnicity' paradigm.

In a paper ostensibly about ethnic minorities and social services, delivered to the inaugural meeting of the TCPS in 1976, Roger Ballard gives an exposition of the 'ethnicity' paradigm of cultural pluralism and, inadvertently, discloses certain aspects of why 'culture' is of such concern to psychiatrists, social workers and other members of the 'caring' professions. His starting point is that white practitioners perceive black clients' culture as a 'problem'. This, argues Ballard, is itself a problem, a negative impediment to the provision of a welfare service, and is seen to arise as a consequence of the practitioners' lack of knowledge of the culture of the 'ethnic' client:

> The fact that members of ethnic minorities organise their lives in culturally distinctive ways *must necessarily cause problems for practitioners* who come into contact with a new group for the first time . . . Whether they realise it or not they [practitioners] step, like Alice, into an unfamiliar world. Once across the ethnic boundary, which may, confusingly, be shifting and invisible, they can never be quite sure whether things really mean what they seem to . . . *Indeed, in the absence of a knowledge of the distinctive internal ethnic rules and logics, it may be impossible to tell whether an item of behaviour is normal or aberrant.*[41]

Ballard goes on to argue that without a knowledge of how a diversity of different cultures distinguish normal from abnormal the welfare agent is 'professionally handicapped': 'In so far as his specialism [i.e. psychiatry, social work, counselling] demands that he [the practitioner] should take into account the social and cultural worlds in which his clients live, he needs to make a response to ethnic diversity. *If he does not, his practice is inadequate in purely professional terms.*'[42]

The concern to clarify cultural difference is animated by the need to ensure the ethical standards on which the welfare professions are based and upon which policies of universalist provision and 'equal treatment' for all clients (or 'consumers') are also based. Ballard warns that failure to distinguish normal from pathological in the 'ethnic' client may lead to poor communication and misunderstandings between the two, and that the 'ethnic' client may receive a 'second-class' standard of treatment as a result.

Ballard acknowledges that in the absence of such proper cultural knowledge, ethnocentric stereotypes may arise and these too are criticized for the way they can undermine the ethical claims of professional agents: 'It is easy to slip . . . into regarding distinctive minority cultural patterns themselves as being problematic and pathological . . . it is all too easy to slip into a perception of the cultural worlds of others as an irrational product of sheer ignorance. Action based on such premises *does no more than demonstrate the social power of the pratictioner.*'[43] This is revealing because it introduces the question of power into the relationship between client and practitioner, patient and doctor. Above all, it is an important admission that white professionals are not just innocently ignorant of 'other cultures', but that they operate particular stereotypes of black people as 'problem clients' precisely on account of cultural differences.

The implication of Ballard's exposition is that white practitioners are so deeply confused about the normal and the abnormal in non-Europeans that they 'pathologize' normal cultural expressions of personal and emotional distress as prima facie evidence of mental illness. The effect of this is to psychiatrize cultural difference. Ballard goes on to suggest that, when a white social worker lacks an undersanding of the cultural expression of the black client, the client's talk about his or her experience of distress in terms of magic, the supernatural, witchcraft and religion is misinterpreted or medicalized as schizophrenia:

> such communications may seem bizarre and deluded, evidence perhaps of schizophrenia . . . Outsiders who lack the necessary cultural competence may not only be baffled by what they hear, but may proceed to struggle to quite inaccurate conclusions about what is happening. *It is much easier to diagnose schizophrenia than to try and come to terms with the culturally specific symbolic systems within which the patient is expressing himself.*[44]

This reveals aspects of the politics that underpin the transcultural analysis. First, Ballard makes it explicit that psychiatric services need to 'take into account' the ethnic diversity of Britain's mentally ill populations and suggests that a 'specialist ethnic service' may be required.[45] But equally important is his rationale: psychiatrists need to understand the cultures of ethnic patients in order to maintain professional codes of ethics inscribed in the ethos of the medical and welfare professions. Ballard acknowledges the 'unfortunate consequences' of misdiagnosis for the black patient, but appears to give greater emphasis to the fact that such misunderstandings threaten to undermine the relations of power, authority, and consent between professional and client. The priority given to the needs and interests of the white professional suggests that the discourse of transculturalism is geared, at least in the first instance, towards the 'hidden' agenda of professional interests.

Second, Ballard's exposition centres this problematic of professionalism within the terms of 'culture' as an object of knowledge. He raises two related questions about the ignorance on the part of white practitioners and the issue of ethnocentric stereotypes that 'blame' black people's way of life as the cause of the problems encountered in diagnosis. But here again, Ballard is preoccupied with the negative effects of stereotypes on the effectiveness of doctor–patient communication. The implication is that stereotyping is an impediment to the treatment of the individual whose individuality is negated by such assumptions.

Third, within the problematic of 'ignorance vs knowledge', Ballard shows that the transcultural 'solution' for problem-areas in the encounter between race and psychiatry consists primarily of information and education for white professionals about the cultures of their 'ethnic' clients. Through such an educative reform of professional's attitudes to black clients, transculturalism seeks the elimination of misunderstandings and faulty communication. Again, the transcultural problematic is oriented towards professionals.

The point of application of the transcultural project is narrowed down to the space between doctor and patient. This relationship is the site on which problem and solution are posed in terms of culture, knowledge and communication. The research of the 1960s also posed the problems of psychiatry's encounter with 'race' in terms of culture as an object of knowledge. As noted already, what distinguishes contemporary research and debate is that the problematic of cross-cultural communication complements and parallels the fundamental assumptions of cultural pluralist policies in other practices of the welfare state. It combines with the policies of 'multiculturalism', 'ethnicity' and cultural pluralism that have become incorporated into education, social work, youth work, community work, social services and other agencies of the welfare state during the 1970s.[46] 'Breaking down barriers to communication' defines 'culture' as the key to the solution of structural problems arising from the encounter with 'race' and racial difference. Ballard explicitly shows that transcultural psychiatry situates itself within this framework of social-policy assumptions:

> The challenge here, which applies to a whole series of fields besides medicine, is one of *establishing communication and understanding* at a whole range of levels: between doctors and patients, between social workers and their clients, and all those who provide personal social services, whatever the professional and cultural provenance of their therapeutic models. The barriers can only be broken down if all the various parties agree to attempt to understand what others are saying and doing, however absurd and untenable this may seem to them at first sight.[47]

It is possible to discern a shift from a quantative preoccupation with differential rates of psychiatric morbidity among migrant and settler groups, towards a more qualitative concern with the cultural and psychological universe of the individual 'ethnic' patient encountered in the clinical setting of diagnosis, examination, interview, observation and treatment. This shift articulates a set of professional concerns in a problematic similar to other social-welfare practices organized by a 'culturalist' policy framework.

Transcultural psychiatry and the 'ethnicity' paradigm

Transcultural psychiatry argues that patterns of differentiation and discrimination exist in the perception and treatment of black mental patients. Its major concern with misdiagnosis revolves around professional concerns with ethics in so far as the negative effects of ignorance and ethnocentrism are held to undermine the ethos of the medical profession. The elimination of 'misunderstandings' is sought at the point of doctor–patient interaction through an awareness of cultural difference.

This is to professionally equip the white practitioner to identify, classify, treat and manage forms of mental distress manifested in black people. The over-arching objective of transcultural psychiatry is the *normalization of the professional psychiatrist's relationship with the 'ethnic' patient.* Let us consider how the central conceptions of culture, cultural difference and 'ethnicity' function in relation to the practical problem-areas located by the problematic of communication.

The white doctor

For transcultural psychiatry 'culture' entails the comparison and differentiation of a plurality of social groups, often called 'minorities'. Jamaicans, Nigerians, Pakistanis, Italians, Turkish Cypriots, Muslims, Rastafarians, Pentecostalists, Hasidic Jews, and more, can each be assimilated to the category of 'ethnicity' defined as a minority social group differentiated from a putative 'ethnic majority' on account of cultural criteria. The inclusiveness of 'culture' facilitates the deployment of different ways of specifying difference: national, regional, linguistic and religious 'differences' are each assimilated to 'ethnicity'. Transculturalism brings a heterogenous range of diverse population groups into the gaze of the psychiatric system. It renders difference visible, not on account of biological attributes, but on account of 'culture'.

This mobile schema for ethnic differentiation is anchored to psychiatry through the concern to distinguish normal and pathological. Ethnic diversity is incorporated into the psychiatric system in order that the role of specific cultural values, beliefs and symbols in the manifestation of distressed behaviour can be clearly identified by the practitioner, and their effects included in the diagnosis of mental illness. Although the category of schizophrenia has been in the foreground, transculturalism applies its culturalist schema to a wide range of medical conditions. Its objective is to relativize the process of medical perception, examination, observation and interview operative in diagnosis. Each of the five essential chapters of Rack's manual for the psychiatric recognition of ethnicity consists of careful delineations of 'cultural pitfalls' in the clinical recognition of depression, anxiety, mania, schizophrenia, paranoia and hysteria.[48] The 'pitfalls' in question are those aspects of 'culture' that confuse and confound the expectations of the practitioner. The different ways in which ethnic groups organize their familial and kinship relations, their gender and sexual relations, their modes of child-rearing, and their ways of explaining their distress are all brought into the remit of psychiatric surveillance because they are identified as 'cultural factors' relevant to mental health and illness.

It is those aspects of ethnic culture that embody conceptions of the self, the soul and the psyche in contradiction with conceptions embodied in the Western tradition of medical science that are of particular interest to the transcultural enterprise. Religious and spiritual systems such as Islam, Pentecostalism, and Rastafarianism are seen as the most problematic aspects of 'ethnicity' and hence most in need of clarification for the white practitioner. The case history that introduces Littlewood and Lipsedge's major work demonstrates how the culturalist problematic objectifies 'other cultures' into a datum of 'positive knowledge' to be clinically deployed in psychiatric practice.[49] 'Calvin Johnson' was diagnosed schizophrenic because his references to Jah were misunderstood as evidence of delusion, and his references to the police (who brought him into the psychiatric system) as Babylon were misinterpreted as signs of paranoia.

Ethnicity is thus objectified into a form of knowledge that can be integrated into the repertoire of medical education and training. At this level the strategic objective of an 'ethnic dimension' to psychiatric provision, the 'Why?' of transcultural psychiatry's interest to 'increase awareness and understanding', depends on a system of representation of cultural difference that brings a whole range of national, regional, linguistic, religious and behavioural criteria to bear on the diagnostic process. This is an educative project for the reform of practitioners' attitudes to ethnic patients as well as the enhancement of their competence. This 'new' knowledge of ethnicity is to be deployed in the doctor–patient relationship.

Historically, institutional psychiatry has not always been interested in doctor–patient communication, any more than it has staked an interest in the 'culture' of its subjects. According to Armstrong's account, psychiatric interest in this topic is a recent development brought about by the major transformation in the therapeutic rationale of the hospital in psychiatric provision.[50] The nineteenth-century model of the 'asylum' in which the mentally ill were to be exiled from society 'for their own good', was radically reversed by new, mobile technologies of medico-psychiatric intervention such as chemotherapy and psychotherapy. The hospital was opened on to society by the model of the 'therapeutic community' and an expanded range of populations and social groups (children, the elderly, ex-servicemen) came to be defined as 'at-risk' of mental illness. Within the new configuration of institutional arrangements for the identification and treatment of mental abnormalities, the doctor–patient relation assumed importance because it was valued as an element of therapy. By the 1960s it had become an integral part of the medical education of psychiatrists. The Todd Report of the Royal Commission on Medical Education in 1964 argued that: 'there is a great deal more (to doctor–patient communication) than simply asking a series of pre-scribed questions and checking the accuracy of the answers. Students must be aware of the factors which impede or distort communication, factors such as limitation of vocabulary, cultural attitudes and social prejudices.'[51] Within this tradition, contemporary transculturalism operates as a potential strategy. The concern with culture as a 'barrier' or 'boundary' to effective communication can be seen as an expression of professional concern with the maintainance of the given relations of power, authority, consent and compliance in the encounter with the black patient, the ethnic subject.

As a strategy, transculturalism's central concern with the doctor–patient relationship could be understood as a concern with the relations of power and authority invested in the relationship. If 'culture' is objectified at one level to make diagnoses more accurate, at another it functions to differentiate the ethnic patient as an individual. 'Culture' acts as a means of making individual differences relevant to the psychiatric encounter with the black person.

The black patient

Although diagnosis appears to be the site within which trans-cultural psychiatry questions the competence of the white practitioner, the concern with doctor–patient interaction extends to the area of treatment. Transculturalism seeks to enhance and extend the practitioner's knowledge to the point of *inter-subjective empathy and identification* across the barriers of cultural difference. More than the provision of supplementary knowledge to eliminate stereotypes, it proposes a modification of the subjective attitudes of the white doctor so that he/she does not misrecognize the black person as a problem, but instead recognizes the black patient as a 'person with a problem'. Black people should, it is argued, not be seen as 'social problems' but as 'people who 'have' problems': the disadvantaged. Rack argues that the culturalist know-how that transcultural psychiatry seeks to promote will enable the white practitioner to become 'part of the picture' in the diagnostic process:

> Crossing some unmarked boundary, the practitioner finds that he is, himself, part of the picture . . . He has not only identified the problem, *but identified with the problem*. The more closely the client's world resembles the practitioner's own world, the more familiar it is, the more easily this step is taken. *But the more different the two worlds, the harder it is to make the identificaton.*[52]

Transcultural identification and empathy is the precondition for psychotherapy with black patients. While Littlewood and Lipsedge are isolated in stating the case for 'ethno-psychotherapy' as a programme, their arguments can be interpreted as a radical restatement of this common transcultural theme of effective communication through intersubjecive identification. Their view that the symptom bears 'meanings' and that mental illness is itself a social communication shifts the focus of the transcultural project beyond 'objective' knowledge of ethnic diversity, towards a 'subjective' ability to enter into the culture of the patient in order to use psychological techniques, psychotherapy, for the treatment and management of mental distress. At this level 'ethnicity' paradigmatically defines membership of an ethnic group or population as the relation that constitutes the individual's sense of *identity*. Psychiatric concern with culture is now rearticulated around an interest in the effects of 'culture' on personality and, in particular, in the cultural specificity of different means of 'coping' with psychological stress.

The concept of stress used in association with therapeutic concern with the individual identity of the patient are aspects of the 'social psychiatry' that has emerged since the Second World War;[53] both are absolutely central to the 'ethnicity' paradigm for social-welfare practices in general. A concern with the *psychological* dimension of ethnicity is a central feature of the formation of discourses in education, social work, youth service, counselling, and personal social services, which all address themselves to issues concerning 'race' through the culturalist system of representation of difference.[54] Littlewood and Lipsedge's framework for the psychotherapeutic interpretation of 'meanings' in black patients' symptoms, predicated on the view of the illness as a response to stressful external social conditions, rejoins this broader paradigm of culturalist representations. The 'meanings' they decode in the symptoms appear to amount to 'alienation', defined in the sociological tradition of Durkheim as a sense of existential dread masked by illusory and false beliefs that enable individuals to psychologically cope with conditions of existence that produce uncertainty and *angst*. This underpins their categorical assertion that, 'the West Indian in Britain is both alienated and anomic: he lives in a world of social acts taken for reality which are not of his own making.'[55]

The concern with black peoples' personal struggles in coping with stressful social circumstances makes possible the deeper penetration of the 'ethnic psyche' with the objective of rendering it more manageable and governable. Their framework for psychotherapy makes individual differences relevant to psychiatric examination, assessments and interventions. I suggested that the concern with ethnic religion was part of a search for a more accurate differentiation between culture and mental illness; but a similar delineation of cultural difference, at a psychological level, also appears to underpin this area of concern with 'identity' as a principle of psychiatric differentiation:

> Why have we talked so much about the importance of religious beliefs for the West Indian community? Religion is also a fundamental way of looking at the world in India, Pakistan and Bangladesh. For Asian immigrants and their children, however, it is becoming less and less significant . . . For the West Indian community Fundamentalist religion has been at the centre of an attempt to acquire a British identity, an attempt whose failure has also been articulated in religious concepts.[56]

This view shifts the focus from 'alien' cultures to 'alienated' personalities: *'ethnicity' becomes the principle for the individualization of cultural difference.*

Littlewood and Lipsedge's views are based on a set of questionable assumptions about the significance of religious practice and belief in the Afro-Caribbean community that define the importance of 'religion' in purely psychological terms.[57] Ethnicity and difference are psychologized. Their framework of 'alienation', the product of psychotherapy and an identification between doctor and patient, makes 'ethnicity' a principle of subjectification. Foucault's historical studies of modern forms of power – invested in institutions such as the school, the prison and the hospital – suggest that the 'individual' is not a given, but is constructed and positioned by the fabrication of power and knowledge:

> The [medico-clinical] examination as the fixing, at once ritual and 'scientific', of individual differences . . . clearly indicates the appearance of a new modality of power in which each individual receives as his status his own individuality . . . the examination is at the centre of the procedures that constitute the individual as effect and object of power, as effect and object of knowledge. With it are ritualised those disciplines that may be characterised in a word by saying that they are a modality of power for which individual difference is relevant.[58]

From this point of view, psychiatric concern with the individual identity of the patient locked into the clinical space of the doctor–patient relation represents a form of management and government seeking as its ideal objective the 'subjectification' of mental illness.

David Armstrong has suggested that in the modernization of power-relations invested in the institution of psychiatry, the former stigmatization and objectification of the patient by the doctor was radically transformed: 'Besides listening to and observing the patient, the doctor had to be self-aware: 'What is my attitude? Am I understanding the situation from the patient's point of view, or from mine alone? What is my reaction to his behaviour?' In short, the interview had to examine both the patient's and the psychiatrist's words and actions.'[59] Although the transcultural concern with the 'identity' and individuality of the ethnic patient has not been formalized to a great extent, the demands for cross-cultural identification and self-awareness on the part of the white practitioner (the pre-condition for more personalized intervention) are clearly enunciated by its leading figures themselves:

Although both anthropology and psychiatry originated in the study of people designated as *aliens*, they can offer a sensitive awareness of the relationship between observer and observed. While we have tried to situate our own theories within the relativistic framework we have applied to others, we are still white, male, middle-class doctors discussing the private experiences of patients who are frequently black, female and working-class – part of what Michel Foucault calls the monologue of reason about madness.[60]

This self-reflexive emphasis on sensitivity and awareness indicates the presence of a strategy of 'subjectification' in which the knowledge of 'ethnicity' will lead to a new degree of self-consciousness on the part of the white practitioner *vis-à-vis* the encounter with the black patient.

At this point, the culturalist system of representation of differences functions to bring the encounter with the black subject in line with the professional ethos of efficient, therapeutic, doctor–patient communication. The project of transcultural psychiatry constructs a culturalist framework of knowledge that objectifies the 'culture' of the black patient and subjectifies that 'culture' in order to make the individual personality or identity of the patient relevant to psychiatric intervention. Its culturalism expands the range of points of psychiatric intervention and deepens the mode of intervention by 'individualizing' the subject. The liberal and humane themes of the project do not reach as far as seeking a fundamental change in the nature and functions of psychiatric provision. Rather, they propose an adjustment, a modification and a reform of the ethnocentric dimensions of the clinical encounter.

The black psyche as a site of struggle: towards an alternative agenda

Writing in the 1940s at the interface between the colonized psyche and the colonial system of psychiatry, Fanon also recognized the importance of doctor–patient communication: 'Twenty European patients, one after the other, come in: "Please sit down . . . Why do you wish to consult me? . . . What are your symptoms?" . . . Then comes a Negro or an Arab: "Sit there boy . . . What's bothering you? . . . Where does it hurt, huh?" . . . When, that is, they do not say: "You no feel good, no?" '⁶¹ Fanon's starting point was not 'cultural differences' between the white doctor and the black patient, rather he started with the question of power, created by historical and social relations and effected in the domain of psychiatry and medicine. His politics of psychiatry sought to describe how forms of 'racial' oppression created forms of psychic and emotional distress among the oppressed and how the dominant system of psychiatric provision in turn perpetuated such oppression in its treatment of black, 'colonial', subjects.

Fanon's political framework may no longer be wholly adequate for the post-colonial forms of racial oppression in a society such as modern Britain, but his fundamental premise that the black psyche was a battleground of contradictory forces may still serve to provide a base for a critique of transculturalism and for the construction of an alternative agenda for a political analysis of race and psychiatry.⁶² Given the marginalization and exclusion of the subject of 'race' from the concerns of white left politics of psychiatry, Fanon's work may still yield the conceptual resources for rethinking the questions raised by black peoples' experience of the psychiatric system in contemporary Britain.⁶³

Closer to home, the ground-clearing work of Errol Lawrence and Pratibha Parmar offers a useful frame of reference for an analysis of how race-relations function as power-relations in the psychiatric institution. They demonstrate ideological connections between the culturalist system of representation in the 'ethnicity' paradigm within sociology and the ways in which 'culture' is used in the political discourses of the centre and the right to represent the black presence in British society as other, as a threat, a problem and a burden. In between the commonplace racism of discourses on 'alien cultures' and the academically respectable culturalism of 'ethnicity' studies, Lawrence and Parmar discern a range of stereotypes that operate in the encounter between black people and the welfare agencies of the state.⁶⁴ These are stereotypes of Afro-Caribbeans as aggressive, excitable and truculent; maintained by being played-off against images of Asian people as meek, passive and docile. Lawrence and Parmar's analyses of these culturalist stereotypes suggest that what is common to the different formations of discourse on race is a *pathologization of cultural differences*. What is at stake is that the culturalist framework of ethnic pluralism as political and social policy accommodates the ideological rationale for practices that absolve welfare institutions from their racism and their failure to ensure 'racial equality' by 'blaming the victim' and locating 'causes' of social problems in black people's ways of living.[65]

We have seen that transcultural psychiatry organizes debate on race and psychiatry within such a culturalist system of representation and that its parameters are defined by professional concerns that focus on the total 'way of life' of the black patient in order to make more efficient diagnostic examination and psychiatric treatment of mental distress. We also saw that at the heart of its project is a concern with 'telling the difference' between normal and pathological, seen to be problematic because of cultural differences between doctor and patient. An alternative analysis might focus instead on how institutional racism manifests itself within the power-relations invested in psychiatry. This could begin with the question of *the medical stereotyping of black patients based on the confusion between the normal and the pathological*. The issue of misdiagnosis could be reformulated from this point of view. Rather than begin with the cultural meaning of symptoms and confine analysis to doctor–patient interaction, we need to look at the structural conditions of the encounter in diagnosis, the interaction between the psychiatric system and the black subject. Diagnosis in such a view is just one point in a circuit of relations between a whole range of welfare and state agencies implicated in the referral and admission of mental patients. Given that the culture of British racism nurtures the stereotype of Afro-Caribbeans, for instance, as loud, volatile and aggressive, we would ask, What role does such a stereotype play in the perceptions of distressed behaviour seen to be in need of psychiatric attention? If the decision to admit is not based primarily on medical grounds but on account of the potential 'dangerousness' of the patient if not admitted, then to what extent is the diagnosis of schizophrenia a 'self-fulfilling prophecy'?[66]

Although these questions can only be posed at this stage, it is relevant to remind ourselves that the category of schizophrenia has been called into question throughout this century and is something of a headache for psychiatry's self-image as a scientific and medical enterprise. Today even figures such as Wing and Clare – who can hardly be regarded as 'anti-psychiatry' – have criticized the category and struck a distance from it on the basis of its questionable validity.[67] The very ambiguity of the category means that it may serve as a convenient 'container' for the psychiatric treatment of various problematic and disruptive behaviours that escape classification in other medical (or legal) categories.

In order to ask what function medico-psychiatric stereotypes of black people play in the provision of psychiatric services, we need to insert the issue of power into the debate. From this viewpoint, the key issue of schizophrenia and misdiagnosis, discussed by transculturalism in terms of the confusion between 'culture' and mental illness, may be regarded as psychiatry's contribution to the 'pathologization of cultural differences' in the political context of ethnic pluralism. By organizing around issues of mental health and illness the Asian, Afro-Caribbean and other black communities are now taking initiatives that challenge, in concrete ways, the hegemony of this culturalism. These are important challenges and many political choices and priorities remain to be clarified in these growing struggles around the 'health' and 'illness' of the black psyche.[68]

5

Psychotherapy of work and unemployment

Peter Miller

Work, it is argued, can cause neurosis; so too can unemployment. Work is the site of exploitation according to some;
yet when absent it is demanded as a right. My concern in this
essay is to look at the apparent paradoxes that emerge in this
intersection of the economic and the psychiatric. Through what
mechanisms and to what effects does the personal and the
family life of the individual become a matter of concern to
productivity? Or, to put it the other way round, how is it that
the individual's relationship to society's productive apparatus
becomes posed as an issue affecting mental health? The emergence of this concern in the early decades of the twentieth
century is a process to which psychiatry and psychology both
contributed. My concern here, however, is less with principles
of demarcation than with looking at the transformations of the
way in which the individual's relationship to his/her work is
understood. In a series of moves, the avoidance of neurosis,
the attainment of full mental health and, finally, the maximal
fulfilment of the self, have come to be regarded as inseparable
from the activity of production. In this process the disciplines
of mental health and the world of production have both undergone significant changes.

In the twentieth century, psychiatry has extended its sphere
of intervention well beyond the asylum. In conjunction with
other professions, particularly social work and psychology, it
now addresses itself to the task of the supervision and government of social life. This is not a matter of the heroic capture

of a new sphere of intervention. It takes the shape of a delicate infiltration that has made the supervision and government of human individuals closely dependent on evaluations couched in terms borrowed more-or-less directly from psychiatry. The world of employment is a crucial site through which such intervention develops.The individual's relationship to employment, and unemployment, is one of the principal 'surfaces of emergence' of the modernized psychiatry of everyday life that has replaced the carceral psychiatry of the nineteenth century.[1]

To ask what is at stake in this psychotherapeutics of employment and unemployment is to raise a number of theoretical questions. It may help to identify these before we proceed. A first one concerns the way in which we are to interpret psychiatry's status as a political science. What type of existence does psychiatry have as an interlinked complex of conceptual, professional and institutional interventions on social relations? One way of dealing with this is by saying that psychiatry is a discipline that has a rather weak epistemological threshold,[2] that it is permeable to non-medical norms, in particular those concerning the relationship individuals have with their productive activity, or with their life whilst in enforced idleness. This is a specifically twentieth-century concern. Of course, in earlier centuries the potential idleness of the worker inside the enterprise and outside had been recognized. In the twentieth century, however, this deviation on the part of the worker from norms of productivity has come to be posed in psychiatric and psychological terms, as has also the effect of the deprivation of the wage relation on the individual. These issues have come to be interpreted in ways that depend on knowledge of the family and the personal life of the individual. Employment and unemployment are crucial spheres through which the sociability of the individual, the stability of his/her family life, satisfactions and dissatisfactions, come to be viewed as issues that bear on productivity, and that affect the contribution of the individual to society's productive output as a whole. With this development, the social and the economic intermesh to an increasing extent

A second issue concerns the ways in which psychiatry is to be understood as a positive mode of intervention in the economic sphere. This is a matter of looking at the ways in which the meaning of employment and unemployment comes to be reformulated in terms of mental health. There are two distinct elements here. One concerns the economic significance of psychiatric interventions on the person. The relevance of this is that as a mode of operation on the human machine, psychiatry is thereby also a mode of operation on the productive machine.[3] In so far as the relations of production of our society are dependent on the supervision of human individuals, to formulate the relations of the individual to his/her work in terms of mental health is to intervene in the economic sphere. To maximize the functioning of the human element of production, to increase individual satisfaction and improve mental health, is also to maximize economic returns. Psychiatry and psychology have, across the twentieth century, produced a constant series of interventions within the process of production. The psychiatric and the economic in this respect have become indissoluble. The other issue here concerns the effects that the introduction of psychiatric expertise produces on the integration of individuals within the social relations of production. The economy itself undergoes modifications as a result of psychiatry's concern with the world of employment. The specific issues around which this takes place are varied. They bear not just on the more obvious questions of neuroses partly brought about by working conditions or by employment. They also concern issues such as forms of access to employment (selection methods and criteria); forms of promotion at work (appraisal methods); vocational guidance; interventions directed at the unemployed in periods of recession, in particularly the young unemployed (youth training); and industrial rehabilitation. Psychiatry, in close association with psychology, has addressed all these issues. Through such interventions the individual's relations with the world of production come to be redefined on their behalf in a series of constantly refashioned images – efficiency, motivation, participation, co-operation, group relations, personal satisfaction and much else besides.

A third issue concerns the way in which psychiatry's encounter with the world of employment illustrates a theoretical and practical premise underlying twentieth-century psychiatry. This is one it shares with psychology, namely that the subjectivity of the person is an entity that is perfectible. Subjectivity is not an inert, a given of human life, but can be acted upon, modified and improved. Moreover, the individual's personal life, happiness and unhappiness, anxieties and fears, are not exclusively his/her own affair. They have effects both on others and on productivity. This leaves open various possible solutions – we can seek to affect them by adjustments either to the individual or to the relations of production. Whichever is chosen, however, it has the effect that personal existence is relocated through this intersection of the economic and the psychiatric as a matter for an army of technicians of the soul. Once it becomes clear that the personal intrudes on the economic in terms of reduced efficiency, increased absenteeism and accident rates, the personal ceases to be a private matter. It comes to be redefined as a concern of the employer, and also of the state. As psychiatry shifts in the early decades of this century from a strictly carceral activity to an intervention in normal social relations, an ethics of living emerges that comprises an insistence that the individual should live his/her life as best as possible and should be given assistance to do so. No longer should we be left alone with our dissatisfactions and unhappiness. The pursuit of optimum mental health comes to provide a minimal unity to the project that is twentieth-century psychiatry. The workplace and the dole queue are two of the principal sites through which this new concern with mental health emerges.

My concern in this essay has little to do with psychiatry conceived as a carceral activity. I am concerned with a psychiatry of the minor disorders, a psychiatry of mental health rather than mental illness, a psychiatry whose boundaries with psychology are indistinct. This psychiatry, to bastardize a term, is a genuinely *social* psychiatry, one that acts on the bonds that link the individual with the social relations of production through which they live. It is a psychiatry that is benign in its aspirations of making people happier in their work, less likely to injure themselves, more likely to be suited to their work, and more able to 'cope' with unemployment. It is a psychiatry that operates primarily by a promotion of the principle of subjectivity to a position of central importance in the life of the individual. It is a psychiatry with its own preconstructed laboratory in the shape of the workplace and the dole queue. It introduces a principle of differentiation of the individuals within the enterprise – between the more and the less able, those in better or worse mental health, those more or less likely to disrupt production or cause accidents, etc. It also has the effect of promoting the relational and interpersonal dimensions of economic life to a position such that they acquire a significant degree of autonomy and self-perpetuation *vis-à-vis* the demands of production. Conveniently for capital, it is also a psychiatry that is constructed in such a way as to be congruent with the imperatives of productivity that define our society. In this respect it offers a principle of adjustment into the mechanisms through which individuals inhabit their relations of production. The economic link between worker and boss undergoes a modification as profitability and the subordination of the worker are redefined as a matter of social solidarity and mental health.

The emergence of a therapeutics of employment

We see, during the 1920s, a shift in psychiatry's sphere of intervention from the asylum to the community, and an enlarged conceptual framework that comes to embrace the normal population.[4] The world of employment is a crucial site through which this concern with the milder forms of mental distress emerges. There is, I suggest, a significant inter-dependence between the shift in the practical, conceptual and institutional basis of psychiatry, and a newly emergent concern to understand and operate on the mental health of the worker and the unemployed. This interdependence can be viewed as bringing about a transformation in the objectives, con-ceptualization and regulation of economic life. The trans-formation takes place both inside and outside the enterprise, and has three characteristics which are particularly significant. First, it addresses the relationship individuals have with their selves in their work. The worker is viewed as having a personal life that continues into his/her productive work, and that influe-nces it. He or she therefore becomes an individual with a mind, with fears and anxieties. This can be seen in the emergence of concerns with questions of monotony, fatigue, attentiveness, motivation and morale. Through such concerns an attempt is made to promote a congruence between the needs of pro-duction and the self of the worker. Second, it brings into view the relationships individuals have with other workers – their colleagues, superiors and subordinates. Questions arise here about the solidarity of both the enterprise and the small group as social forms, and about the importance of the informal life of the enterprise more generally. The possibility of governing such dimensions of economic life emerges as a new terrain to be investigated. Third, it focuses on the interdependence now identified between the worker as a productive machine and the worker as a person with a family and home life. The preoccupation here is with ways in which departures from specified norms in a worker's home and personal life can disrupt his/her work performance.

What is at issue in this new attentiveness to the behavioural norms of the worker is more than simply a further device for increasing productivity. Doubtless this is a concern that animates the entire history of the capitalist enterprise. Doubtless too the new promoters of mental hygiene sought to convince the bosses of their utility in this respect. But there was something specific in the preoccupations that emerged in the inter-war years. This was the establishment of a new practice and conception of the worker which had as its objective to ensure that the bond linking the individual to the enterprise, and also the individual to society, should no longer be narrowly economic. The ambition of this new psychotherapeutics of employment and unemployment has been to supplement the wage relation and the power of the boss by a personal bond that links individuals to themselves in their work, to their co-workers and bosses, and to society as a whole. The personal existence of the worker comes to be constructed as a domain of immense interest to both the employer and the state. And with this a change occurs in the conceptualization and objectives of citizenship.

Scientific management, or Taylorism as it has been called after its best-known proponent, emerged before the First World War.[5] The transformation brought about by this, in conjunction with other techniques such as standard costing, was to reduce the human activity of production to a sequence of minute physiological activities governed by a logic of efficiency.[6] The work of Taylor, along with others such as the Gilbreths, had the effect of interposing between the boss and the worker a plethora of calculations that were to regulate the individual's activity. Scientific management treated the worker as a brute – the person with a mind had not yet been discovered. It took the motivations of the person to be purely economic, and its only tactic was to issue commands held to derive from the imperatives of the productive apparatus. This had the effect of displacing the source of discipline from the will of the boss to the technical requirements of a productive apparatus regulated according to the dictates of efficiency. Scientific management was unable, however, to address itself to the task of regulating the subjectivity of the worker.

It was during the First World War that certain shifts were to occur that opened the way for a departure from scientific management. The war was an inventive and destructive apparatus of mammoth proportions. It gave a stimulus to a psychotherapeutics of employment in three principal directions. One of these concerned selection. Vast numbers of individuals had to be selected for military service of varying types. There was, one might say, the proletarian job of actually killing people. There were also the scientific-technical tasks such as using listening devices for locating enemy submarines. How was one to allocate individuals to such tasks? The answer was to identify the different aptitudes and levels of intelligence each required, and fit these to an individual.[7] One had, that is, to individualize the difference between persons, and to ensure that appropriate tasks could be found for the different aptitudes. A second issue concerned the experience of war and the discovery of the war neuroses. As with the question of selection the figure of C. S. Myers was important here also.[8] Working with the Army Medical Corps and against majority medical opinion, Myers insisted on the psychological nature of what was then called shell-shock. This was, he argued, a psychoneurotic disturbance rather than certifiable lunacy, a physiological disturbance, or simple cowardice (see chapter two on this point). This had the effect of broadening the options as to what to do with such individuals. Instead of them either being certified as insane or shot for desertion, they could be treated. A third issue that arose during the war concerned the discovery that there was a 'human' dimension to the activity of production. The war added a new imperative to the existing capitalist one of profit. Production had to be increased dramatically to ensure that the killing could continue. With this stimulus the productivity of the munitions workers became a major preoccupation.[9] The question became one of how long people could keep working without damage to their health, without losing concentration, and without causing accidents. A psychology of individual differences led those such as E. Farmer and his colleagues to introduce the term 'accident-proneness' to show that liability to accident differed from one person to another, and that a personal study of the individual made it possible to predict in part those most liable to cause accidents.[10] There developed a concern also with more mundane issues such as bench layouts and the bodily movements they imposed on the worker. In differing degrees all these developments registered the same point – that the mental state of the worker was a concern of productivity.

This was the beginning of a movement that was more fully developed in the 1930s and that gained a firm hold on thinking about the enterprise after the Second World War. This was named 'the human factors' school; Myers described what he meant by it in the following terms:

> Of the four main determinants of industrial and commercial efficiency – the mechanical, the physiological, the psychological, and the social and economic – the psychological is by far the most important and fundamental. Intelligence in foreseeing demands and in improving industrial conditions, and a sympathetic understanding of the standpoint of others, are much more 'productive' than mere capital or mechanical labour. The physiological factors involved in purely muscular fatigue are now fast becoming negligible, compared with the effects of mental and nervous fatigue, monotony, want of interest, suspicion, hostility, etc. The psychological factor must therefore be the main consideration of industry and commerce in the future.[11]

This concern with the human factor, formulated here in terms of psychology, provided the means by which the subjectivity of the individual could be opened up as a concern of productivity.

The First World War had provided an ideal laboratory in which could be developed a host of new technologies of the individual. These were, however, only weakly formulated. The individual as conceptualized within the activity of production at that time was still little more than a bundle of physiological and mental attributes that were seen to demand consideration if the optimum output of the human machine was to be achieved. The opening had been made though, and further developments were to occur in the inter-war years. To begin with there was a consolidation of the discoveries of the war years – the formation of a psychotherapeutics of the individual worker. Represented institutionally by Myers' National Institute of Industrial Psychology (NIIP), this psychology of individual differences was to consider issues such as the physical movements of the worker, rest periods and lighting conditions. But it was also to develop a more direct interest in the mind of the worker – sources of irritation and worry, vocational guidance, and a more general concern with attitudes.[12]

The psychology of individual differences was, however, soon to be superseded. During the late 1920s and 1930s a concern emerged with what can be called the relational life of the enterprise. Prompted by problems of absenteeism and high labour turnover, the mental condition of the worker came to be defined in terms of the individual's relations with his or her colleagues and bosses. The enterprise was seen as composed of informal work-groups and of social-psychological networks, all of which had an effect on the mental health of the worker. The figure of Elton Mayo is central here.[13] His first major study reported in 1924 and was concerned with labour turnover. It was, however, the studies carried out at the Western Electric Company's works in Chicago under Mayo's supervision between 1923 and 1932 that provided a symbol for the change that was taking place. The essential message of these studies was that group relations – the informal life of the enterprise – were more significant than physiological variables such as lighting and rest pauses. This much is usually identified in the secondary literature.[14] What concerns me here is not the 'discovery' in itself, but how it provided a new terrain upon which could be investigated the mental health of the worker in all its dimensions. The relations between the individual and his/her co-workers, the individual and his/her work, could now be viewed not simply as explicable by reference to a bundle of physiological attributes. One could begin to look at the worker as enmeshed within a web of relational networks that comprised the human life of the enterprise. The previously unobserved and unformulated minutae of interactions between individuals became worthy of study and supervision. The attitudes the worker had to his/her work became legitimate objects of study. Mayo's early study had pointed to 'a disequilibrium within the individual and between him and his work'.[15] By 1983 he was able to affirm that the focus should be on the vast network of interpersonal relations that was given the name 'the group'. It was the implication of the individual within the group that was to become the focus of concern for management after the Second World War.[16]

The problem groups presented, however, was one of access and regulation. How was one to gain knowledge of and supervise an entity which, by its very nature, was resistant to observation and control? The answer was deceptively simple. It took the form of a simple technique – the non-directed interview which later was to become almost a metaphor for all interpersonal encounters at work.[17] Direct questions such as 'Do you like your boss?' tended to provoke antagonism or stereotyped responses. Non-directed and neutral questions, with the interviewer listening rather than talking, allowed the person the possibility of revealing his/her genuine feelings and grievances. This had the advantage of providing access to those dimensions of industrial life hitherto obscured, and in itself it supplied a rudimentary therapeutics. Airing one's grievances can have beneficial effects on one's morale. Such a message was to be well understood, with the non-directed interview in all its forms becoming a significant mode of intervention on the relational life of the enterprise.

Mayo was not just a researcher, however. He also devised speculative theories and remedies for the evils he detected. His concern was the Durkheimian problem of social solidarity under an increased division of labour. Durkheim had recognized that the state was an inappropriate organ 'to penetrate deeply into individual consciences and socialize them within'.[18] He argued that mechanisms that would secure the integration of the individual into society were needed: 'A nation can be maintained only if, between the State and the individual, there is intercalated a whole series of secondary groups near enough to the individuals to attract them strongly in their sphere of action and drag them, in this way, into the general torrent of social life.'[19]

Mayo's answer to the disintegration of industrial civilization had strong similarities with the Durkheimian formula of the occupational group. Interdependence was to be achieved through the face-to-face colleague work-group, through linking the work-group to management, and through linking management to the wider society.[20] Social solidarity would be promoted in this way, both inside the enterprise and in society at large.

It was during the inter-war years too that the 'maladjusted worker' was to be identified in the USA. Vocational maladjustment as a reflection of emotional maladjustment was used to describe the wide variety of disturbances of personality that affect individual adjustment in every phase of life.[21] The adjustment of the individual requires an integration of conflicting tendencies to the demands of the activity in which he or she is engaged. Emotional maladjustment follows from a conflict in the individual of impulses that are incompatible with one another. Emotional maladjustment breeds dissatisfaction and thwarts the search for happiness and success. Personal dissatisfaction with one's work produces the vocationally maladjusted individual.[22]

Manifestations of the milder emotional maladjustments are seen as including petty jealousies, mild forms of self-pity, lack of cheerful co-operation, fault-finding, hard-boiled tactics and labour agitation, and desire for undue attention, feigned bravery, and foolhardiness as a retreat from fears. The more serious emotional maladjustments include frequent change of jobs, extreme reticence and withdrawal, tired feelings, spasmodic and irregular application to the tasks of the job, day-dreaming, deficiency in range and power of attention, distractibility, extreme irritability, nervous indigestion, nausea, abnormal fears, fear neuroses, feelings of being spied upon, watched or followed, hearing voices and other miscellaneous symptoms.[23] The significance of such factors was considered to be enormous. It was estimated that one half of the amount expended annually because of labour turnover was spent on the replacement of emotionally maladjusted workers; the effectiveness of approximately half the working force was considered to be disturbed by either minor or major emotional maladjustment that required intensive analysis and training.[24] Included among workers suffering from personality disturbances were those who had never 'grown up' – whose experiences, instead of maturing and ripening, had simply carried the faulty characteristic of adolescence into adult life, producing the underdeveloped, inadequate, difficult, poorly integrated or unstable workers, commonly called 'job misfits', or 'work failures', 'mediocrities', or 'ne'er-do-wells'.[25] 'Unstable personalities', 'faulty attitudes', 'irrational thinking' and 'pessimistic reverie' were all to come under observation in this new concern with the maladjusted worker.[26]

In Britain the significance of emotional disturbances in creating maladjustment was studied by Smith, Culpin and Farmer.[27] In a study of 'telegraphists cramp' – an occupational disorder – they found that of 41 cramp cases examined, 75.6 per cent showed symptoms that would lead, quite apart from the cramp, to the diagnosis of minor mental disturbances or mild psycho-neurosis characterized by anxiety, obsessions, or hysteria. In 26 cases the symptoms were considered to be of a serious nature. The difference between the individuals suffering from psycho-neurotic symptoms and those free from these symptoms was brought out well in a summary of the characteristics of the different types. The individual free from such symptoms:

> finds his work interesting, and looks forward to getting on at it – goes in for sports or hobbies – is sociable, enjoys being with his fellows – if shy at first with strangers becomes less so with experience – respects authority but is not overwhelmed by it – can be observed without undue emotion, has no particular fear of the dark, noises, etc. – doesn't worry about his work when it is finished – sleeps well – can go at an easy pace in telegraphy – can hold his own opinions with and against his fellows – can realize himself in relation to others reasonably. An approximation to this we should call normal, particularly if combined with a healthy physique and cheerful expression.

The psycho-neurotic however:

> thinks the work interesting, but is doubtful whether he is making progress – is never sure of himself – worries when he has done a thing as to whether it is right – is conscious of being watched in trains, buses or restaurants – goes back to make sure he has done what he thinks he has – likes to check his work many times – dislikes all games and social activities – doesn't feel at ease with people – irritated and frightened by authorities – speculates on the possibility of the floor giving way or the building falling down – upset by noises – always wants to rush at dots. Such a type we should class as psycho-neurotic and under the conditions of telegraphic work we should anticipate the development of cramp.[28]

The discovery of the 'human factor' in industry provided a norm around which individuals' relations to their work, other workers and their selves could be evaluated. The 'maladjusted' or 'emotionally disturbed' individual, unable to tolerate the stresses and strains of particular tasks, provided a means by which to identify the parameters of the normal worker.

The emergence of a therapeutics of unemployment

The economic and the psychiatric sphere do not intersect only between the walls of the enterprise. Rather it is the worker's personal relation to his/her employment that supplies the key to a therapeutics of productive activity. The absence of such a relation, in the form of unemployment, becomes as significant an issue as its presence. If the economic links between the worker and the enterprise are supplemented by a concern with the worker's mental health, then it is only appropriate that the latter concern should be maintained even when work ceases. We might say that this was the principle behind what can be called a therapeutics of unemployment, which emerged in the 1930s with the onset of mass unemployment.

The phenomenon of unemployment as a condition defining the person had only been identified in the 1890s.[29] In the 1930s a new conceptualization of unemployment emerged that complemented the therapeutics of work within the enterprise. The dole queue replaced the enterprise as the laboratory for the new preoccupation with the mental health of the worker. The ex-worker or the young person who had not yet become a worker became the new object of concern. This new therapeutics was one in which the severing of the employment bond was seen to have profound effects on a person's mental health. Stress, depression and anxiety came to be linked to the status of being unemployed. This was seen, in turn, to have severe effects on family life, disrupting its normal pattern and affecting spouses and children alike. From this a series of rationales were to develop for interventions directed at the unemployed person and their family. The project that underlay these schemes was one of seeking to engender in the unemployed person a motivational commitment to their personal life that would maintain them in a state of good mental health.

What is so striking about this new conceptualization of unemployment is the way it tends to make the maintenance of mental health dependent on being employed. Whilst account is taken of variation between individuals who experience unemployment, the removal of the employment relation came to be viewed as an irreplaceable psychological deprivaion. Compensation might be attempted since the loss was not absolute and irreparable, but this could only ever be partial. And, what is perhaps most important, whilst the economic deprivation was not ignored, the loss was construed primarily as affecting the mental health of the individual. This had the effect of adding a new and additional dimension to the phenomenon of unemployment. No longer was it exclusively a question of social administration or economic policy.[30] Both might still be relevant, but they were to be supplemented by a concern with the personal: unemployment came to assume a human face.

There were two main dimensions to this new preoccupation with the mental health of the unemployed person. One of these centred on youth as a specific object of concern, and took the form of programmes of instruction and training for the young unemployed. The second was a more general concern with the psychological consequences of unemployment and its effects on family life. The first addressed the individual who was in danger of not becoming a worker, of not becoming integrated within the discipline of work. The second addressed the individual deprived of employment, and sought to delve into the intimacies of his/her personal and family life. Together, what these dimensions demonstrate is not a basic concern to simply *do something* with or to the unemployed. They were not a natural response to the phenomenon of unemployment. They represented rather a specific form of conceptualization of unemployment as having psychological effects such as stress, depression, and the disruption of family life.

Unemployment comes to be posed as more than a simple economic deprivation, the removal of a wage. It is seen as the removal of those stimuli that maintain the individual and, by extension, his/her family in full mental health and with a full motivational commitment to that series of minute projects that constitute the life of the person. With this development the economic tie that links individuals to capitalist society comes to be accorded a new dimension. And whilst this cannot be viewed as a transformation of capitalism into a different economic system, it does have the effect of introducing a significant inflection into the functioning of that system.

At issue here is not just a revitalized version of the Protestant Ethic or of the desire of the capitalist state to inculcate habits of labour discipline. Nor is it a simple expression of humanitarian concerns. Of course such factors may be relevant, but they do not serve to wholly explain these new concerns. There was a novelty in the way in which the whole question of employment came to be posed in the inter-war years, first in attending to the worker in the enterprise, and then to the unemployed individual. In both cases this novelty lay in a new perception of the individual's relationship with the economic sphere as a relation that entailed norms of conduct and mental functioning. When the individual appeared to be departing from such norms, interventions into his/her personal life were called for.

The concern with the young unemployed was best exemplified in its institutional embodiment. This took the form of what came to be called 'dole schools' or, in official terms, Juvenile Unemployment Centres and later Junior Instruction Centres.[31] First established in 1918 and reorganized in 1930, these centres sought to 'give boys and girls a real interest in life'.[32] Offering primarily practical activities – wood-work and metal work for boys, cookery and dress-making for girls – the centres clearly had as one important aim to prevent demoralization and to promote an ethic of work. With unemployment viewed as a threat to the operation of economy and society, the centres had a preventative, negative quality.[33] But in addition to this pragmatic controlling objective of keeping young people off the streets and attempting to prepare them for work there was a distinctively psychological dimension to the manner in which the objectives of these interventions came to be conceived. This entailed a new and wider set of conceptions of the psychological relationship that the individual maintains with his/her productive activity. This was not just a matter of work discipline conceived as the subordination of the individual to the logic of the stop-watch. It entailed a more positive conception of discipline that can be characterized under the term 'technologies of the self' (see the discussion in chapter 2).[34] This refers to the various practices and discourses through which the individual comes to recognize him- or herself as a subject and to regulate his/her life according to certain norms and criteria of conduct, a set of conceptions about what one should expect of one's work, and the ways in which one's mental health is affected by the absence of employment.

This shift away from a notion of discipline that comes from above to one that should ideally come from young people themselves can be seen in the recommendations for the choice of supervisors for the Juvenile Instruction Centres. As Bell was to argue, 'The wrong type, as experience has proved, is "the old sergeant major", the iron disciplinarian.'[35] One should not seek to impose discipline from without, but cultivate it by starting with the self-discipline that arises from personal commitment to certain activities: 'The secret in the JICs is to start with the interests of the young folk and work up from them. Even the toughest of lads can display interest when a paint box is given to them.'[36] The disjunction between the operation of the different measures provided and their declared objectives should not obscure their significance. The latter were central in establishing the principle that employment should comprise not just a wage but a personal bond linking the fulfilment of the worker as a subject to his/her productive activity.

The second dimension to the newly emergent therapeutics of unemployment concerns the effects of job loss on the worker and his/her family. The psychologization of unemployment is more pronounced here. The onset of mass unemployment in the 1930s is accompanied by an avalanche of studies undertaken by a wide range of social scientists, including psychologists, psychiatrists and sociologists.[37] These studies all sought to render visible the effects of unemployment on the mental health and social functioning of the individual. Family life, sexual activity, anxiety levels, attitudes towards the future all came to be opened up as legitimate spheres of study and intervention for the social sciences concerned with the mental health of the unemployed person.

This concern was not psychiatric in the sense of a restricted interest in identifying the varied mental pathologies of unemployed individuals. In many cases it was even stressed that what was at issue was not genuine neurosis.[38] What occurred was, rather, a permeation of psychiatric knowledge and competences into modes of judgment and interventions towards the unemployed. So, whilst specific psychiatric disorders may not always have figured in such studies, psychiatric modes of investigation for the detection of minor psychiatric disorders were deployed in a more generalized evaluation of mental health, emotional stability, and so forth.

There is a striking uniformity to the conclusions reached in the various studies of unemployment. One general conclusion concerns the subjective experience of being rendered unemployed. An initial phase of *shock* is quickly followed by a burst of *optimism* as the newly unemployed person seeks to find work on the assumption that this is a possible and realistic option. A third phase of *pessimism* follows as the unemployed person meets with failure in his/her search for work. As the search continues he or she becomes increasingly pessimistic about the chances of finding a job again. The fourth and final phase is one of *fatalism* as the now demoralized individual accepts the logic of the situation. Job-hunting activity ceases, and the individual adapts his/her style of living to the constraints of permanent unemployment.

I do not wish to dispute the appropriateness of such a characterization of the effects of unemployment on the individual. Unemployment clearly has disastrous effects on morale and attitudes as well as on the economic dimension of personal existence. It would be hazardous to suggest a way of separating these different aspects. It would also require a more thorough examination than is possible here of the different processes by which employment has been constituted in our society as one of the most regulated dimensions of our existence. This would entail consideration of the boundaries that have been drawn around it in terms of such issues as regularity (the hours worked), its total duration across the life of the individual (the historically variable period between youth and retirement), and gender (the exclusion of women from certain activities and the construction for them of a different principle of work).

My concern here is more restricted. It centres on what this new interest in the psychological effects of unemployment has signified. For what emerged along with it was a vast project of investigation into the entire life of the unemployed person. Concern with the mental health of the unemployed became a principle for studying the organization of their daily activities, their commitment to these activities, their eating habits, sexual relations and overall outlook on life. Indeed the entirety of the minutae of the life of the individual and his/her family became a legitimate object of scrutiny. This was carried out according to a measure of norms of mental functioning. To study such phenomena researchers were to literally move into the homes of the unemployed in order to better scrutinize them.[39] They were to observe the unemployed on street corners. And they were to do this in terms that placed the personal relation to employment as the norm around which we should evaluate the lives of individuals.

This produced some interesting paradoxes. For instance,

when the unemployed finally reached the fourth stage of unemployment – that of fatalism – they were often found to be
satisfied with the new equilibrium their lives had attained.
They would, in short, declare that they were content with their
lot. But for the researchers this declared happiness could only
function as the sign of a profound deprivation and a malaise
with life. One cannot, it would appear, be truly content with
such a low level of motivational commitment to life, and in
particular to the employment relation.[40] The only exception
here was the unemployed woman, depicted as an exception by
virtue of the implied essential masculinity of employment.
Whilst unemployment produced a generalized impoverishment
of the living environment, it was held to produce differential
effects on men and women. In general, and despite suffering
as a result of job loss, women were considered to adapt better
since they still had the imperatives of child-care and maintenance of the home. The subject for whom employment was
a necessary condition for the attainment of mental health was
a gendered subject – male.

Mental hygiene in wartime

During the inter-war years a concern with the mental health
of the worker came to be viewed as intimately related to the
wage relation. The pursuit of mental health within and through
one's employment became established as a legitimate end to
be sought. With this development an enlarged conception of
the objectives of the economic sphere was to emerge. Whilst
the goal of optimizing productivity remained unchallenged,
the mechanisms through which it was to be achieved were
reinterpreted according to specific conceptions of mental
health. Productivity was to be maintained in the face of problems such as absenteeism, high labour turnover and high accident rates. But there was more at issue than simply responses
to the imperatives of productivity. What emerged was a modification of the employment relation itself. Put simply this was
from one in which the wage was the sole link between worker
and enterprise, to one in which the worker was bound by a
complex of psychological and social ties. Rather than a wholly
external relation between the individual and his/her work, the
new objective was one in which employment was to provide a

source of meaning, with the effect that if a worker were to be deprived of employment he or she would be potentially more liable to anxiety and depression. If the issue is seen as one of discipline, it is a self-discipline in which the individual's relationship to him- or herself and to his/her co-workers are paramount. These twin objectives can be viewed as a psychotherapeutics of the individual worker and a technology of the social relations of the enterprise.

I have sought so far simply to chart the emergence of these two themes in the inter-war years. Since then they have been redefined a number of times. The Second World War in particular provided a considerable stimulus to the expansion of psychiatric practice *vis-à-vis* the goal of productivity. This promoted psychiatric expertise to a central role in the government and supervision of the lives of human populations. In turn, this hinged on promoting two key issues – the relationship individuals have with their selves, and the relations they have with their fellow soldiers or workers. This was a new technology of the person and of his/her integration within the group. Although the beginnings of such a technology can be detected before the war, it was only during and after it that it emerged in a consolidated form. Along with this development was the formation through the war of new working relationships between psychiatrists, psychologists, social workers and administrators. The war gave rise to new ways of understanding the selection and apportioning of individuals to specific activities; the personal experience of war, particularly in relation to psychoneurotic disturbances; and a more generalized concern with group relations, morale and motivation.

One area in which this new role for the concern with mental health can be seen was the field of selection. In the First World War the British army had a 'consulting psychologist' and a number of neurologists, many of whom in fact were psychiatrists.[41] The experience of the war, and afterwards in the Ministry of Pensions' special hospitals and clinics for servicemen, led to the establishment of clinics for civilians. It was argued that there was a large problem of civilian neurosis that had until then been almost untackled (see the discussion in chapter two on this point). The only special hospital for neurosis before the First World War was the Lady Chichester Hospital at Hove. After the war, the Tavistock Clinic was founded in 1920 for out-patient psychotherapy. The Maudsley

Hospital, which was built before the war and then used as a military hospital, assumed its full functions for civilians shortly afterwards. From then on an increasing number of clinics and special hospital out-patient departments were opened.

In Britain the knowledge gained of the neuroses and their effects on the individual and the groups to which he or she belonged was only slowly applied to such matters as selection. In the USA developments were much quicker and more extensive. During the First World War they applied modern psychological methods to the problem of selection. Germany was also quick to apply elaborate selection techniques permeated by the latest psychological knowledge. At the outbreak of the Second World War there was, however, no psychological or psychiatric screening for the general recruitment of the armed forces in Britain. The psychiatrist saw only those individuals whom the personnel selection officers thought might possibly be unstable or in some way out of the ordinary in terms of mental health. Individuals were siphoned off after the routine examinations of the National Service Recruiting Boards, which were civilian boards run by the Ministry of Labour. Even so, in an average intake, psychiatrists were asked to see something in the region of 15 per cent of the whole intake and to advise about disposal or posting, or in some cases hospitalization.[42]

At the start of the war the only psychiatrists recruited for the British army were two consultants, one with the British Expeditionary Force in France, and one in Britain itself. Extra psychiatrists were brought into the army early in 1940, but by then they faced large numbers of unsuitable recruits. The process of weeding these individuals out was then begun. Many were discharged as unfit for service. A variety of intelligence tests was brought into use by the different psychiatrists. Rees was to comment later that perhaps it 'was this flood of inadequate and dull men' that 'forced us to do something about selection'.[43] All the early selection procedures had to be operated by psychiatrists simply because there was no one else to do it. A new and generalized concern with recruits was beginning to develop, in which psychiatrists and psychologists would combine their expertise in an effort to differentiate the human material presented to them.

There were a number of dimensions to this new concern with differentiating individuals according to their suitability for specific types of activity. One was the need to weed out that class of human material considered defective in its mental capabilities. The 'dullard' was identified as one category likely not just to underperform, but to be prejudicial to the war effort. He might malinger, develop anxiety, or simply fail to comprehend orders. In various ways he would be a consumer of manpower rather than a contributor. Dullards formed a social-problem group. The solution of what to do with them was found in unarmed sections of the pioneer corps.[44] Every man in these sections was investigated psychiatrically. They were assigned to live in hostels and carry out agricultural work. In such a setting they were placed with those considered to be their equals, and here they were supposed to find a new community and companionship.

Routine employment and group solidarity was deemed to provide a formula for those of low intellectual ability, one which was considered to have implications for peace time as well as war. The concern with selection was not, however, simply a negative one of eliminating human material deemed defective. There was also a positive concern to identify the different types of good-quality individuals, and to fit them to the tasks for which they were most suited. Exacting tasks required individuals of high quality: 'Armoured regiments cannot be manned by men of inferior physique or inadequate mentality, and elaborate radio-location plants are not usefully operated save by intelligent men or women.'[45]

In the USA, the army maintained a continual screening process designed to eliminate men considered psychologically incapable of withstanding the stresses of combat duty. This began with a preinduction psychiatric examination to determine whether or not potential draftees were psychologically fit for military service in general. Screening was continued throughout the various stages of precombat training and was extended into the period when men had already been committed to combat. The screening was carried out primarily by psychiatrists.[46] Their usual procedure was to examine the men in a clinical interview in order to detect behavioural disturbances. Although directed primarily toward eliminating psychotics, pre-psychotics, psychoneurotics, and psychopaths, the process sought more widely to identify any individual who showed signs of inability to tolerate anxiety.[47] The different stages of the screening procedure served to distinguish between those it was felt were not worth training because their emotional disturbances seriously interfered with adjustment to the army, and those who could be trained but were considered unfit for combat duty. It was in this context that the Neuropsychiatric Screening Adjunct (NSA) was developed, a test based on a large-scale research study that comprised questionnaire responses of psychoneurotic patients in army hospital wards and the responses of a cross-section of soldiers in the USA.[48]

There were, one might say, three categories of candidates unsuitable for the army. First, there were those people who were useful members of the community, and whose utility and capacity for self-support would be reduced or destroyed by service in the army; second, there were those who would certainly break down with psychotic or seriously psychoneurotic disabilities, with harmful effects on morale, solidarity and discipline; third, there were those who would do well under military training, in some cases better than in civil life, but who could not be discharged back into civil life because of the likeliood of their developing disabling personality disorders. The task of psychiatry that emerged was to ensure that all three of these categories were excluded from the army.[49]

It was in the area of officer selection that psychiatrists were to have the opportunity to demonstrate their abilities in Britain. It was frequently observed that psychiatric factors were often responsible for producing inefficiency in officers. The psychiatric breakdown rate among officers was high. Some had even been in receipt of disability pensions for neurosis since the First World War. Many had been clearly inefficient on psychiatric grounds for some time before being sent for a psychiatric interview. Equally, there were a number of men from the ranks who were newly commissioned yet had a history of psychopathy which should have excluded them. The cause of neurotic breakdown was taken to be that the men were unable to carry the extra responsibility that accompanied their increase in rank. This did not mean, however, that they would not have been suitable for efficient cotinued service in the ranks. The implications here were evident. Psychiatric expertise was needed to differentiate those capable of functioning efficiently at officer level from those who should remain in the ranks.

Once it was established that the mental health of the potential officer should be given as much attention as his physical health, the way was open for psychiatric forms of argument and investigation to be used in the selection of officers. Experiments were started to discover possible techniques for the rapid selection of large numbers of candidates. In one experiment candidates were given a group intelligence test, a short questionnaire, and an hour-long psychiatric interview. Temperamental and personality factors were examined by, among other methods, an electrical 'chest expander', that gave the candidate an increasing electric shock as they made their maximum pull on the springs. The result of these experiments were apparently viewed as encouraging.[50] Clearly defined neuroses were indentifed with a high degree of certainty, whilst minor phobic disturbances and personality deviations proved less easy to detect.

The felt success of these original experiments can be measured by the decision to set up an experimental War Office Selection Board, from which emerged an elaborate system covering the whole of the country. The staff of each board comprised an experienced regular officer president, a deputy president, three military testing officers who would be line officers of some experience, one or two psychiatrists and a psychologist. The team was to carry out an assessment of the whole person from then on and it had to take serious account of psychiatric modes of judgment in the selection of officers. Selection was a team process, albeit one in which the psychiatric contribution was of considerable importance.

The prophylactic tasks of psychiatry through such means as selection were highly significant in the introduction of new principles for assigning individuals to tasks. Treatment for the effects of battle experience also led to innovations. The crucial problem here was 'battle neurosis'. The concern was both with the effects of battle in producing anxiety neuroses in an individual, and the danger that this might 'infect' other men in the unit. What is intereting here is the line that came to be drawn between neurosis and cowardice. For it was not just a matter of psychiatrists reinterpreting cowardice as a medical condition. Deliberate evasions of dangerous front-line duty remained outside the preserve of the psychiatrist, which was restricted to cases where the individuals displayed the physical signs of anxiety. An important determinant of the amount of breakdowns that occurred was the kind of war situation the men were in. The nearer the fighting approximated to the trench warfare of 1914–18, the higher the incidence became. Being attacked by particular dreaded weapons, in combination with conditions of personal isolation and lack of sleep, led to breakdown rates of 10, 15 or even 20 per cent. One way of treating breakdowns in battle was divisional rest centres close to the battle zones and from which men would return to duty within approximately a week. Prophylactic sedation was also often used for men near to breaking down.

The most powerful innovation of war psychiatry, however, was the elaboration of a technology of group solidarity. The integration of the individual into a fighting unit was not simply a matter of personal commitment. Group discipline was at issue also; indeed it was paramount. But discipline understood as a system of punitive measures was only to be used as a last resort. Discipline should firstly be accepted freely. As Rees was to state: 'It is therefore part of our job to see that the soldier understands and accepts discipline voluntarily and welcomes it and, indeed, prides himself upon his participation in the activities of a well-disciplined unit. While morale is a vertebral column that keeps us erect, discipline by itself is only a corset which can for a while hold a man erect.'[51]

Discipline is not an alternative of good morale. The two form part of an overall mechanism of group solidarity. And this, in turn, is dependent on three main factors: 'adequate war aim and purpose, a sense of one's competence and value, and the feeling that one matters as an individual in a group of other similar people'.[52] It is the last of these that is central here. The principle developed was that understanding, welfare, individual care and responsibility for each person in the group was the best prophylactic against antagonisms that might destroy morale. It was explicitly stated that this was not just a principle applicable for military purposes. Simple mental hygiene of this type is as relevant to civilian industry as to the services. Low morale and lack of cohesion is almost certain to lead to high rates of absenteeism. Attempts to counter this can take various forms. During the war psychiatrists helped in designing radio programmes and films for specific problems. Out of these varied interventions a whole new enterprise of prophylatic psychiatry began to take shape.

The issue of group solidarity was also a prominent object of concern in the studies and experiments conducted on the American army. A massive series of studies was conducted by the research branch of the US War Department's Information and Education Division. This was published after the war in a series of volumes by a team of sociologists and social psychologists.[53] The concerns of these studies spanned the social sciences, ranging from psychiatric studies, through the social psychological, to the sociological. One of the most enduring findings concerned the relations betwen the individual, the primary group to which they belonged, and the large organization of which they formed a part. The studies supported the view that officers and enlisted men alike attached little importance to idealistic motives such as patriotism and the aims of the war. Combat troops were often highly critical of the war and of the deprivations it produced. The key role in maintaining morale and efficiency was shown to derive from primary group relations. The group, with its close interpersonal ties, served two principal and interdependent purposes – the setting and enforcing of group standards of behaviour, and the supporting and sustaining of the individual. Whilst the war as a national objective provided 'a set of generalised moral predispositions',[55] inner cohesion derived 'not simply by a series of commands controlling the behaviour of soldiers disinclined to respect the symbols of formal authority but rather through a system of overlapping primary groups'.[56]

The relational life of the enterprise

During the inter-war years an enlarged principle of mental health had developed. No longer was it a matter of just treating those individuals who departed from reason. A concern with the neuroses emerged – disabilities that could affect any one of us. This shift blurred the frontiers between the normal and the pathological. One no longer had to enter the 'other' side to require the ministrations of psychiatric expertise. A further shift occurred after the Second World War, partly as a result of the experiences of the war, and partly as a result of innovations that had commenced earlier. This was a growing concern with *positive* mental health in the workplace. There remained a concern to identify various classes of 'defective' individuals. But there also developed a preoccupation with optimizing the mental health of all individuals in their relation to their work.

There remained a concern with the individual worker and the incidence of neurosis. Tredgold highlighted the different effects of neurosis on production.[57] First, there was the amount of work directly lost through absence. Second, was the effect of neuroses on wastage in production, as a result of the inefficiency of those who remained at work, but did not give their best. Tredgold was to comment on this aspect: 'In firms where much more depends on the behaviour of the individual, so much more production can be lost by workers going slowly, or by being moody and failing to concentrate.'[58] The third effect was on the rest of the firm, on the steady reliable workers. Often, Tredgold remarked, supervisors 'would prefer the neurotic to stay away altogether.'[59] Interventions entailing counselling and a range of other specialized forms of interview were to develop. These interviews took as their focus the individual and the relation he or she maintained with the working environment.[60]

There remained a concern with questions of motivation and morale, and with absenteeism and industrial accidents.[61] The latter emphasised not individual characteristics but the integration of the individual within the group. It was not, however, a matter of simple continuity. After the war there developed a terrain of mental hygiene which had been enlarged and transformed by the intervention of psychiatric competence in personnel matters. This terrain was not to be dominated by even the psychoneuroses and milder character disorders: 'A much more important consideration than this is the necessity to further, by every means in our power, positive enjoyment of mental health.'[62] The prescription was simple: 'It consists in the protection and development at all levels of human society of secure, affectionate and satisfying human relationships, and in the reduction of hostile tensions in persons and groups.'[63] The concern which emerged was with *positive* mental health, perceived as a question of the ways in which populations of human individuals should be governed under the new post-war era.

One author posed the following question: 'What has the mental hygienist to say to the controversy between the advocates of social security "from the womb to the tomb" and the protagonists of a more rugged approach who see in such measures a danger to independence, enterprise and incentive to effort?'[64] His answer was to recommend mental hygiene as a strategy of government that could help to resolve the conflicts between the individual and the group:

> All of us have yet to assimilate the notion of the community, of which the leadership is, as it were, the ego. That is to say, management or government is a specialized organ for integrating and carrying on the affairs and external relationships of the given group . . . (. . .) The main problem, then, is to bridge peacefully the gap between the individual and the group through the replacement of anxiety-arousing pressure ('fear' and 'want') by insight based on friendly participation. This technique applies at all levels, in the home, in education, in industry and in politics and is essentially the same techique as that used in modern psychotherapy.[65]

The responsibility for promoting the health of a society was seen to reside not in its medical services but in its social practitioners – managers, politicians, teachers and other leaders of human groups. Encountering mental health within the contexts of the workshop and the school they were in a better position to respond earlier than the doctor. From within the complexity of social existence the relationships of the working group were to emerge as the context in which individuals were to derive emotional and intellectual satisfactions. As Tredgold remarked, 'It is not a question of deciding whether or not a worker has neurosis – it is whether he is at his maximal mental health, happiness and efficiency, or a fraction below it . . . Quite apart from the time absolutely lost by neurotic illness, there is some wastage from incomplete effort when health and efficiency are not at the maximal.'[66]

The question of neurosis in industry had been studied by many during and shortly after the Second World War. One study that involved psychologists, psychiatrists and social workers found that 10 per cent of its sample had suffered from definite and disabling neurotic illness. A further 20 per cent had suffered from minor forms of neurosis during the course of six months. Neurotic illness was held to have caused between a quarter and a third of all absences through sickness. Tredgold commented that these findings 'sound a clear challenge to a country the survival of which is constantly to depend on its power to produce.'[67] He continued, however, in a more critical manner. The report had noted that 'the circumstances outside the factory, which were associated with a high incidence of neurosis, are characterized by unsatisfactory human relation-ships. The more obviously unsatisfactory the human relation-ships, the closer the association.'[68] Tredgold considered this attention to the worker's attitude to his work and to his home to be valuable. But overall the report was lacking, he felt, in dealing 'so little with the personal relationships of the worker with his supervisors, fellows and subordinates at work.'[69] Whilst difficult to measure, these were an important aspect of the total situation.

The new concern with promoting positive mental health was pre-eminently a social concern. Whilst many of the techniques and concerns focused on the individual, this was generally in terms of his/her impact on the group. But there was also a distinctive preoccupation with the relational life of the enter-prise. It was this that provided a new technology of the human resource in the two decades following the Second World War. Of course 'the group' had been discovered in the late 1920s, particularly through the renowned Hawthorne investigations.[70] But it was only after the war that a deluge of studies and practical interventions occurred that took as their focus the nexus between the individual and the group.

The relational life of the enterprise supplied the focus for a vast range of concerns. Even leadership, which might be regarded as a 'personal' quality *par excellence*, came to be reinterpreted in terms of the significance of the group. It was viewed not as a single quality possessed by some and not by others, but as the effectiveness of an individual in a specific role within a specific group united for a particular purpose.[71] Selection, previously regarded as a matter of identifying certain qualities inherent in the individual, became under Bion a matter of interpersonal relations (see chapter two on this point). Commenting on the principle of the 'leaderless group', a technique developed for officer selection, Bion was to remark on its more general significance:

> The essence of the technique . . . was to provide a framework in which selecting officers . . . could observe a man's capacity for maintaining personal relationships in a situation of strain that tempted him to disregard the interests of his fellows for the sake of his own . . . The problem was to make capital of this emotional field in order to test the quality of the man's relationship with his fellows.[72]

The 'leaderless group', rather than placing the person on a spectrum of individual differences, located him or her firmly in the complex of interpersonal relations of the group. Such techniques were not just theoretical constructs but had practical implications in schemes such as the Unilever Company's management development procedures.[73]

The Tavistock Group, comprising psychiatrists, psychologists and anthropologists, represents in many respects the emblem of this concern with optimizing the mental health of the individual through the relational web of the enterprise. The Tavistock Clinic, a voluntary out-patient centre for psychotherapy, and its post-war sister insititution, the Tavistock Institute of Human Relations, together had a profound effect on the conceptualization of the significance of group relations for enhancing the functioning of the enterprise.

A study of industrial accidents carried out by the Tavistock Institute utilized this relational grid as a mode of explanation. There is a limit, it was argued, to the reduction in accidents that could be achieved by alterations in the physical environment, such as guarding or protecting machinery. As noted above, the intial response to the question of industrial accidents had been to seek to identify the personal characteristics of individuals involved in accidents, from which had emerged the notion of 'accident-proneness',[74] a personal attribute normally identified *post-hoc*. However, during the 1950s the argument emerged that accident-proneness should be understood not as an individual but as a group characteristic. The understanding of accident proneness 'should be widened to take into account the social aspects of the relationship of people to their work . . . Accidents are social as well as personal events and, in industry, happen by virtue of the fact that the people concerned are members of some kind of work organization.[75] Accidents came to be presented in this way as group characteristics. They were understood in terms of their 'absence effects'. Accidents could be viewed, it was argued, as a means of withdrawal from the work situation through which the individual could take up the role of absentee in a manner acceptable to him- or herself and to the employing organization. Sickness and accidents, both falling within the class of events called absence phenomena, could be viewed as motivated absences. In this new interpretation the worker is not seen as exposed to a physical environment apt to 'attack'. Rather, the emphasis is on the fact that the propensity of the physical environment to attack him could be reduced if his working relations improved. As with the other preoccupations of the time that concerned connections between mental health and employment, the central focus here was on the integration of the individual within the social life of the group.

Towards the contractual self

From Pinel onward psychiatry has concerned itself with the self-regulating capacities of the person. The notion of cure has always entailed a certain conception of regulated subjectivity. The boundary between reason and unreason coincided with the division between a fully functioning subjectivity and its absence. The task of psychiatry was to help the mad person cross the frontier. As this boundary becomes less rigid, and as psychiatry has come to operate increasingly on the normal mind, the task of psychiatry has been redefined to include the promotion and cultivation of an optimum functioning of subjectivity rather than simply its restoration. One's subjectivity might become slightly damaged, or it may be functioning below optimum capacity. In such cases we now have recourse to a variety of technologies that derive more-or-less directly from psychiatric competence and expertise. Such interventions include prophylactic adjustments of the social relations to a range of institutions to minimize the risk of damage and to maximize the promotion of healthy subjectivity. In the twentieth century the adequate and, more recently the optimum functioning of the individual's subjectivity has been redefined in terms of its relation with the activity of production. In turn, the wage relation has been transformed into the employment relation, a much wider principle in which the mental health of the worker becomes of increasing importance. I have attempted above simply to follow some of the contours of this new terrain, from the early developments in the interwar years to the preoccupation with the individual/group nexus after the Second World War. Even if the coincidence of work and happiness is a myth, as an objective it helps to strengthen the link between personal satisfaction and increased productivity.

Today we have moved far beyond the preoccupation with the individual/group nexus. A new political vocabulary is dominant, in which the individual is called upon to draw on the resources of the self rather than those of the group or the state. This vocabulary has emerged as a powerful political philosophy, and one which has profound practical implications. As a principle for the regulation of societies it accords well with the new psychiatric vocabulary and interventions. It would be foolish to try to provide this interrelation with a causal principle. The important point indeed is not to establish causality, but to register the shift that has occurred from a concern with group solidarity to an entrepreneurship of the self. We might tentatively suggest that there is an interdependence between a new political culture based on an economic entrepreneurship of the self and the new psychological culture founded on a psychological autonomization of the individual's subjectivity. Group solidarity has the potentially harmful effect of increasing the dependency of the individual on the immediate group or on society more generally. The employment relation tends to foster this dependency. However, what is currently taking place is a refashioning of the link between the individual and society. Whilst care is taken that it should not be severed, the onus of responsibility is being shifted from that of society to the individual. It is not surprising in this context that the notion of the self operative in psychiatric and psychological discourses should be modified. It is in this context that we see the rise to prominence of the contractual self.

In nineteenth-century capitalism the relation between worker and employer was defined as that of a freely entered contract. The concern in this century with the mental health of the worker uncovered an operative principle that conflicted with this contractual freedom. Group solidarity was found to be an immensely resistant material through which workers formed bonds with each other. One can see the emergence over the last two decades of a new principle that provides the ideal accompaniment to the economic contract between worker and employer. This is a contractualization of the psychological bonds linking worker and colleagues, worker and boss. Instead of groups bound to one another by relations of solidarity, what emerges to prominence is a series of encounters between persons that take place on a constantly shifting and *ad hoc* basis.

The promotion of the contractual self attains its most developed form in relation to the problem of unemployment. In the mid-1970s as unemployment began to increase dramatically, and as the sacred principle of full employment receded further and further into the distance, a concern developed with the psychological effects of unemployment. There is a formal similarity in the concern with the mental health of the unemployed person between the 1930s and the 1970s. There is a further avalanche of writings on the effects of unemployment on the mental health of the individual and his/her family. The same four-stage model of the experience of unemployment is utilized in both periods. But there are significant differences also. The first lies in the effect produced by some three decades of full employment. The previous period of mass unemployment did not follow a generation in which full employment became an accepted condition of the economy. Nor did it follow a period of some half a century during which the world of employment came to be promoted as the sphere of full psychological health and rewarding interpersonal relations. Banal as these factors may be, they are no less significant. Until the late 1970s, in both an individual and a social sense, full employment had come to be established as a condition of economic and psychological health.

A second difference concerns the conceptualization of unemployment and the nature of the interventions aimed at the unemployed, in particular the young unemployed. This group has received the most attention. And in the measures addressed to them, in addition to the crude attempts to control and keep them off the streets, there is a further dimension. This concerns essentially the 'attitudes' of the young. Unemployment for the young is redefined as a *transitional* phase in the *life* of the individual. Whereas previously one could apparently pass without effort from adolescent to worker, today the individual seems to need to adapt psychologically to the world of work. There is more at issue here than a distasteful tactical ploy to obscure the real level of unemployment. There is a transformation taking place that seeks to shift the onus on to the individual. The essence of the new vocabulary that accompanies this transformation can be found in the word 'adaptability'. Training should be directed, it is argued, towards making the individual adaptable. This adaptability is not just toward different possible jobs. It is towards a generalized adaptability of the person to the different experiences life may offer him/her. Just as the individual should learn to 'cope' with the demands of a particular job, so too he or she should now learn to cope with unemployment. The rehabilitation of long-term prisoners and mental hospital patients provides a model here for the social and life skills taught to the young unemployed.[76] The contractual self provides the foundations for a new concept of the person, a new image of the economy, and a new image of the relations between them.

Let me return in conclusion to the paradox with which I began. If work drives you mad, and unemployment does so too, why should we not turn the issue round? Instead of allowing work to be subordinated to the wage relation, might we not construct an image of work that makes it subservient to the needs of the person? This argument is not new. There is the old socialist vision and demand for the right to work, which still finds weak echoes today. For Marx in particular the notion of production was inseparably bound up with the realization and fulfilment of the labourer as a subject. There is a much more limited demand that recently achieved a certain currency. This hinged on a criticism of work processes and demanded that we pay attention to the quality of working life. The implication here is that we should seek to transform not the foundations of production but the nature of work processes. And there is a third line of argument through which an attempt is made to give unemployment a *positve* value. We see here those such as Illich reversing the socialist demand and calling for the 'Right to Useful Unemployment'.[77] And we hear also a psychiatrist arguing that people have rights to be unemployed just as they have rights to be employed.[78]. In their widely differing ways all three critiques commit the same error. They fail to recognize the extent to which their demands seek to promote a principle by which the self is to be regulated through engaging in productive activity. Although the definition of productive activity is different in each case, the self is to be regulated in each through a commitment to such activity. The first proposes a fundamental transformation of production relations as a means of enabling the fulfilment of the labourer as a subject. The second seeks to reform production so as to provide greater satisfaction through employment. And the third seeks to transform unemployment into a kind of work, with the notable difference that the wage is absent. We might view this most recent stage as a final dominance of the psychological principle of work over the economic principle. This optimization of the functioning of the person is to be achieved in each case through a form of occupational therapy generalized in its application to the entire population. Mental health as a goal for all has been welded together with work for all as an objective of society. The difference we are witnessing today is that the provision of such work and the rewards that flow from it are promoted as a personal responsiblity rather than the responsibility of the state. Perhaps we might benefit by separating the notion of work from the concern with the self and the optimization of mental health. There may, after all, be a liberation of the individual that does not consist in the release of their subjectivity through productive activity.

6

Law, rights and psychiatry

Nikolas Rose

Since the early 1960s, psychiatry has come under a sustained attack articulated in the language of rights, liberties and justice. It has been argued that many aspects of psychiatry violate or ignore the rights of citizens and that mental-health law is in need of fundamental reform to enshrine and defend these rights. Such strategies have not been motivated merely by a concern for formal legal propriety. They have argued that substantive weaknesses and harms in the current provision of mental-health services can be traced to their lack of concern for the rights of individuals – sane or sick – and that substantive improvements in the lot of the mentally disordered will follow from a recognition of their rights.

Rights strategies have won significant victories. In the USA, court cases in many states from the mid-1960s onwards established a number of procedural and substantive rights within the psychiatric system. In England and Wales, the provisions of the Mental Health (Amendment) Act 1982, consolidated into the Mental Health Act 1983, are widely considered to have followed from the reforming campaign conducted in the language of rights by MIND (the National Association for Mental Health) from the mid-1970s.

In this essay I will argue that there are fundamental limitations to such rights strategies for mental-health reform. They disguise problematic political objectives and depoliticize debate over the organization of psychiatry. They are based on a mistaken analysis and evaluation of both law and psychiatry. Rather than empowering patients, they reorganize relations between different forms of professional expertise – medical, legal and social. The language of rights seeks, and fails, to resolve contemporary disquiet over the ethical basis for legitimate social authority. Despite their apparent differences contemporary psychiatry and rights-mindedness share a rationale for the contractualization of subjectivity.[1]

Violating civil rights

Rights campaigns for mental-health reform from the 1960s on were grounded on a fundamental challenge to the powers allotted to psychiatric expertise in contemporary society.[2] Mental-health systems were criticized from this perspective on at least four levels. First, it was claimed that there were fundamental violations of rights in the ways in which persons who were guilty of no criminal offence could be deprived of their liberty by detention in mental hospitals, and the ways in which decisions were made as to when, or whether, they should be released. Second, the conditions in which such persons were detained, and the administration to them of intrusive physical or pharmacological treatment without their informed consent, paid insufficient attention to their basic rights. Third, the lack of availability of non-custodial forms of care, habilitation or rehabilitation for mentally disordered persons made incarceration a first rather than a last resort, and denied those in need of health and social provision the services to which they were entitled. Fourth, the civil and juridicial disqualifications suffered by those resident in mental institutions, in particular those that denied them the elementary political right to vote and that placed barriers in the way of their access to the courts, also constituted an unjustifiable infringement of civil rights.[3]

Rights campaigners drew upon a variety of sources in developing this critique of the psychiatric system. We need to attend to these sources if we are to be able to assess the social and political rationale of rights strategies. The first, classically formulated in the nineteenth-century liberalism of John Stuart Mill, was a critique of state paternalism.[4] This argued that state power could only be legitimately exercised over members of a civilized community against their will in order to prevent harm to others. An individual could not rightfully be compelled to do something, or to forbear from doing something, because it would be better for him to do so, because it would be wise or right in the opinion of others, or because it would make him happier. Even if motivated by a sincere concern for their welfare, compulsory treatment of mentally ill people who posed no threat of harm to others was, therefore, illegitimate.[5]

Such a critique of compulsion in psychiatry became even more potent when refracted through the prism of anti-psychiatry. For the apparent benevolence of psychiatry could now be construed as illusory, its treatments harmful and its institutional regime degrading, dehumanizing and damaging. Far from curing the sick, psychiatry contributed to the creation of a group of disabled individuals dependent upon professional expertise and unable to function in the world outside the asylum. And, far from being scientific, the knowledge claims of psychiatry were bogus. State and psychiatry colluded in upholding the myth of *parens patriae*. This implied that compulsory interventions were undertaken for the good of the suffering individual. But, in fact, psychiatrists were engaged in a moral enterprise of control, rationalized and legitimized through the appeal to a specialist body of esoteric knowledge. This critique of psychiatric power was joined both by the radical left and the radical right; for each, the activities of psychiatry constituted an illegitimate expansion of the coercive authority of the state.[6]

This criticism of psychiatry linked up with a third theme: opposition to the expansion of the interventionist 'welfare state' articulated by post-war neo-liberals.[7] This drew upon the doctrine of 'the rule of law' as established in the jurisprudence of the nineteenth century, which purported to provide an ethical rationale for the exercise of state power and a means of evaluating any particular instance of it.[8] At its most basic, the doctrine of 'the rule of law' implies that the regulatory activities of state-empowered agencies should be constrained by a system of publicly declared codes, applying equally to all citizens, declared in advance and not operating *ex-post facto*. Such a system, it was argued, allowed citizens to voluntarily adjust their conduct according to such rules or to knowingly, and hence culpably, court a sanction. Individuals were to be deprived of their liberty only if a case could be proved that they had, beyond a reasonable doubt, commited a definite, illegal act. Such a finding should take place in the ordinary courts of the land, or at least, by a judicial determination before a tribunal where judgment was nade by a power independent from the state, utilizing a procedure governed by due process. This entailed such features as the presumption of innocence, the right to know the charge, hear the evidence, make representations on one's own behalf, be represented by an advocate and make appeal against conviction.

To adhere to the doctrine of the rule of law is to reject the basis of much of the social power that psychiatry has accrued over the last century. For central to the rule of law is the principle that a person can only be held responsible for what he or she has done as an individual. Persons cannot suffer penalties because of who they are, on account of what they might do, or because of acts that have been committed by others like them. The doctrine rules out interventions that purport to benefit individuals who may be thought to suffer but who have not committed crimes, and sets limits upon the power of the state to intervene into the lives of its citizens to prevent them committing dangerous or unlawful acts in the future.[9]

Yet a fourth theme was conjoined in this opposition to 'therapeutic justice'. This was a disquiet voiced both by lawyers and welfare reformers about the consequences of the growth of discretionary authority. Discretionary authority was the antithesis and negation of the rule of law. It had flourished within the bureaucratic systems of social planning, state management and welfare in the regulatory systems that developed in the USA and Britain in the twentieth century. Social legislation had vested in administrative and professional agents the power to make significant decisions about individual cases guided only by very broad and vague legal criteria. Hence such decisions were made according to *ad hoc*, *ad hominem*, variable and subjective criteria, whilst justice demands that they be made according to formalized, publicly available rules that apply equally to all persons, and that specify in precise terms the appropriate outcome for given circumstances.

The granting of such discretionary authority was based on a belief in the objectivity and scientificity of specialist knowledge, and a trust in the neutrality, consistency and fairness with which such knowledge would be applied to particular cases, Critics of discretionary power cast doubt upon these beliefs, and pointed also to the absence of proper provisions for hearing evidence and arguments pertinent to such decisions, and for appealing against them. Hence they demanded that rules be laid down to 'legalize' the decisions professional and administrators make, and that forums of adjudication be set up in which such decisions could be made subject to formal adjudication governed by legal reasoning, that is, 'judicialized'.[10]

This aspect of the argument against discretion harked back to the earlier doctrine of the rule of law, but there was a second significant aspect. This hinged upon the notion of entitlement. Discretion, it was argued, makes the recipient of a benefit or a service dependent upon the judgement, and hence the benificence, of someone in authority over them. It thus smacked of charity or gratuity, placing potential recipients of services in the demeaning role of mendicant, opening them to risks of stigmatization, deterring them from access to services. But when discretion is eliminated, and entitlement to resources is specified in public rules, then access is by right, with dignity and without stigma. And where public authorities are inefficient, dilatory or recalcitrant in providing statutorily specified resources to individuals, the courts may be used to enforce their compliance with the law. Hence, it was claimed, rights arguments could be used not merely defensively, to protect individuals from unwelcome state intrusion upon their privacy and integrity, but also as demands, to direct social resources to specific types of provision.[11]

The wrongs of psychiatry

The first and most obvious target of attack was the use of so-called 'police powers'.[12] Police officers with no expertise in diagnosing mental disorder had been allocated powers to compulsorily incarcerate individuals, not on the grounds of the illegality of their conduct but of its undesirability. Had they been suspected criminals, such persons would have been provided with far more safeguards than they were as potential mental patients. The claim that such action was in the interests of the individual detained was seen as merely dissimulating a wish to preserve social order and public tranquillity. Hence proposals were advanced to safeguard the rights of such persons to liberty, to limit police detention to cases of imminent danger to the person or others, or to cases where behaviour would render the person liable to arrest.

But removal to hospital under police powers was only the extreme example of a general problem that rights strategists identified in procedures for determining detention in mental hospitals. In the USA, legal disquiet over the legitimacy of psychiatric detention was first raised within the criminal courts. Here it posed the question of the distinction that did or should exist between confinement in a penitentiary and confinement in a hospital. In the Baxstrom case, in 1966, the Supreme Court declared that the involuntary commitment of a prisoner to a forensic ward of a prison hospital was illegal: a further 992 inmates of the prison hospital in question were transferred to ordinary hospitals or discharged.[13] The judge in another case declared that a criminally insane person who had been detained in hospital for four years – four times the maximum sentence he could have received for the offences in question – should have been treated and cured. He proclaimed that such persons had a right to treatment; mental institutions where treatment was not given were no more than prisons.[14]

From 1970 onwards, the implications of such legal interventions into the mandate of psychiatry were taken up within the system of civil commitment to mental hospitals. Academic lawyers and their students conducted numerous investigations into the grounds and conditions of civil detention of mental patients. In the USA, the bulk of admissions to mental institutions was through the mechanism of judicial commitment. This required a petition asking for an examination of the mental health of the proposed patient, the examination of the person by one or more medical practitioners, and a hearing at which evidence and testimony was heard and where the court had to be satisfied that the criteria for commitment – usually those of danger to self or others – were met.[15] But despite this judicial process, critics argued that commitment proceedings were frequently a sham, merely rubber-stamping medical decisions. These were often based upon the most cursory examination and frequently depended upon inaccurate reports of behaviour and unsubstantiated hearsay; such opinions were not presented and justified in court but merely expressed through the ritual incantation of the legally required formulae. These investigators and lawyers argued that, as a result of such abuses of elementary rights, many persons had been detained in mental institutions for decades on the basis of trivial breaches of social norms, and they sought to use the courts to challenge such rights-violating practices.[16]

Additionally, further rights violations were added to these initial abuses: the absence of formal review of the cases of detained persons or effective mechanisms of appeal against detention; the confinement of detained persons in conditions that would not be tolerated in the prisons; the subjection of such individuals to regimes such as 'token economies' that would be proscribed as cruel and unusual punishment within the criminal justice system; the forced administration of treatment – often hazardous or of unproven efficacy – without the informed consent of the patient.[17]

In the cases brought during the 1970s, the American courts gave support to these challenges to the powers of the psychiatric system in the name of rights.[18] Judges declared that individuals had a right to treatment in the 'least restrictive' settings, implying that commitment to a mental institution should be a last and not a first resort. They declared that individuals had a right to the constitutional safeguards of due process wherever there was the likelihood of involuntary detention, whether on the grounds of crime, juvenile delinquency or mental incompetence. Hence individuals had a right to procedural and substantive protections during the civil-commitment process, and a right to protection against indefinite detention in a mental institution following a finding that they were incompetent to stand trial. The courts did not accept that the jurisdiction of the law ended at the door of the institution, to be replaced by that of psychiatry. They proclaimed the rights of detained persons to certain standards of care, and to receive treatment as opposed to mere detention, and declared that they had a right to refuse treatment given to them other than with their express and informed consent, after consultation with others of their choice.

In order that this panoply of rights should be effective, and not merely paper rights, courts established a number of different enforcement and monitoring mechanisms. These included ombudsmen to receive and report complaints, lay advocates located within the mental institutions themselves, human-rights committees, often with extensive powers to scrutinize institutional practices and compel changes, special review panels and special masters who could examine hospital procedures, make specific recommendations for change and audit their performance.[19]

Since the 1960s, it might thus appear that rights campaigners have scored a remarkable series of victories, making the judicial apparatus the arbiter of the terms and conditions of exercise of psychiatric power, with the aim of overturning long-standing harms and abuses inflicted upon a socially powerless group and furthering the interests of actual or potential mental patients. We shall return presently to consider how far these aims have actually been achieved.

Legality and psychiatry in England and Wales

The procedures for admission to mental hospitals in England and Wales were very different from those that obtained in the USA, as was the public face and express philosophy of the psychiatric system itself. At the start of the 1970s, over 80 per cent of admissions to mental hospitals were informal, that is to say they had been accomplished without certification by a medical practitioner, through the joint consent of the proposed patient (or his or her legal guardian) and the hospital authorities. Such patients – and they accounted for over 90 per cent of those actually resident in such hospitals at any one time – were legally free to withdraw their consent at any time and hence to leave the hospitals.[20]

The preponderance of informal admissions to hospital under the 1959 Mental Health Act represented the victory of a strategy that began to take shape in the 1930s (see chapter 2). The Lunacy Act of 1890 sought to enshrine legal safeguards against the illegitimate detention of sane persons by corrupt doctors. It established a set of formal procedures involving petitions for the admission of persons into lunatic asylums supported by medical certificates, with a judicial functionary – a Justice of the Peace or a Judge in Lunacy – as the arbiter of whether such a petition should succeed. Further, it consolidated and extended the degree of judicial scrutiny over the internal world of the asylum, requiring regular inspections by Lunacy Commissioners, limiting the use of restraint, and allowing patients to send unopened letters to certain persons in authority.[21]

By the 1920s, the focus of social concern had shifted from wrongful detention of the sane to the harm resulting from hindrance to early treatment of the mentally ill. It was argued that public policies for mental health should model themselves upon the preventive social medicine that had been deployed to counter the ills of the infant mortality, the poor physical condition of youth, tuberculosis and sexual diseases. Legal formalities deterred early treatment of mental disorders and hence actually exacerbated the damage done by mental illness by allowing it to worsen untreated. Such legal requirements as certification created fear and stigma attached both to the mentally ill and to the institutions that treated them. Further, these measures were unnecessary, creating a wholly artificial separation between mental and physical disorder when the two were inextricably and essentially linked. Hence the Mental Treatment Act of 1930 reframed provisions within the language of medicine. It permitted voluntary admission in certain circumstances to what were now called mental hospitals, and promoted the development of modes of non-custodial treatment, such as out-patient clinics and after-care, that were not amenable to legal constraints (see chapter 2).

The very title of the Mental Health Act 1959 testifies to its objective of promoting mental health as a personal responsibility and a national resource. When it abolished judicial involvement in civil commitment proceedings completely, and disbanded the Board of Control, only diehard libertarians questioned the vesting of so much power in a medical profession whose authority and judiciousness was hard to doubt.[22] The Act both confirmed and contributed to the move away from compulsion in admission to hospital for psychiatric treatment. The medical profession was the obvious sector to make the decision to use compulsion to admit the decreasing minority who could not, because of the nature of their illness itself, recognize their need for specialized help. The Act framed their powers in the broadest of terms, allowing medical judgment to ascertain if a person was suffering from a mental disorder that warranted detention in a hospital. It enabled such detention if it was considered to be in the interests of the patient's health, as well as where it was necessary for their safety or the protection of other persons.[23] The Act did not consider it necessary to establish any specific mechanisms for appeal against such medical decisions, and did not provide for general judicial review of detention. Whilst it did establish Mental Health Review Tribunals, these were to provide the opportunity for a professional review of only a small number of cases and had only limited powers to discharge.[24]

The 1959 Act was part of the general move towards open-door policies within mental hospitals and the integration of psychiatry within the institutions, practices and rationale of general medicine. By the early 1960s, British mental-health services were priding themselves upon their enlightenment, and regarded themselves as models of 'community psychiatry' to be emulated by 'progressive' mental-health professionals in other countries, especially the USA.[25] A few individuals did, nonetheless, express disquiet about the powers alloted to the medical profession, the social and moral judgments entailed in diagnoses of mental illness, and the consequences of this for the legal rights and civil liberties of patients.[26] But it was not until the early 1970s that lawyers became significantly involved in mental-health reform. At this time MIND was campaigning with NCCL (the National Council for Civil Liberties) for a representation scheme to strengthen patient's rights. But when MIND appointed Larry Gostin, an American lawyer who had worked in the mental-health rights movement in the USA, as their first full-time Legal and Welfare Rights Officer, and later as their Legal Director, rights-mindedness came to define the form and limits of British campaigns for mental health reform for a decade. In a stream of pamphlets, papers, conference speeches, evidence to official committees and in test cases brought in the British and European courts, it was argued that many aspects of the mental-health system denied or violated the rights of the mentally ill, and that legal means should be used to right such wrongs.[27] There were three principal themes: limiting psychiatric power; promoting community mental-health services; and empowering the recipients of psychiatry.[28]

Limiting psychiatric power

The first element in the critique of the powers allotted to medicine under the 1959 Act concerned the respective powers of psychiatric and judicial expertise in commitment decisions. It was argued that the criteria of the Act were unnecessarily broad and ill-specified. In particular, given the absence of a definition of mental illness, the Act effectively allowed detention merely because medical practitioners thought it desirable. In place of such loose, subjective criteria, 'whose interpretation is purely a matter of individual medical opinion', it was proposed that an apparently more objective test – that of dangerousness – be substituted. 'Only grave and genuinely probable future harm to others should form the basis of compulsory admission, and this prediction should be based upon recent overt acts.' This was to allow decision makers to make an independent evaluation of the views expressed by psychiatrists, based upon empirical evidence.[29]

This disquiet concerning the criteria for detention was based upon a more fundamental distrust of the claims of psychiatry to an authority based on scientific expertise. Drawing on both psychiatric and sociological literature on diagnosis, doubt was thrown on both the capaciy of psychiatrists to make reliable diagnoses under ordinary clinical conditions, and on psychiatric competence in the prediction of dangerousness.[30] Hence, it was argued, medical recommendations provided an inadequate safeguard against illegitimate detention. The solution proposed was not the reinstatement of judicial commitment, but the transformation of Mental Health Review Tribunals.[31] When these tribunals were introduced they were not intended to consider the legality of the initial detention, but to provide a forum for a kind of therapeutic case conference. The vast majority of patients did not apply for a hearing; much time often elapsed between application and hearing; the atmosphere was anything but adversarial. Further, certain information could be kept from the patient, and the psychiatric report upon which the decision was usually based might not be available even to the patient's representative. Hence, it was argued, such tribunals did not effectively safeguard patients' rights; they served to legitimate medical powers rather than to ensure that doctors could objectively justify their judgment.

The strategy sought to turn such tribunals into forums within which the legality of psychiatric judgments of the need for detention could be scrutinized, and their objectivity and justification evaluated. Tribunals, it was argued, should provide the opportunity for full and fair hearings, using traditional judicial procedures and standards in accordance with the requirements of natural justice in order to safeguard the natural rights of the person. They should be independent of hospital and medical authorities, operate with clear procedural guidelines, include the right to an appointed representative, a proper statement of the reasons for detention, the right to question relevant witnesses and authorities and for the patient to bring forward expert testimony on his or her behalf.[32]

A second element in the challenge to medical authority concerned events within the world of the institution itself.

Echoing American precedent, non-medical mechanisms within the psychiatric system were proposed, that would monitor clinical practice and prevent rights violations.[33] A Committee on the Rights and Responsibilities of Staff and Patients of Psychiatric Hospitals (CORR) was to be set up, operating at both regional and national level. Any practices that allegedly violated the ethical or legal rights of patients or staff were to be referred to this committee. It would have the power to scrutinize practices and to require their supervision, modification, or cessation. Within the hospitals themselves, an advocacy system was proposed, with advocates to monitor rights violations and provide advice and advocacy wherever they occurred. Amongst the rights of in-patients were to be rights to treatment, habilitation, exercise and a right to an individual treatment plan that specified problems, goals, timetables, responsibilities and criteria for release, and that was continually reviewed.

Further, again based on American precedents, certain legal safeguards were proposed to govern the administration of a very wide range of treatments deemed 'suspect': those given without the knowing and willing consent of the patient, treatments involving noxious or aversive stimuli, surgery, electroconvulsive therapy, hormones, experimental drugs, physical restraint, seclusion, or any other irreversible or unpredictable treatments. In these cases it would be CORR, not the responsible physician, who would determine whether the treatment should be administered – whether, for example, the patient had given valid consent, whether the treatment and treatment plan were acceptable and necessary, and whether treatment was being carried out in the least restrictive conditions necessary to achieve the purposes of admission.[34]

This project for a massive displacement of psychiatrists from their clinical authority was grounded in a profound suspicion of both the curative claims of psychiatric treatment and of the capacity of the profession itself to regulate its activities in the interests of its patients. Neither unquestionably scientific, nor trustworthily humane, the clinical mandate of psychiatry was to be subordinated to a judgment made in terms, on the one hand, of constitutional rights and, on the other, of lay beliefs and values. In short, psychiatry was to be de-professionalized.

Promoting community mental-health services

This fundamental challenge to the professional authority of
psychiatry underpinned the second theme of the 'new legalism'.
This sought to promote the development of non-medical forms
of treatment and to divert as many persons as possible from
entry into the medically controlled psychiatric hospital. Three
elements were involved here. The first was to increase the
powers of social workers in the admissions procedures, bols-
tering their legal role and status to establish their independence
from psychiatry and their capacity effectively to contest medical
judgments concerning admission. It was to take the form of
requiring an evaluation of all prospective patients by social
workers, not to seek signs of mental illness, but to see if there
were alternatives to in-patient care.[35] This would facilitate the
use of non-medical care, for the social worker was only to
authorize commitment to hospital if it fitted the criterion of
'the least restrictive alternative'. The use of the coercive power
of the state was only justified if it was the least invasive of
personal liberty that was necessary to achieve valid public
objectives. Social workers should refuse to authorize admissions where there were 'less restrictive' community settings in
which treatment could be provided – the assumption being that
environments could be ranked along a dimension of invasion
of liberty, with compulsory detention in a psychiatric hospital
about the most invasive of all.

Establishing a right to treatment in the least restrictive
setting, together with the body of statute, administrative regulation and common law, would enshrine a legal entitlement to
certain types and standards of provision, that could then be
used as a basis for action in the courts. It 'would require the
Government to create a full range of community services . . .
[and] require the social worker . . . to refuse to make an
application where the person could be supported at home or
in a non-institutional setting'.[36] Coupled with the obligation
placed on local authorities and health authorities in respect of
after-care, such entitlements were seen as a powerful means
of shifting the focus of mental-health services away from the
psychiatric institution. The courts could be used to make local
authorities direct resources to community services, and allow

the development of effective remedies – judicial, administrative or financial – where entitlements created by statute were ignored. It was the concept of legal entitlements that provided the basis for the claim that the new legalism could do more than fetter the powers of doctors and react to abuses; it could ground a progressive strategy for change in the structure of the psychiatric system itself.

Empowering the recipients of psychiatry

Whilst the strategy sought to shift the balance between medical and social expertise, it was not conceived as merely a rejigging of professional authority. The mentally disordered were not to remain powerless supplicants dependent upon the discretion of authorities. Empowered by entitlements, and utilizing the mechanisms of the law, they could demand and obtain their rights. Hence they would aquire the capacity, and the responsibility, to effect change in their own condition. Thus the third theme of the rights strategy was the removal of the civil and juridicial disablements of the mentally disordered.[37]

Patients in mental hospitals automatically lost many of the rights that should accrue to all citizens merely as a result of their admission. Residents of mental hospitals could not be entered on the electoral register where the hospital was situated and lost their right to vote there. Persons liable to be detained under the Act were denied a driving licence. Patients suffered a loss of welfare benefit, were disqualified from jury service and might have their mail withheld. Perhaps most significant were the impediments that hindered the recourse of mental patients and those acting on their behalf to the courts of justice. A preliminary hearing in the High Court was required for any case brought in respect of performances under the Mental Health Act; there was immunity from prosecution unless there were substantive grounds for the belief that the person acted in bad faith or without due care.[38] These provisions, which dated from the Lunacy Amendment Act of 1899, were designed to protect doctors from vexatious litigants. But, it was argued, they were used by the courts to provide a blanket protection to staff, and prevented the use of the law to safeguard the basic rights of the patient to protection from assault, let alone the provision of adequate standards of care.[39] Restoring the civil and legal competence of patients would not only challenge entrenched paternalistic attitudes to the mentally ill, but would also enable them to exercise legal and political pressure to enforce their rights. Enfranchisement would enable the patient to directly enter the political domain; access to the courts would allow the patient to obtain redress for detention or treatment that infringed legal or human rights.

The wrongs of rights

This appears to be a powerful and coherent strategy for reform of the psychiatic system, using the language of rights and the mechanisms of the law to turn the prolific literary, academic and radical criticisms of psychiatry into a real and sustained challenge to medical power. It aims to constrain the powers of professionals over those subject to them, to redistribute authority away from medicine, and to promote a new way of thinking about and acting towards the mentally disordered. Yet it is surprising that a mental-health reform campaign in Britain should have been conceived in these terms, and have gained the momentum which it did. Psychiatric practice in Britain makes only limited use of compulsory powers, and government and professions have been explicitly committed for over a quarter of a century to minimizing the role of the mental hospital and developing a 'community psychiatric service' (see chapter 2). Further, legal mechanisms and concepts of rights have a very different role in the British political context from that which obtained in the USA, where the legal environment provides encouraging conditions for rights strategies.[40] In the late 1960s, many progressive American lawyers promoted such strategies of welfare reform with limited success, in the belief that legal means provided a way of mobilizing and empowering disadvantaged and oppressed groups, and that radical lawyers had the expertise to spearhead a campaign to bring the power of the government and its bureaucracy to account.[41]

The British environment is considerably less favourable to rights campaigns. No written constitution establishes rights, and thus appeals to rights either have to concern themselves with duties and obligations expressly imposed upon authorities by statute and common law, or appeal beyond the law to domain of moral or social rights that have, as yet, no legal standing.[42] Indeed, theorists of welfare in Britain have used the notion of rights in a rather different way from that understood by lawyers. They have tended to conceive of social rights as claims that, in a particular social and cultural context, are regarded as legitimate obligations by public, politicians and administrators, and as resources used in guiding policy and decisions. Such rights were not primarily conceived as justiciable entitlements attaching to persons and not predominantly safeguarded through the law, but were held in place by established institutional rules and principles, and sustained by a judicious combination of public accountability, professional supervision and appeals procedures.[43]

Further, legal arguments, techniques and functionaries have generally been regarded as inimical to the sensitive and humane operation of welfare services, decreasing flexibility, subordinating the aim of individualized justice to bureaucratic central control, introducing unhelpful adversarialism and, far from empowering clients, rendering them passive and bewildered in the face of criteria and disputes that focus upon esoteric issues in the interpretation of labarynthine legal rules, and seem to have nothing to do with their needs.[44] Such an evaluation underpins much of the opposition to 'legalism' in mental health, most visibly represented in Kathleen Jones' standard history of the mental health services in England.[45]

Nevertheless in the 1970s, partially inspired by the American experience, British welfare reformers increasingly adopted the language of rights, seeking to utilize courts and tribunals in a test-case strategy to establish rights and challenge discretion in the allocation of benefits, and to reform the law in such a way that entitlement to benefit was specified in clear public codes.[46] MIND was in the forefront of these campaigns for law reform, seeking to test the extent of patient's rights in the British courts – with largely negative results – and in the European Court of Human Rights – with rather more success – in order to enforce changes in domestic law.[47]

The principal success of the campaign was considered to be the major reform of mental-health legislation in 1982 and 1983. Whilst many of the proposals discussed above were not adopted in the Act, nonetheless significant shifts did occur.[48] Social workers' involvement in admission procedures was made obligatory, their levels of training were to be raised, and they were required to satisfy themselves that detention in hospital was, in all the circumstances of the case, the most appropriate way of providing the care and medical treatment of which the patient stands in need.[49] Whilst there was some tinkering with the specifications of those subject to the provisions of the Act, the grounds for detention remained substantially the same, and the proposal to substitute a criterion of dangerousness was not accepted. The time delays before application to a Mental Health Review Tribunal were reduced, and automatic reviews were introduced for those who did not apply; the powers of tribunals to discharge were also increased.[50]

Constraints were introduced on the use of certain classes of treatment, requiring the consent of the patient and/or consultation with other parties and second medical opinions, although the proposals to transfer power over such decisions from clinicians to a lay committee were rejected.[51] As far as entitlements were concerned, the success of the strategy was limited, with the Act merely specifying a duty of after-care in respect of patients detained for treatment or entering hospital from the criminal justice system.[52] No provisions were made for any advocacy system or committee on rights but, following the classical pattern of inspectorates favoured by British public law, a Mental Health Act Commission was established to keep the care and treatment of both detained and informal patients in mental hospitals under review.

Whilst clearly increasing the extent to which psychiatric practice was to be governed by procedural rules and subject to formal review, the Act was not formulated in terms of rights, and certainly did not constitute a fundamental challenge to medical power and the clinical authority of psychiatry. Hence, on the one hand, it has been castigated for its failure to effectively enshrine rights and control psychiatric power.[53] On the other hand, it has been condemned for reviving legalism, imposing inflexibility, hampering access to treatment, exacerbating antagonisms between patients and doctors, diverting psychiatrists from the business of medical care, and wasting scarce resources better directed to the improvement of services.[54] What can be learned from these events about contemporary psychiatric society?

Disputing expertise

Since the 1960s, the social authority accorded to professional expertise has come under scrutiny across a range of fields and from a variety of political perspectives. The powers and capacities of 'experts' in social work, applied psychology, medicine and psychiatry have been questioned on a number of grounds. The practical utility of expert knowledge has been doubted. The truth status of its knowledge claims has been disputed. Criticisms have been made of the effects of the powers of expertise upon the social responsibility and personal autonomy of those subject to it. Scepticism has been directed at the assumption that a knowledge of medicine, psychology, psychiatry or whatever necessarily equips the professional with the capacity or the justification for making the social and moral choices entailed in, say, removing a child from its home, discontinuing life-support to a malformed neonate or incarcerating an individual who is behaving in a troubling manner. The attack mounted upon the authority of psychiatry in the name of rights is clearly an element in this more general social disquiet concerning the role of expertise.

Rights strategists argue that the powers accorded to psychiatry in the determination of civil commitment are based upon a mistaken belief in the scientific objectivity of psychiatry.[55] They claim that diagnoses in psychiatry are not 'objective' but 'subjective'. This is because of the nature of mental disorder, the fact that objective correlates of a diagnosis – demonstrable organic lesions, abnormalities of cells or tissues, physiological or biochemical malfunction – are rarely present. Similarly, objective physiological pathways for such conditions have not been established, nor are there clear accounts of the mode of action of psychiatric treatments. This empiricist critique of psychiatry is misguided. The notion that diagnosis of non-psychiatric illness is an objective matter of the demonstration of organic malfunction is clearly ill-founded. Concepts of health and illness vary greatly between cultures.[56] Within and between cultural groups there is considerable variation in the readiness of individuals to construe personal discomfort as illness.[57] All clinical medicine involves the application of socially, historically and culturally variable norms of health and sickness to particular cases.[58] Hence, if psychiatry is to be denied its clinical mandate on the grounds of the culture-bound nature of its conceptions of health and illness, the same would apply *a fortiori* to all clinical medicine.

Further, the process of diagnosis in clinical medicine involves far more than a simple recognition of a set of observable phenomena. The identification of symptoms involves the organization of certain physical characteristics of a patient and features of their history into meaningful patterns. This is made possible through the use of specific forms of reasoning learned through apprenticeship in particular systems of knowledge and practice. The organization of phenomena into symptoms is not prior to and independent of diagnosis; it is part of the diagnostic process. Indeed, investigations of diagnosis in clinical medicine show that it is resistant to rational reconstruction, either at the level of its formal codes or at the level of its types of reasoning.[59]

Clinical medicine is not, however, 'subjective'. Clinical judgment is not a personal matter. Clinicians are initiated into a structured and stabilized mode of perception and interpretation through their lengthy training. The claim for exclusive competence made by the skilled clinician that underpins the status and power of medicine is based upon the fact that diagnosis can only be made in consequence of such an apprenticeship. The inability of clinicians to formulate diagnostic protocols that would be intelligible to non-doctors does not undermine their claims to professional status – it is the very basis of this claim.[60]

The doubt thrown upon the scientificity of psychiatry because of the lack of established organic pathways for illness or treatment is also naive. Many conditions currently diagnosed in non-psychiatric medicine have no known organic correlates. Many diseases now considered to have a biological foundation were characterized long before their mechanisms were worked out. If clinical medicine were to limit its treatments to those where there was a clear knowledge of organic pathways, most available drugs and techniques would have to be rejected. And the same criticism would have to apply to the forms of help most favoured by rights campaigners – counselling, psychotherapy, and so forth – that have seldom attempted to produce scientifically falsifiable theories of aetiology or treatment.

The critique of the objectivity of psychiatry that is deployed in the rights campaigns is supported by evidence as to the low reliability of psychiatric diagnoses – the low levels of agreement between trained clinicians on specific diagnoses of non-organic disorders under ordinary clinical conditions.[61] But these criteria cannot distinguish psychiatric medicine from non-psychiatric medicine, where diagnostic reliability is similarly low.[62] Further, the selection of evidence is tendentious, emphasizing certain studies, explaining away those providing evidence of much better reliability in diagnoses of the major conditions of schizophrenia and manic depression, and seeking to dismiss the improvements in diagnostic concordance that can be achieved through improved definitions, training and interview technique. Indeed the aim is not to support demands for improving the education of medical professionals, for more sophisticated discussion of diagnoses, or for changing the practical conditions that affect diagnosis, such as time, caseloads and staffing. The criticism seeks not to improve psychiatry but to debunk its truth claims, and hence displace it from its privileged clinical position.

This debunking has come to focus upon the capacity of psychiatrists to predict dangerousness. In the USA a judgment as to dangerousness – to self or others – is fundamental to most decisions to detain a person who has committed no crime. In Britain, dangerousness is not given such a central place in legislation; indeed the term itself seldom appears. Nonetheless, beliefs about and prognoses of dangerousness are certainly significant in decisions to detain a person in hospital, and in the judgments of Mental Health Review Tribunals. Civil libertarians have explicitly sought to promote the dangerousness standard as an apparently objective criterion for confinement, to substitute for the subjectivity of psychiatric diagnosis.

Despite the fact that mentally disordered people are, as a group, no more dangerous than the population at large, there is much evidence that psychiatrists massively over-predict the dangerousness of patients, often falsely predicting four harmless persons as dangerous to every one accurate prediction.[63] Yet this should not be used as the basis of a critique of psychiatric expertise. Other methods of prediction have proved similarly fallible, seldom achieving better than two wrong predictions of dangerousness to each correct one.[64] Further, dangerousness is neither a clinical category nor a personality type. Whether or not a particular individual will perform dangerous acts in the future cannot be extrapolated from an analysis of the person concerned or their past history, for it depends on a host of indeterminable interpersonal, social and environmental circumstances. Such judgments will always have to be based on insufficient evidence and will have to be made by fallible individuals subject to conflicting social pressures and personal anxieties.[65]

Rights campaigners argue that alternative modes of judgment are to be preferred to psychiatry, and that they would better protect patient's rights. They seek to shift the locus of judgment to legal or quasi-legal forums – Mental Health Review Tribunals – and to have them made according to the techniques of legal reasoning with the safeguards of due process. Such a strategy justifies itself by appealing to the belief that legal reasoning provides a more just, equitable, objective, neutral and accurate mode of judgment than psychiatric reasoning; hence the latter should be subordinated to the former. Yet a cursory examination of legal argument dispels the claim that it is an unparalleled means of rationally and objectively reasoning from rules to decisions.

First, it is clear that existing tribunal reviews of psychiatric decision-making do not, in fact, manifest the virtues that are claimed for legal judgments.[66] The decisions of such tribunals are often made in ignorance of the law, in the light of mistaken beliefs about the law, or in spite of legal criteria. Tribunal members are influenced more by therapeutic goals than by the application of the legal rules – that is to say they are less concerned with whether the formal criteria for detention have been satisfied than with what would be in the best interests of the patient. In making such decisions, they are necessarily guided by their own beliefs and judgments as to madness, dangerousness and the ethical balancing of containment against liberty. In such difficult and uncertain waters, tribunals do not demote medical expertise but defer to it, no doubt for a variety of reasons. But the consequences of such deference are rather different from those implied by advocates of non-medical knowledge as a defence of patient's rights. Non-medical tribunal members are more likely than doctors to conceive of bizarre behaviour as itself evidence of mental illness, and more likely to associate mental illness with dangerousness; hence it is not surprising that medical members of tribunals are relatively more disposed to discharge than others. The lines of opposition between lay and professional knowledge are more complex than proposed in the philosophy of civil libertarianism.

Evidence concerning the way in which existing tribunals

function has been deployed by rights campaigners to support demands for the increase of legalisation of commitment decisions. We have seen above that replacing the broad and general category of mental illness with the supposedly objective criterion of dangerousness would not significantly reduce the discretionary element in decision-making, although it might aid in the project of disempowering psychiatry by framing criteria in non-medical terms. But discretion in decision-making would not be fundamentally transformed by codifying the rules, increasing the level of legal representation and couching arguments within the rhetoric of the law. Whilst much legal doctrine and legal education presents an image of legal reasoning as a determinate process, studies of legal decision-making over the last half century have stressed the indeterminacy of legal rules, their incompleteness as explanations of decisions in particular cases, and the contradictory ways in which rules can and do justify decisions. In short, they have stressed the subjective nature of legal interpretation.[67]

The opposition between rules and discretion is an internal element within the discourse of the law. Judges or advocates will appeal to either as a tactic in order to urge or justify particular decisions. Indeed, the object of advocacy is less to determine facts than to win cases; advocacy selects its arguments in an attempt to produce one or other of a small number of possible decisions. The suggestion that legal reasoning – unlike psychiatric diagnosis – relies upon 'objective evidence' is thus ill-founded. In law no less than psychiatry, a domain of evidence is constituted in relation to a particular case through an interpretive process. Nor is this domain undisputed, for advocacy of different outcomes will often proceed by seeking to redefine what is pertinent evidence in order to support a particular decision. Hence the disquiet felt by many advocates in cases concerning detention of mentally disordered persons over whether their objective is to construct the facts of the case with the object of securing the release of the individual, irrespective of their condition, or to aim for an outcome which they regard as in their client's best interests.[68]

There are certainly clear differences between psychiatric and legal conceptions of evidence, modes of argument, techniques of judgment and notions of proof, but these differences cannot be evaluated in terms of an opposition between certainty and variability, or objectivity and subjectivity. Both legal and psychiatric instances rest their claim to social authority upon their capacities to make truthful determinations; the appeal to the superior truthfulness of legality does not provide a way of arbitrating between these rival claims for it is a tactic in the competition between them. The move to legalize and judicialize decision-making in matters of psychiatry does not eliminate professional discretion or redress the powers of expertise over those subject to it; it merely shifts discretion and power around the psychiatric system. The consequences of such shifts cannot be evaluated from within an analysis conducted in terms of epistemology.

Liberty vs therapy

The epistemological attack upon psychiatry is frequently conjoined with an ethical attack upon 'therapeutic justice'. This does not depend upon disputing the truth claims of psychiatry, for it argues that even were these well-founded it would not justify paternalism on the part of the state or its mental-health services. As we have seen, the classical doctrines of liberalism are used to support the argument that danger to others should be the only justification for state intervention. The role of the law is not to provide for compulsory intrusions into the privacy of individuals in the name of their best interests, but to defend their freedom, liberty and autonomy. Treatment should be limited to that obtained through contractual relations between freely consenting parties. Rights here have the function of marking out and defending a sphere of private action that is not the business of the state: individuals have 'the right to be different'. A continuity is claimed between the involuntary confinement of the disturbing eccentric, the quarrelsome alchoholic or the socially disruptive derelict and the burning of witches, the pathlogization of homosexuality and the confinement of political deviants in the Gulag Archipelago. Similarly, these arguments oppose the involuntary administration of treatments, not simply because they are hazardous or of unproven efficacy, but on the basis of an individual's right to protection against others invading and entering his or her personality, grounded in a right to privacy, to control over one's own internal thoughts and feeling, and to protection from assaults, no matter how well-meaning their motivation.[69]

Civil libertarianism of this type has been subjected to powerful criticisms. Mental-health reformers have argued forcefully that demands couched in terms of civil liberties are the wrong basis for a political strategy to determine the policies and provisions for mental health or to aid in their development.[70] Such a strategy can constrain and delimit the activities of professionals and react to abuses of their power. At its extreme, it can reduce social intervention into the lives of mentally distressed people to that minimum provided by the sanctions of the criminal law – emptying the mental hospitals and denying the psychiatric enterprise its social mandate. But when it comes to arguing out the types of service to be provided, assessing needs and priorities, determining and resourcing organizational practices, civil libertarianism is impotent.

Psychiatrists have also reacted strongly to this attack upon their clinical function in the name of rights. They have argued that the legalistic fictions of libertarians bear little relation to the actual conditions of psychiatric practice. If acted upon, they would deny patients access to the treatments they need to help them recover, condemning them to lives of suffering outside the hospital if not admitted, or to long-term segregation within it if admitted and not treated. They would also condemn those around the untreated or unconfined ill person – family, friends, doctors, nurses – to misery and possible harm.[71]

Further, psychiatrists argue that, in relation to the refusal of treatment, mental illness is frequently characterized by the loss of precisely that rationality necessary to give informed consent – the capacity to evaluate risks, balance options, select alternatives or assess the motives of others. Patients who refuse medication under the sway of delusional fears, feelings of worthlessness arising from pathological guilt, or a transitory but suicidal depression, are a long way from the legal fiction of a freely choosing, rational subject with rights to personal autonomy.[72]

We should not, however, allow this opposition between civil libertarianism and psychiatry to conceal their common premise. Psychiatry was constituted as a discipline in the same transformation of social and intellectual rationality that gave birth to the concept of the individual free to choose. The very same social, political and intellectual forces that inscribed the slogans of the rights of the individual upon their banners in the late eighteenth and early nineteenth centuries also invented all those disciplinary mechanisms for the systematic management of individuals through actions targeted upon the soul.[73]

Thus the nineteenth century, in Britain, Europe and the USA, was the heyday of the moral, social and economic doctrines of political economy – the market governed by private contracts between isolated individuals motivated by the universal utilitarian calculus of pleasure and pain. This individual was invested by Christianity with a personal soul and relation with God, and constituted in political thought as a free and equal citizen with rights and duties. Yet this was also the individual whose personal characteristics could be systematically manipulated by the techniques of discipline deployed in the new, individualized factories, prisons, workhouses and asylums. Psychiatry was born within these new institutions for the reformation of troublesome persons into moral individuals and responsible subjects. The philosophical doctrines of individual rights and fundamental liberties, and the therapeutic techniques for the reconstitution of malfunctioning subjects arose in the same process of individualization. At the same time as the free individual became the atom of the liberal doctrines of liberty, equality and freedom of choice, the particularities of individuals became the object of social management, of systematic knowledge, of techniques of assessment and technologies of regulation.

The dispute between legalism and psychiatry is possible precisely because they operate with commensurable conceptions of their subjects. They share a conception of the person as consistent in thought and emotion, unified in capacities and beliefs, autonomous in the sense of free from interventions from alien forces or spirits, and having the capacity and responsibility for personal choice. If such individuals exist and are believed to exist in our culture, it is not because of some fundamental and universal attributes of selfhood, but in consequence of specific cultural codes, repertoires of conduct and social supports.[74] Whilst civil libertarians claim the self-evidence of such a subject as the basis in nature for their doctrines of rights, psychiatry utilizes such a conception as the reference point for its ascriptions of insanity. That is to say, it is the inability of persons to conform to or support this conception of a subject that is prima facie grounds for a diagnosis of mental illness. Hence the role of much compulsory civil commitment and treatment in contemporary psychiatry is not to destroy the autonomy of the subject but to construct autonomous subjects – construed as those who can cope without professional support. Much institutional psychiatry seeks to reform those who have lost autonomy, who feel at the mercy of circumstances, of outside forces, of thought insertions or inexplicable mood swings beyond their control. It seeks to re-establish control over uncontrollable aspects of existence, to promote autonomy and encourage the acceptance of responsibility.

Civil libertarianism is, of course, an ethical doctrine that seeks to find a moral basis for the exercise of state power in its appeal to rights. But it is just as consistent to use an ethics of human rights and the freedom of the individual to justify compulsory social intervention into the lives of mentally disordered persons as it is to proscribe it. Contemporary psychiatry accepts the modern conception of the individual and bases its claims for social authority in part upon its capacity to reconstruct and maintain individuals as responsible contractual subjects.

Legalism vs psychiatry?

The interdependencies between law and psychiatry extend beyond their theoretical premises to their reality as instances of social power. There is no fundamental opposition between the legal and the psychiatric sectors, even though their alliance is often uneasy. It is in the courtroom that the antagonism often appears to be most acute. We are all familiar with the ceremonial of the public trial of the monstrous criminal, where a jurisdictional struggle over pathologies of conduct appears to be played out around the popular question 'mad or bad'.[75] But the actual operation of the courts and the prisons has entailed a strategic alliance between the legal/penal and the medico/therapeutic. Penality relies upon psychiatry to provide the rationale and the technology for confinement when the law reaches its limits – in offences without motive, the bizarre, the monstrous and the perverse. For if reason defines the limits of the population subject to legality, legality itself must be insufficient to regulate unreason. Psychiatry depends upon the judicial instance to confer legitimacy on its activities and to provide it with a vital handle on social life. The penal system provides psychiatry with key populations – the criminal, the delinquent – and with sites for its operation, research and expansion. In the mundane operations of the courtroom, in respect of petty offenders, shoplifters and alcoholics, in relation to the penality of women, in the prisons from Grendon to Holloway and in the 'special hospitals', psychiatry and law are welded together in the effectuation of the power to punish (see chapter 8).

Since the early nineteenth century the legal apparatus has played a key role in marking out the territory of psychiatry and establishing the sites where it would find a foothold – not just courtroom, reformatory and prison but also social work and the asylum itself. And the law has defined and legitimated the mandate of doctors over a sector of social pathology, defining the respective powers and relationships between family members, police and professionals in the control of troublesome individuals. Thus statutes passed in the first half of the nineteenth century both imposed a duty on social authorities to establish asylums, created the legal requirement for medical attendance, and established a Commission of legal and medical personnel to scrutinize madhouse conditions. And, in codifying the conditions of commitment to asylums, and requiring judicial involvement in certification, the legislation of the nineteenth century accorded the medical profession legitimate powers over madness in the very same process in which it circumscribed the form and limits of this power.[76]

This enables us to see the 'legalism' of the 1890 Lunacy Act in a new light. The debates leading up to it were critical of medical practitioners and their activities, representing doctors as frequently brutal and often corrupt, colluding with relatives in the incarceration of their eccentric or unwanted kin and subjecting those within their power to cruelty and abuse. But, in directing this concern with 'the liberty of the subject' into a set of codified procedural rules, and in transferring formal responsibility for the decision to detain to a legal functionary, the Act actually contributed to establishing the legitimacy and humanity of medical powers over lunacy. It both freed doctors from the accusation of wrongful confinement and minimized the contentious nature of commitment decisions. Making the criteria for the legitimacy of confinement a formal rather than a substantive matter turned a potentially disputatious process into a matter of following routine and predictable administrative procedures. Such rules function to shield those who operate them from accusations of arbitrariness or self-interest, testifying to a process operated '*sine ira et studio*' – without hatred or passion.[77]

The prominence of the contemporary rights critique of psychiatric powers certainly attests to a new erosion of the legitimacy of medical control of madness, but whatever its programmatic rationale may be, the consequences of rights strategies do not amount to a simple reduction of such power, but rather to its reframing and reorganization. Such moves contribute to the modernization of psychiatry. They free it from those aspects of its social role that cast doubt on its legitimacy and, simultaneously, extend the ambit of psychiatry through the links thus established with other sectors of social power. The limitation upon the use of psychiatric institutions as holding facilities for those whose only 'illness' is that they are a 'danger to society' contributes to the relegitimation of psychiatry, allowing it to re-establish its humanistic and curative vocation, through the transfer of this troublesome and unprepossessing element of the psychiatric population to other institutions – such as the prisons – within which psychiatry can exert power without taking responsibility.[78] Similarly, the use of mental hospitals as repositories for those whose only 'illness' is an inability to cope with the demands of life outside casts doubt upon the therapeutic potential of psychiatry. Here, rights advocacy has contributed to the 'decarceration' of such patients, their transfer to non-medical professionals and voluntary organizations, or their eviction from bureaucratized social care into the private sector or the domestic domain.

The social reality of rights advocacy is thus entirely consistent with psychiatry's self-modernization. It contributes to the relocation of the mental hospital within an expanded psychiatric system, the reduction of the numbers of in-patient beds and the discharge of long-stay patients, the minimization of compulsory detention, the utilization of non-medical institutions for the containment of those parts of the psychiatric population not amenable to therapy, and the promotion of mental health as a social goal and a personal responsibility (see chapter 2). Far from being irreconcilable antagonists, legalism and psychiatry are mutually dependent and reciprocally supporting.

Entitled to psychiatry?

The promoters of rights strategies in Britain explicity sought to distance themselves from a libertarian opposition to psychiatry and claimed that the aims of their campaigns were to improve mental health services not shackle them. In particular, they claimed that the doctrines of rights and entitlements could provide the basis for furthering substantive policies – the promotion of psychiatric services 'in the community' and the transfer of patients from mental institutions to such services. However, considerations both practical and conceptual suggest that such a claim is ill-founded.

The most significant consequences of such a transformation of provision were thought to flow from the right to treatment in the least restrictive settings. As we have already seen, it was argued that this right could be derived from the principle that the use of compulsory powers must always be the least invasive of personal liberty necessary for the achievement of valid public objectives. It was claimed that this established an entitlement that would require the government to provide a full range of non-institutional forms of treatment and that such an entitlement could be used as the basis of actions in the courts to enforce such provision.[79] But experience in the USA shows such a belief to be absurdly optimistic. There, as we have seen, litigation has persuaded the courts that the constitutional rights of the mentally ill are manifold. But the consequences of these developments have been equivocal. Legal mechanisms have proved competent at the limiting of civil commitment, the closure of wards, the discharging of patients from hospital and upholding the 'right' to refuse treatment. In the American context, where some 80 per cent of hospital admissions were under compulsion, the consequences of the rights movement have thus been considerable, especially in conjunction with a more general movement for de-institutionalization supported from a range of different political positions.[80]

But when it comes to the positive changes upon which the strategy bases its claims for progressive mental-health policy reform – improving buildings, staffing levels and proficiency, conditions, standards of conduct or treatment regimes, or providing the 'alternatives to institutionalization' – the results have not been promising. In the USA the courts can use a wide variety of mechanisms to try to implement their decisions and monitor the outcomes. But, nonetheless, the legal apparatus has not, in general, proved to possess effective mechanisms for specifying, enforcing or monitoring changes in substantive provisions. In many cases the proposed community facilities were not planned, funded or implemented.[81] The majority of those patients de-institutionalized were merely transferred to other institutions, frequently in the private sector, often run for considerable profits, usually providing an environment more 'institutional' and less stimulating, congenial, secure and private than the much criticized asylum. Hence the numerous articles arguing that the effects of such a strategy were that mentally ill people were 'dying with their rights on', decarcerated through the self-righteous actions of the civil libertarians only to wander the streets and accumulate in the ghettos, exploited by private landlords, without care or assistance, enjoying formal but not substantive liberty.[82]

In Britain, the strategy of utilizing the courts to enforce substantive changes in patterns of spending by health and social service authorities will be even less successful. Whilst some rulings of the European Commission of Human Rights have led to the allocation of resources to improve hospital conditions, no indigenous body of constitutional rights exists to appeal to.[83] The British courts have occasionally overturned decisions of authorities to refuse benefits, but in general they are reluctant to usurp the power of the legislature and the executive in determining the nature and pattern of state provision.[84] At a time when the volume of the rhetoric of community care at the professional and political level is only matched by the lack of resources directed to it at the organizational level, the belief that the courts can be used to enforce such an allocation is somewhat naive. Indeed we are already seeing a reversal in the ways in which the social problem of psychiatry is being constructed, with exposés of appalling conditions for the de-institutionalized and non-institutionalized mentally disordered people in Britain being deployed by various professional groupings and political factions in order to support their demands. Yesterdays 'scandals' of the institution have already been replaced by todays 'scandals' of the community.[83]

The problems of a strategy based on rights and entitlements are not confined to its inability to deliver the social resources it promises. They flow from fundamental characteristics of the politics of rights. To argue for a right is to make a claim that the satisfaction of a perceived need be regarded as a legitimate obligation by a government or its agencies. But different claims may be formulated in terms of rights, and these may be contradictory or compete for attention or resources. For example, the 'right' of a patient to refuse to enter hospital may impose 'duties' upon their relatives who have to tolerate bizarre behaviour and provide nurturance at the expense of their own 'rights' to liberty. Such relatives might, with some justification, claim a 'right' to measures that would promote the rapid recovery of their loved ones and their return to social and interpersonal competence. Persons in the community can, and do, claim their 'right' to be left in peace from bizarre and frightening behaviour. Governments or taxpayers might claim a 'right' to take measures that would promote the maximum efficiency of a system of psychiatric care and the rapid restoration of disabled individuals to a condition where they can exist without additional social support. Moral philosophers have devoted considerable attention to how rights may be ranked in order of priority, whether rights can conflict and, if so, how such conflicts might be resolved. But such questions are unresolved and the debate over them is, in a literal sense, interminable. Hence the appeal to rights can provide no effective means of substantiating demands that particular claims are valid and should have priority over others. The doctrines of rights and entitlements cannot resolve the issue of whose 'rights' shall prevail; it merely dissimulates the grounds upon which choices are made.[86]

Whether the language of rights is deployed in respect of individuals or in attempts to formulate theories of collective rights, its reality is to disguise the moral and political grounds upon which interests are construed to exist and their satisfaction demanded. For example, by utilizing the courts to establish a right and to demand that it be met, rights strategists are seeking to direct resources to those groups they are currently supporting, at the expense of others who have no such advocates. For a court to order improved conditions or set specified standards according to which an institution ought to be run, or for a court to demand that a state authority establish certain provisions in order not to infringe the constitutional rights of its citizens for treatment in 'least restrictive' settings, effectively constitutes a legal arrogation of discretion in choices as to allocation of funds amongst competing priorities. The appeal to rights substitutes legal rhetoric for political argument, and grounds an attempt to shift powers from the political apparatus to the legal apparatus; paradoxically it depoliticize the debate over priorities in the allocation of resources and over different mechanisms of social regulation.

Nowhere is this more evident than in the way in which rights campaigners have sought to promote community mental-health services. They have argued that the minimization of the use of the psychiatric institution and the promotion of mental health services 'in the community' is a consequence of the recognition of the 'right' to treatment in the least restrictive settings. This appears to be based upon an evident fact: that detention in a psychiatric institution is the most restrictive of all the forms of provision for the mentally distressed. But this depends upon the criteria according to which 'restriction' is evaluated. Many different criteria may be offered as candidates: physical confinement, intellectual confusion, emotional relationships, personal happiness, productive activity and so forth. It is not self-evident that existence in hospital, in physical comfort and institutional stability, is any more 'restrictive' than the 'liberty' to remain in one's own home unable to reach the shops because of anxiety or depression, visited once weekly by the 'community' psychiatric nurse. Nor are local-authority group homes, or private establishments, necessarily 'less restrictive' than hospitals – even when they are 'in the community' in the sense of being in the same administrative area as that where the inmate once lived. This shows the impossibility of resolving questions about the nature of provision – let alone its efficacy or preferability – in terms of an appeal to rights. It also illuminates the politics of rights strategies, for the psychiatric reforms urged in the name of the least restrictive alternative did not flow from the discovery of a right. On the contrary, the 'right' was invented as the ground for the desired outcome. In a disingenuously circular process, the rights are produced by extrapolation from demands which they are then used to justify. The language of rights disguises a social judgment and a political strategy – to curb the professional powers of psychiatry and hence reduce the role of the institutions controlled by the psychiatric profession. To forward such a strategy by appealing to a right appears to remove the necessity for the basis and implications of this judgment to be argued out and evaluated. The political implications of this strategy should be opened up for scrutiny, not masked in the self-righteous discourse of rights.

Rights strategists in Britain advocate a reduction of the powers of medicine, and treat as self-evident the virtues of increasing the discretionary powers of the professions of the social, and the apparatus they control – 'the community'. Yet at the very time when a welcome is being extended to the increased role and powers of social workers in the field of mental health, the knowledge claims and professional motives of the welfare apparatus are being scrutinized and challenged in child-care policy and the juvenile courts. Whilst one group of critical legalists castigate social work as a means for scrutinizing and enforcing social norms, the new legalists of mental health seek to allocate it new powers in mental-health services. Rights-based strategies do not transform the relations of dominance between professionals and those subject to them, but redistribute status, competence and resources amongst the professionals of unhappiness.[87]

Rights, psychiatry and the contractual self

There are fundamental limitations in the rights strategy for mental-health reform. This is not to say that the law has no place in political campaigns. The mechanisms and forums of the law may allow symbolically significant 'guerrilla' assaults on particular practices and institutions. There may be tactical reasons for using legal means to challenge particular instances of power. Changes in the law may be one element in a programme of effective social reform. But there are basic weaknesses in a strategy that seeks to translate moral and political objectives into the particular technical form of rights and entitlements. Legality is merely one mode of regulation and body of professional expertise amongst others, neither conceptually more rigorous, nor necessarily more effective in bringing power to account.

The example of rights strategies for mental-health reform lends support to a long-standing socialist suspicion. Socialists have long argued that notions of rights are welded to liberal moral humanism and an aspect of the ideology of bourgeois individualism. They have claimed that demands for rights accept the illusions that liberty and equality can be obtained in the sphere of distribution whilst ignoring fundamental inequalities and coerciveness at the level of production. They have drawn attention to the incompatability of rights arguments with socialist beliefs in the need for collective and social struggles for liberation. They have argued that notions of rights, liberties and justice are incapable of conceptualizing the objectives of struggles to transform the conditions of production and appropriation of the surplus, to democratize enterprises and social institutions, or to challenge structural features of power as opposed to individual abuses. And they have warned that struggles for rights might actually impede such a strategy, through supporting the mistaken belief that a right recognized in law is a power effective in reality – the substitution of symbolic for genuine victories.[88]

Recently, a certain ambivalence has entered this left opposition to rights. The example of mental-health reform suggests that here, at least, there is some virtue in orthodoxy. There might be an argument for the tactical use of the language of rights because of its consonance with the common sense of Western social and political thought. But such language provides no means of formulating objectives for substantive reforms or for implementing such reforms. It is not effective in the calculation of priorities or the resolution of conflicts, for conceptualizing or defending freedoms, for characterizing or evaluating decision-making processes, for regulating or improving them, or for analysing or transforming the powers of expertise over those subject to it. It sidesteps the ethical issues, by smuggling in an unanalysed morality concerning the value and attributes of humans and the rules of just conduct. It evades the political issues by its inability to confront the question of the distribution of scarce resources and by disguising the politics of its own utilization of legal mechanisms for the exercise of political power. The problems of psychiatry cannot be analysed, the interests of the mentally disordered furthered, or a politics of mental-health reform grounded from within the language of rights.

Rights discourse gains its contemporary potency because it promises to resolve a number of problems that trouble modern social thought. Arguments in terms of rights propose to answer political questions about the power and obligations of the state, moral questions about what is proper human conduct and technological questions about how all these matters might be best socially regulated and scrutinized. Rights-minded critics find psychiatry guilty on all three counts. But there is, paradoxically, a startling level of congruity between the rationale of rights and that of our contemporary psychiatric system.

Rights suggest a way of resolving moral uncertainties about the way we should behave. The issues around which rights arguments have been deployed – such as those concerning doctors terminating the life of damaged infants and children, children removed from their homes by social workers, or the incarceration of those whose thought and conduct are bizarre – act as dramatic forums within which deep moral concerns are symbolized and played out. In a society without shared beliefs, and with no authoritative instance to resolve questions of moral conduct, such questions have been sidestepped for some fifty years by allocating the responsibilities for them to scientific expertise – seeking to resolve moral dilemmas through an appeal to the true knowledge and wise judgment of professionals. We can speculate as to why expertise is now under attack. The discourse of rights, with the proprietorial subject as its atom – autonomous, private, entering into relations with those around it by means of a free contract in which each party has its entitlements and its responsibilities – does indeed appear a minimal line of defence for troubled times. But, despite the self-defeating attempts of theorists of collective rights, concepts of rights are inimical to the language of collective solidarities. It is a sign of our times that one has to remind oneself that it is possible to think of an ethics without rights, perhaps framed in a language of duties and obligations, of social support given not because it is a right, but because it would be virtuous to give it, or politically correct to give it, or because it would make the giver a better person. It is worth remembering that other grounds for morality exist than those in which humans are to be valued only in so far as they get what is due to them.[89]

We have seen that there are remarkable similarities between the individual presupposed by the discourse of rights and the individual whose maintenance is the objective of contemporary psychiatry. At the risk of oversimplification, we could say that they each work in terms of a contractual notion of the self. The objective of producing and maintaining autonomous selves able to cope without formal social support may seem unquestionably good, especially when bolstered by the appeal to a mythical community of private individuals within which such selves would exist – outside the responsibilities of both government and psychiatry. But we might remind ourselves of two alternatives. The ideals of community promoted both by the moral treatment of the last century and by the contemporary therapeutic-community movement certainly led to the development of profoundly moralizing institutions, but they also make thinkable a mode of support and care for distressed people that locates them within a matrix of emotional and practical affiliations, and that sees autonomy as a problem and not a solution. In a somewhat similar manner, the communitarian, mutual-aid approach of Geel in Belgium, maintains the mentally distressed in a system of family placements, linked together by structured collective support mechanisms.[90] My intention is to recommend neither, merely to point out that each is difficult to conceptualize within the horizon of the contractualization and autonomization of both rights discourse and contemporary psychiatry.

The popularity of rights arguments attests to a way of seeking to resolve the political issues of the obligations of, and limitations upon, the state. In this recontractualization of the relations between state and citizens, an attempt is made to demarcate a sphere of social and personal relations that are not the legitimate concern of social authorities. No longer is the state construed as having an overriding duty to use its powers to protect a set of moral values, or to advance the happiness or well-being of its citizens. Rights seek to establish and police a border between a public domain that is the concern of the state and a personal domain that is the space of private choice and contractual relations. The role of the state is to regulate the public sphere; it may cross this boundary only when it is obliged to do so, that is to say in respect of a contractual obligation it owes to a citizen. Within the domain of the personal, life is to be regulated by private choice and contractual mechanisms. Not, of course, that this means spontaneity and liberation; in the sphere of privacy, individuals seek to adjust the reality of their personal lives to the images offered up to them of happy families, personal fulfillment, self-realization, sexual pleasure, and 'the quality of life' (see chapter 2).

Again, one is struck by the similarities between the objectives of rights arguments and the mechanics of contemporary psychiatry. One can point, on the one hand, to the proliferation of the psychotherapeutic technologies of marriage guidance, child rearing, sexual difficulties and the problems of everyday life and, on the other, to the ever-increasing demand for pharmacological products to assuage personal unhappiness. The contemporary psychiatric system operates predominantly through free choices made in the personal domain, in which mental health is both a private objective and a personal responsibility; the promotion of the self is conducted through the voluntary enlistment of help from skilled technicians. Opposition to the 'coercive' aspects of psychiatry has been central to its modernization, together with promotion of voluntary responsibility for one's own mental health; no wonder this distinction between the public and the private cannot provide the means for an analysis of the political functioning of the contemporary psychiatric system. The politics of rights maintains as a social objective 'mental health for all', merely seeking to free it still further from its coercive connotations and urge it on us as a private value. But perhaps, instead, we might try to conceive of a politics which sought to disengage the issue of personal fulfilment from that of mental health.

7

The category of psychopathy: its professional and social context in Britain

Shulamit Ramon

This essay examines psychopathy as a psychiatric classification in Britain during this century, especially since the Second World War. It looks at the meanings attached to the category and the perceptions of those thought to be psychopaths. This category is particularly important in that it reflects significant interactions between social context and professional knowledge. It will be argued that the category of the psychopath was rediscovered in professional circles during the war, and that its social adoption solved a number of contradictory features that came to the fore during the war and its aftermath. The essay traces the processes through which psychopathy came to be professionally defined and the interventions made in relation to this category. It investigates the concurrent approaches adopted by politicians, and the legal framework they have approved.

In this investigation, a number of questions are posed. First, what is meant by psychopathy in terms of description, aetiology and prevalence? Second, how did psychopathy come to be interpreted as a psychiatric disturbance? Third, what were the relationships between developments in psychiatry and parallel developments in society; in particular, what was the impact of changes in psychiatric policy in general upon the specific attention given to psychopathy? Fourth, how was the category of psychopathy utilized within the legal system, both in the Mental

Health Act of 1959 and in the new Mental Health Act of 1983? The essay considers these issues over the following periods: the nineteenth century; 1900–45; 1954–9; post–1959.

Professional descriptions and definitions of psychopathy

Descriptions of psychopathy concern the behaviours that are assumed to be the manifestations of this illness, whereas definitions of it concern the essence of the classification and the ways in which it is to be differentiated from all other psychiatric categories. In the psychiatric literature, psychopathy was first 'discovered' as a category of mental disorder by Pritchard in 1835. Its main indicators were described as irresponsible behaviour that occurred without the presence of any established form of mental illness 'the moral and active principles of the mind are strongly perverted or depraved; the power of self government is lost or greatly impaired and the individual is found to be incapable not of talking or reasoning upon any subject proposed to him, but of conducting himself with decency and propriety in the business of life.'[1]

Psychiatric textbooks between 1900 and 1940 mention the category, but accord it no more than a few paragraphs. It is only after the Second World War that a chapter on psychopathy appears for the first time in a major textbook, namely Henderson and Gillespie's *Textbook of Psychiatry*, despite the fact that Henderson had been working on the subject for some time and had published a book on psychopathic states in 1939.[2] Nonetheless, in 1954 the first edition of *Clinical Psychiatry*, which was to become a major British textbook in the fifties and sixties, grouped psychopathy with neurotic states and did not suggest that it was potentially a major and distinctive category of mental disorder.[3]

The *description* of psychopathy has remained much the same from 1835 to the present day with only minor variations. In 1909 Kraeplin spoke about the excitable, unstable, impulsive, eccentric, anti-social features of the behaviour named psychopathy. In 1930 Partridge wrote about the explosive, excitable, aggressive, sexually perverted psychopath, as well as of the insecure, depressive and weak-willed psychopath. Since 1939 it has become fashionable to follow Henderson's classification of psychopaths into three types: the aggressive; the

inadequate; and the creative. And although the list of characteristics provided by Cleckley is considerably longer, in essence
it remains the same.[4]

Equally, the *definition* of psychopathy has changed little
from 1835. However available definitions have been recognized
as unsatisfactory; so much so that, as late as 1944, Curran and
Mallinson entitled their chapter on psychopathy 'I can't define
an elephant but I know one when I see one'.[5] The only
innovation up until the 1970s was Cleckley's suggestion that we
should view psychopathy as a semantic psychosis.[6] However, in
his wish to 'unmask the psychopath', Cleckley appears to have
overlooked the fact that the behviour of psychopaths does not
demonstrate any known psychotic symptom. Indeed others,
especially psychoanalysts, classified psychopathy amongst the
neuroses, as a character disorder – a severe neurosis with an
innate background.[7] This wavering between a large number of
psychiatric classifications attests to the difficulties psychiatry
has had in making sense of psychopathy.

A number of causal explanations have been proposed for
psychopathy. These can be divided into two main areas. First,
there are those that propose an organic basis for the condition,
such as malfunction of certain brain mechanisms or a lowered
state of cortical excitability.[8] Second, there are those that
suggest a psychological basis, such as inability to form relationships, based on emotional deprivation during critical periods
in childhood, an inability to develop conditioned fear
responses, or to make connections between past events and
the consequences of present behaviour.[9]

Psychiatry has had difficulties in adjudicating between these
competing explanations. There is only one longitudinal study
that follows people who became classified as having psychopathic features from childhood to adulthood.[10] This demonstrated that these individuals had suffered several types of
deprivation in childhood, including the absence of a father
figure, erratic behaviour by their mothers and poverty. Within
psychiatry it is acknowledged that, in the current state of our
knowledge, none of these explanations can be regarded as
more .than tentative hypotheses.[11] Thus West wrote, in 1968:
'in the absence of any generally accepted theory as to cause,
or any agreed criteria of definition, psychopathy must remain
an imprecise, descriptive label, dependent upon the habits of
clinicians and administrators.'[12] However, for those of us who

are not that happy with a total dependence on the habits of clinicians or administrators, the uncertain basis for the identification of this category must remain a serious cause for concern.

Beyond this self-declared problem of definition and causal explanation, the question of prevalence is equally problematic. The current statistics published by the Department of Health and Social Security combine personality disorder and behavioural disorder, making it impossible to tell how many individuals were diagnosed as belonging to one or the other group of disorders. In 1979, there were 15,241 such people in our psychiatric wards. Of these 6,743 were male and 8,498 were female. There was a downward trend in these figures in comparison with 1976, when 18,564 people were so classified: One can only speculate whether the reduction in numbers represents transfer to another setting, such as prison, or whether it implies that the diagnostic category is now used less by psychiatrists. It is also noticeable that there has been a change in the sex ratio since 1970. Up to that time, men received this diagnosis more frequently than women, but the position has now been reversed.[13]

Certain other significant points concerning the prevalence of psychopathy emerge from the literature. It is estimated that 20 per cent of the prison population could be placed within this diagnostic category. Further, more than half the residents of special hospitals are classified as suffering from psychopathy or personality disorder.[14] The professional literature characterizes the psychopath as likely to be working class, aged below 35 and male. But this literature has given little attention to the issue of class differences, and has explained the age distribution in terms of the effects of reaching maturity. The issue of gender has, however, received some attention. Guze has argued that men and women exhibit similar behaviours, but that in women this is diagnosed as hysterical personality, whilst in men it leads to a diagnosis of psychopathy.[15] Guze claims that these differences in ascription of diagnostic labels arise from cultural biases. The changes in sex ratios might appear to confirm his hypothesis, suggesting that as women achieve more equal status with men, so more of them are ascribed the label of psychopathy.

One aspect of the social distribution of psychopathy has yet to be charted. There is, to date, no information on the ethnic distribution of this diagnoses that would allow a judgment as to whether ethnic minorities are more likely to be diagnosed as psychopaths than white people manifesting similar behaviour.

Before 1945

Social reactions to the psychopath in the nineteenth century

Socially undesirable behaviour that seems, at least to the observer, to be largely self-defeating was, of course, acknowledged by the human race long before 1835. It is as old as collective existence itself. At times people behaving in this way were seen as intentionally bad, as 'weak' people who gave in easily to temptation. The turn in the nineteenth century, towards interpreting such behaviour in psychiatric terms, signifies the shift towards the exclusion of certain types of asocial behaviour from social life. Such behaviour was first interpreted from a clinical-somatic viewpoint, and later a clinical-psychological perspective was added. Socially undesirable behaviours that seemed to lack a profit motive of any type were more likely to be seen as indicative of psychiatric disturbance than as criminal activity.

The overall move towards an encompassing clinical-somatic approach in psychiatry during the nineteenth century has been amply documented.[16] Despite the lack of evidence for success of the interventions inspired by this approach, its social acceptance was reflected in the ever-growing readiness in the last century to establish large psychiatric institutions, to employ more psychiatrists and nurses, and in the upgrading of the social status of psychiatrists. The development of this clinical approach within medicine has been characterized by a separation of symptoms from their social context, and from the totality of the person.[17] In particular, when deployed within psychiatry, such a process of distancing and dissection enables socially unintelligible behaviour, which becomes socially undesirable partly because of its unintelligibility, to be given a narrow meaning that focuses only upon symptoms. This perspective, with its halo of 'scientificity', fitted nicely into the ethos of social rationality that prevailed in the second half of the nineteenth century.[18]

Developments in social and professional orientations:
1900–45

The major change in the social position of psychopathy occurred during and soon after the Second World War. The following section outlines this change and considers how it came about.

The development of psychological approaches to mental distress in the twentieth century has added to the number of possible explanations at the level of individual behaviour, and to the range of methods of intervention. However, psychologists of different schools have, by and large, adopted the clinical model of individual pathology and the ensuing framework of professional relationships. Thus the new psychological interpretations have remained within the realm of the clinical approach, and doubts concerning this framework have hardly ever been expressed.

Although the experience of the First World War led to a rethink concerning the issue of neurosis, it had no impact on professional or public attitudes to psychopathy. It would seem that the major turning point was the experience of the Second World War. In contrast to the first war, the death penalty for desertion was removed. Further, no public outcry followed the discharge of many civilian psychiatric in-patients for the duration of the war, which resulted from the fact that hospital buildings were required to house wounded soldiers.

It was during the Second World War that the first move was made to initiate a therapeutic-community environment for soldiers, including those who were thought to show psychopathic features.[19] This move was made concurrently by two groups of army psychiatrists – Lewis and Jones at Mill Hill, and Foulkes, Rickman and Bion at Northfield – each adopting a slightly different version. Instead of being put in a military prison, or just being dishonourably discharged, these soldiers were perceived as suffering from a psychiatric disturbance, as in need of therapeutic intervention and as potentially having the capacity to recover and go back to the front. This newly differentiated approach to psychiatrically disturbed soldiers, including those labelled as psychopaths, was still based upon the need for segregation, but also upon the belief in the possibility of resocialization. That is to say, it was believed that such disturbed individuals could be turned into conforming and productive soldiers and citizens.

The emphasis upon productivity as a key element in social cohesion was reinforced during the war on two accounts (see the discussion in chapter five of this volume). First, it was considered to be an expression of the individual's solidarity with the nation at a time of crisis. Second, capitalism had found by that time that group cohesion encouraged factory workers to produce more, and such a knowledge of social psychology was put to use by the army psychiatrists and psychologists.[20]

The Second World War highlighted this issue of cohesion, both calling for, and offering, a higher degree of cohesion than the 'Great War'. This was not only because Britain itself was under direct attack. It was also because the social changes that had been initiated by the First World War were consolidated in the Second, leading to a greater participation of representatives of the middle and working classes in policy-making. This produced a cohesion that was, in turn, called upon during the nation's period of social crisis. In this climate a more positive reception to psychological explanations of socially undesirable behaviour was possible, as was their utilization in practices that sought to promote social cohesion.

Such a readiness to accept a psychological basis for undesirable behaviour might be related to a need to provide an explanation for the high levels of aggression and cruelty that were exhibited by so-called normal people, not only by the enemy but also by our own side. Indeed, atrocities carried out by our own forces required a more convincing and complex explanation than those committed by the enemy. For while the humanity of the other side could be doubted, that of our side could not be allowed to be blemished. By focusing on the individual, psychological explanations of such behaviour shift its source away from social factors. Moreover psychoanalysis, which was the psychological approach that came to the fore in the thirties and forties, located the aetiological basis of behavioural disturbances in the unconscious of the individual as formed in his/her childhood. It could thus be construed, in commonsense terms, as shifting guilt for such behaviour as far as possible from the arena of collective responsibility. It is significant in this context that psychodynamic explanations of national character also emerged during the war and its aftermath.[21] Such explanations attempt to use psychoanalysis to understand the assumed characteristics of the collective, usually via a detailed interpretation of the life of a well-known figure such as Hitler, Luther or Gorky.

However, the psychoanalytic message on its own was not optimistic in terms of potential recovery and early resocialization. In fact, the orthodox psychoanalytic perspective on human aggression, that was formed largely in the wake of the First World War, is gloomy. It emphasizes the innate nature of aggression, and sees such aggression as a necessary defence against death wishes and fears of death.[22] In these circumstances, a psychoanalytic explanation alone could not have appeared useful to those wishing to restore the functioning of the collective. The therapeutic-community approach offered an attractive solution to this problem. It combined a watered-down psychoanalytic approach with the lessons industrial psychology had alredy begun to learn about the psychology of organizations, and added the development of group psychotherapy. By creating a new social environment – rather than by relying on the therapist–patient relationship – the therapeutic community acquired the potential to be a powerful tool of resocialization.

In addition to the development of therapeutic communities, psychiatric expertise was beginning to be used in the army on a wider scale than ever before, especially in the screening and assessment of abilities and personalities of recruits and of those seeking promotion. Although not on the American scale, the British Army became one big psychological laboratory (on this issue see also chapters two and five). There were developments on the civilian front as well. A free general medical service was provided for the first time, and it included a psychiatric service. Further, the mass evacuations of children, and sometimes of parents, led to a greater degree of intervention into childhood by social workers and psychologists, coupled with an increase in conceptual interest in childhood.[23]

In these ways, the period of the war led to a considerable expansion of the psy complex, and to the psychologization of several types of socially desirable and undesirable behaviours. Whilst motherhood and childhood were among the socially desirable events that were now seen in psychological terms, psychopathy was among the undesirable phenomena construed in this way.

The readiness of lay people within parliament to view psychopathy as a category of mental illness may partly be accounted for in terms of the social and cultural changes of the wartime period.[24] But this on its own does not explain why it was regarded as preferable to specify psychopathy as a distinct and separate category within the legislation, rather than to include it within the broader category of mental disorder. Further, while the latter was to remain undefined in the Mental Health Act of 1959, psychopathy was accorded its own definition. The reasons for this will be investigated below.

1945 to the 1959 Mental Health Act

Society and psychiatry

The social decision to view psychopathy not only as a psychiatric disorder but also as a special legal category must be understood in the context of the changing relationships between psychiatry and society in the period following the end of the war. If psychopathy was rediscovered during the war as a way of accounting for maladjustment and aggression, after the war it had the function of rendering intelligible residual asocial behaviour. The necessity for this arose as a consequence of the final disappearance of the poor-law system of social welfare.[25] With the development of the welfare state, and the changes in beliefs concerning the causes of poverty that it exemplified, the systems of classification of recipients of benefit that were associated with the poor laws became obsolete. In the forties and fifties it was confidently believed that poverty would soon be eradicated, and a new sterotype of the poor was developed. The poor were no longer viewed as irresponsible rascals; they were not the authors of their own misfortunes. On the contrary, they were victims of circumstances. Whilst, however, in the majority of cases, it was possible to accept that the poor were not to be blamed for their condition, there were those who appeared not to fit this analysis. Those who did not easily fall within the stereotype of passive victim had to be categorized in a different way.

This was where the category of psychopathy could be used. The behaviours that did not fit the new frameworks, the odd ones out, were now placed within another framework – that of psychopathic non-criminal behaviour. The Mental Deficiency Act of 1913 had included a category of moral defectives that appears similar to that of psychopathy, and this category did not disappear from the law until the 1913 Act was repealed in 1959. But, in that it associated persistent anti-social behaviour with a notion of mental defect, it did not incorporate the new social recognition that there were people who were not defective but who repeatedly behaved in socially undesirable ways. It was these people who were now legally specified and socially administered as psychopaths.

The fifties saw a further change of great significance for the category of psychopathy. This was the period in which the rate of admissions to mental hospitals reached a peak as did the total number of in-patients. This was also the period when hospital superintendents embarked upon a policy of 'open doors'. This was for two main reasons. First, it was a response to overcrowding. Second, it arose from the continuation of the softened view concerning the potential violence of the mentally ill that had emerged during the war.

The open-door policy implied both unlocked wards and a higher rate of discharge than ever before.[26] 'Unlocking the doors' was an attempt to change the image of the hospital from that of an institution primarily concerned with control to one primarily concerned with caring. Discharge implies, on the one hand, a greater belief in the potential for responsibility that can be borne by the ex-patient. On the other hand, it also implies a shifting of the burden of care and control to those who live with ex-patients, and/or provide the services outside the hospital. A that time very few hospitals took care to plan the discharge of their patients properly, or to ensure that the necessary support would be provided outside their gates. It is important to remember that the 'open-door' policy was not based on new techniques of psychiatric intervention. The most recent innovations were those already introduced in the for-ties – namely insulin therapy and electro-convulsive therapy and, for a tiny minority, the therapeutic community. The psychotropic drugs followed the open-door policy, although history has been rewritten in the myth created later by psy-chiatrists, which attempts to make it appear as if these drugs were introduced first and made the open-door policy possible.[27]

Indeed, the growing number of incoming patients could not have lent itself easily to optimistic portrayals of success.

Although the decision to open the doors was taken individually by each hospital and its medical director, the change was generalized throughout Britain in the relatively short period of ten years from 1945–54.[28] We are dealing here not with the choices of individual hospital superintendents, but with a generalized change in approach; this conclusion is supported by the fact that such a change occurred as much in the USA as in Britain. In addition to the wartime experience, several beliefs fed into this assumption that mentally distressed people could live outside the hospital. It was based on the belief that symptomatology and social undesirability could be reduced with existing means of intervention. It also arose from an acceptance of the incurability of most of the mental disorders. And it assumed the existence of a fairly tolerant general public outside the hospital.

The results of the open-door policy appeared to vindicate these beliefs. There was no public outcry and there were even pockets of public readiness to accomodate this marginal group. There was no evidence of an increase in dangerous behaviour such as homicide or suicide on the part of those who were discharged. There was consistent evidence of incurability, if this is judged by the massive increase in the rate of readmissions. And, while the behaviour of the majority of discharged patients did not become socially desirable, it was, on the whole, within the range of the socially acceptable.

There was one group that posed particularly acute problems in this newly forged framework: those who were of normal intelligence yet who manifested recurring agressive behaviour or a high level of behaviour that was socially self-defeating. Although their psychiatric state was assumed to be under control, their level of social acceptability did not improve. Hence this group was considered to require a special categorization and a special treatment. At first sight it might appear that those who came to be defined as psychopaths could have been either psychiatrized or criminalized. Three factors militated against criminalization. First, the growing acceptance of psychological reasoning in accounting for a whole host of criminal activities made it more likely that what would be called for in the case of the psychopath was psychological treatment rather than mere punishment. Second, many of those who were thought to be psychopaths had not carried out any recognized criminal activity; in order for them to be dealt with within the criminal justice system, new categories of criminal offence would have had to be created, such as persistent changes of address or remaining unemployed while employment possibilities were available. Third, there had been a sharp increase in the number of those in prison in the immediate post-war period and, hence, there was no wish to add further categories of potential prisoners to those that already existed.

The options of psychiatrization vs criminalization were never satisfactorily sorted out. The fact that our special hospitals contain, proportionally, more people labelled as psychopaths or classified as having personality disorders than any other psychiatric category, indicates the possibility of resolving the issue between psychiatry and crime by opting simultaneously for both.[29]

With the growing acceptance of a psychologization of the criminal, many more prisoners were identified as having psychiatric symptoms and difficulties. It was argued convincingly that this group of prisoners was getting the worst of two worlds, namely the prison and the psychiatric system. It was, therefore, understandable that there should be a move to shift the burden of at least one such group to any other authority who might be made to accept it – that is, to shift the load from the prison to the psychiatric system. But were the psychiatric services willing to accept the burden of the psychopaths? The short answer is no. Ordinary psychiatric hospitals, which then comprised the bulk of the psychiatric services, were far from keen to take on the responsibility for this special group. With hospitals increasingly moving towards an open-door policy, they had no wish to have such troublesome and trouble-causing persons as their patients.

The suggestion that psychopathy should be included in the 1959 Mental Health Act was not made to the Royal Commission and the government by the majority of professionals in psychiatry. Whilst this proposal was very willingly adopted by the Home Office, no doubt for the reasons discussed above, it came not from the main stream of psychiatry, but from a small minority of psychiatrists – those involved in the therapeutic communities.

Professional reactions to the proposals for change:
1957–9

Not surprisingly, the issue of whether the psychopaths should be included in the 1959 Mental Health Act, and hence become part of the brief of psychiatrists, nurses and social workers, became one of the most frequently debated aspects of the proposed changes in legislation. The literature, in particular the short contributions from practitioners to journals like the *British Medical Journal* and *The Lancet*, indicates much ambivalence, and a clear reluctance to become involved with this group.[30] The ambivalence was attached to concerns over the lack of a clear definition of psychopathy, and to the lack of suitable methods of intervention. It appeared that the existing definitions were unsatisfactory, in that they did not cover the range of symptoms that came under the heading of psychopathy, and did not offer clear guidelines as to when this classification should be ascribed. However, these doubts as to definitions and guidelines for classification were technical; they did not shake the belief of psychiatrists that they were indeed justified in calling something 'psychopathy' and in perceiving somebody as a 'psychopathic personality'. With regard to methods of treatment – the other recurring theme – it was claimed that those designated as psychopaths were not responding to any of the variety of interventions on offer. These included electro-shock, psycho-surgery, the beginnings of the use of psychotropic drugs, and psychotherapy.[31] Again, however, this did not produce any fundamental questioning of the relevance and efficacy of these methods of treatment.

The lack of response by patients was attributed to an apparent lack of motivation to change, and a lack of feelings of discomfort, shame or guilt. Psychopaths were thus less likely to evoke sympathy than most other patients, for they did not themselves appear to be suffering. However, their condition did cause suffering to others. There was agreement that these patients created havoc in the hospital, but this fact was not given as a reason for the ambivalence expressed towards them. One might suspect that one element in this was that to have cited such a reason would have been to go against the ethical commitment to treat any patient in need, whether that need is personal or is defined by society on the person's behalf.

In the absence of guidelines for diagnosis, definitions of the condition and effective methods of intervention, we might well ask what psychiatry can offer in relation to this problem, either to its practitioners or the so-called psychopath. The answer, I would suggest, is not to be found at the level of medical expertise but at the level of social regulation. The psychiatric concept of psychopathy makes possible a way of explaining conduct that would otherwise be socially unintelligible, regulating individuals who do not fit prevailing explanations of social need and their associated welfare systems, and confining persons who would otherwise fall outside the ambit of both the criminal justice system and the psychiatric system itself.

The non-psychiatric professions and the psychopath

Nurses, psychologists and social workers, in the period leading up to the passage of the 1959 Act, had relatively little to add to the reactions of the psychiatrists. Social workers discussed the pros and cons of including the category of psychopathy in the Act. They were not among the professionals looking forward to such a group being incorporated in the legislation and hence in their remit. Indeed, one commentator followed Barbara Wootton in suggesting that the matter should be deferred and that a large-scale study of the issue was necessary prior to legislation.[32]

Psychologists had previously studied psychopathy in terms of personality traits. Those who followed the behaviourist approach saw psychopathy as the outcome of faulty learning of social responses, an inability to internalize social norms, probably based upon some inherited characteristics.[33] They thus saw this group as falling within their jurisdiction, and subject to their professional competence, But psychologists as a group did not react to the proposed legislation. This may have been because they saw themselves as scientists who should be uninvolved in such political matters, or it may have been because of their numerical weakness. In any event, their voice was conspicuous by its absence.

Nurses were, perhaps, likely to be most affected in their daily practice by the inclusion of the psychopaths within the hospital system. If psychopaths were unmanageable – as was argued – then it was the nurses who would have to live with the implications of this unmanageability or work to change it. Yet the nurses' publications of the time, and the formal discussions on the Act in the nursing literature, reveal little interest in the issues involved. Was this because nurses underrated the difficulties due to their lack of experience with this group of patients? Whatever the reasons, we shall see that, by 1975 when the negotiations were occurring over regional secure units, the voice of the nurses was far from muted.

The 1957 Royal Commission and the government's position

Despite the lack of evidence that there was a growing number of people with psychopathic disorder, the Royal Commission that reported in 1957 recommended the inclusion of this category as a distinct classification in any reformed legislation.[34] It did not feel it could offer a definition of the phenomenon, and thought that it was preferable to leave it without one. Nevertheless, the Commission did not hesitate to use the term 'psychopathic personality' despite the fact that it could not define what was meant by it. A global term of this type was not used by the Commission for any other category of mental disorder. As the Commission had no evidence for the existence of such a type of personality, its use of this concept appears like an act of labelling in the classical form – the generalization from one identified detail to a totalized stereotype.[35] In adopting this position, the Commission followed closely the views of the minority of psychiatrists who were keen to include psychopathy in their brief. Indeed, there appears no doubt that the Commission viewed this decision as a progressive and humanitarian step.

The government adopted a position very similar to that of the Commission, accepting the validity of the category and including it in the new legislation. However the government was unhappy about the lack of a definition, and therefore included a definition in the 1959 Mental Health Act that reads as follows: 'In this act "psychopathic disorder" means a persistent disorder or disability of mind (whether or not including subnormality of intelligence) which results in abnormally aggressive or seriously irresponsible conduct on the part of the patient, and requires or is susceptible to medical treatment.'[36] Mental disorder, on the other hand, is defined thus: 'In this act "mental disorder" means mental illness, arrested or incompleted development of mind, psychopathic disorder, and any other disorder or disability of mind; and "mentally disordered" shall be construed accordingly.'[37]

Thus, although psychopathic disorder is perceived as a category of mental disorder, it is still felt necessary to define it more specifically than any other mental disorder, or indeed than the global category of mental disorder itself. Three components of the definition of psychopathy stand out: first, the persistence of the disorder; second, the degree of agressive or irresponsible behaviour; and, third, the likely contribution of medical intervention.

The focus on persistence is an attempt to delineate psychopathic behaviour from infrequent episodes of aggressive or irresponsible behaviour, knowing all too well that all of us are liable to behave in this manner on occasions. Yet although 'persistence' indicates a quantitative evaluation, neither the Act nor psychiatric textbooks provide guidelines on the frequency that should count as a clear indication of persistence. 'Persistence' depends on the discretion of the individual psychiatrist. In the absence of guidelines, the psychiatrist has to rely heavily upon his/her clinical apprenticeship, socio-cultural background and particular beliefs. Given that the ethos, culture and recruitment of psychiatry is predominantly middle class, there are good grounds for suspecting that judgments over the issues bound up with psychopathy will be made in relation to middle-class norms. Where such factors as deviation from norms of employment, sexuality and interpersonal relationships are involved, one is entitled to be somewhat suspicious of how such judgments operate in relation to the working-class psychopath.

Abnormal aggression and seriously irresponsible conduct are criteria supposedly based on both qualitative and quantitative changes from the normal. Aggression is relatively easy to define, as violent behaviour that harms others. Irresponsibility, however, is not so easy to conceptualize, because of its high dependency on social acceptability, which is likely to vary across situations, sub-cultures, gender and social classes. The main role of the psychiatrist in making these judgments is to act as the custodian of morality. It is not being argued here that the psychiatrist can avoid making moral judgments. On the contrary, this function of psychiatry should be explicitly acknowledged and safeguarded, rather than being denied, as it is by the majority of British psychiatrists.

The evaluation of the requirement for, or susceptibility to medical treatment falls more clearly within the brief of medically qualified psychiatrist than do either of the first two components of the definition of psychopathy. Yet the addition of the notion of susceptibility is odd. Usually indicators of the need for medical treatment would be sufficient to warrant such an intervention. The inclusion of the term susceptibility – defined in the dictionary as the readiness of a person to be acted upon or to act – seems to be aimed at providing from the outset a justification for the predicted low level of success of medical intervention in arresting or preventing this type of behaviour. Thus the definition of psychopathy contained in the legislation does not prevent the term being uncertain or contradictory; on the contrary, the uncertainties and contradictions in the notion of psychopathy as a category of mental disorder are clearly highlighted.

Certain other features of interest arise from the terms of the 1959 legislation. The Act stated that those diagnosed as psychopaths below the age of 21 (or 25 if they are already hospitalized) can be admitted on a compulsory order by virtue of the diagnosis alone. This is in contrast with the usual emphasis that compulsory admissions depend on the severity of the disorder at a given point in time. This aspect of the legislation clearly indicates the level of threat from psychopaths that was felt both by doctors and by politicians.

This provision can also be related to the fact that the 1959 Act 'de-designated' hospitals, making it possible for any hospital not only to admit psychiatric patients, but also to refuse them. Admission could now be refused on the grounds that the hospital lacked suitable provisions or methods of treatment for a potential patient. The framing of the provisions for compulsory admission of psychopaths can be construed as an attempt by the Ministry to ensure that hospitals considered very carefully the implications of refusing to admit young psychopaths. We will return in a subsequent section to see how this attempt to constrain the decisions of hospitals worked in practice.

The reaction of Members of Parliament

In the House of Commons, MPs unanimously thought that the

introduction of the category of psychopathy into the legislation was enlightened, and appeared to regard it as a step on the ladder towards a more humane approach to such persons. This view was shared by MPs who were generally critical of the psychiatric services; it is in line with the general view of the 1959 Act as a very progressive piece of legislation. Not one MP dissented from this view, or raised the possibility that there were dangers in the inclusion in this legislation of provision for compulsory detention in mental hospital of people whose behaviour may not be socially acceptable, but who, nevertheless, are not insane. MPs were aware of such risks. Dr Summerskill pointed out that the suffragettes might have come to be perceived as psychopaths, but did not go so far as to suggest that anti-Nazi fighters in Nazi Germany would also have qualified, had the category been available at the time.[38] Nevertheless, Dr Summerskill herself spoke enthusiastically about this new addition to the list of mental disorders.[39]

Mr Iremonger, representing the prohibitionist Scottish voters, expressed clearly the strong element of social judgment of those defined as contained within the category: 'It is that of the changeling and the waif. They are not so different from those who, in these days, pathetically and fantastically refer to themselves as the "beat generation" and "rebels" and all that sort of thing.' He was also one of the few MPs who linked psychopathy to a specific aetiology: 'There seems to be one thing which all these people have in common, they are incapable of forming real, lasting and valid relationships with the rest of society.'[40] Psychologization went hand in hand with moral condemnation, despite its objective of absolving people from responsibility from their asocial activities.

The one MP who was also a psychiatrist specializing in working with psychopaths highlighted the difficulty in definition and the relative failure of intervention. Yet at the same time he too perceived the inclusion of the category in the Act as a humanitarian step.[41]

It would seem that this belief in the humanitarianism of the new legislation was a reaction to the perceived inhumanity of the alternative prison environment. If MPs believed that from now on psychopaths would be placed in therapeutic communities, as the minority group of psychiatrists would have liked, then such an alternative might appear more attractive and humane than prison. But MPs knew that very few such communities existed, and that for the majority of psychopaths an ordinary psychiatric hospital would be their likely final destination. The same MPs who criticized prolonged hospitalization and professed their belief in community care still maintained that, for psychopaths, hospitalization was a progressive step. Not one MP publicly admitted that compulsory admissions were prescribed for psychopaths because of a fear of their dangerousness rather than a wish to treat them humanely.

It was only in the House of Lords that opposition was voiced to this innovation, albeit by a minority led by Baroness Barbara Wootton. On the basis of her experience as a magistrate, and her scepticism concerning the growing psychologization of social life, she argued that psychopaths should be treated as people able to exercise will and control. Therefore if they offended they should be tried; if found guilty they should be punished for their unlawful behaviour. When not offending, they should be left to themselves: they should not be detained or treated as psychiatrically disturbed people. This was a clear and explicit recognition of, and opposition to, the extension of the jurisdiction of state regulation in general, and psychiatric jurisdiction, in particular, that the new legal category of psychopathy exemplified.

Wootton laid the blame for spreading the belief in psychological reasoning upon social workers, rather than psychoanalysts, psychologists or psychiatrists. This is surprising, given the small numbers of psychiatric social workers at the time and their low social status compared with psychoanalysts and psychiatrists. Furthermore, she appears to have equated 'medical treatment' with a psychodynamic or psychoanalytic orientation, despite the fact that only a minority of psychopaths were treated within such a framework, while the majority were treated in hospital settings with drugs. However, despite her eloquent arguments, the majority in the House of Lords was unmoved, and remained in line with the position adopted in the Commons. It would seem that, by 1957, Wootton was culturally out of step with the majority.

Since 1959

The theory and practice of professionals

A review paper entitled 'The psychopath and his treatment'

by J. S. Whitley was selected for republication in a collection recommended by the Royal College of Psychiatrists in 1976.[42] We may thus consider it to be an authoritative view on the subject at that time. Dr Whitley has been, for some time, the director of the Henderson Hospital (formerly Belmont), where he has continued Maxwell Jones's tradition of working with psychopaths in a therapeutic community. He reminds us that the most salient features of psychopathy are: first, persistent non-conforming behaviour by the individual; second, his/her lack of awareness that this behaviour is seriously at fault; and, third, that the abnormality cannot be readily explained as resulting from the 'madness' we commonly recognize, nor from 'badness' alone. He concludes that 'the many definitions of psychopathic disorder that have been given bear evidence to the inadequacies of the medical concept . . . the composite definition makes no mention of illness, although definitions conclude with the statement that the condition is to be regarded as an illness.'[43]

Both Scott and Walker have commented that whether such people are treated as ill or criminals depends upon the preferences of society rather than upon convincing evidence for the first or the second option.[44] If Dr Whitley were to have heeded such advice, his first task would have been to consider why our society has chosen to view psychopaths as ill. However, he neither adopts, nor mentions such a perspective. Instead, a summary of aetiological positions, assumed to be scientifically based, is presented. These positions include: the physical approach – hereditary basis, organic disease of the brain; the psychodynamic orientation – psychopathy as an extension of neurosis or as an immature personality; and the sociological approach. Whitley considers this latter approach to be a view of psychopathy as a form of deviancy caused by a psychological deficit; he does not, therefore, examine sociological perspectives on psychopathy, but psychological perspectives that label psychopathy as deviant.

Whitley's account of treatment includes physical methods, individual therapy, group therapy and therapeutic communities, but this discusson continues with no recognition that the implementation of social and medical treatment is based upon a prior decision to view psychopathy as an illness. Doubts are expressed as to the value of physical methods, which Whitley judges to be of very limited value. Equally psychotherapy is of limited use because of the massive defensive behaviour of the psychopath. But Whitley is also aware of the limited effectiveness of the therapeutic community approach, which is suitable only for the 'creative' type of psychopath, or those most similar to neurotics.

The effectiveness of all available methods of intervention is summarized thus by McCord and McCord: 'Psychotherapy offers little hope – other approaches seem even less promising . . . incarceration alone . . . does not seem to change basic personality trends; organic treatment has shown few, if any, beneficial results.'[45] Whitley accepts that prognosis is poor. Despite the finding that the overt anti-social behaviour often diminishes in mid-life, it would appear that the destructive qualities in older psychopaths are expressed instead inside the family circle.[46]

The psychiatric profession seems to continue to struggle and fail with the ambiguities inherent in the concept of psychopathy and in methods of intervention for so-called psychopaths. Nevertheless, no one within the camp of psychiatry has expressed the view that these difficulties might indicate that this category has no place within psychiatry.

Psychologists are the main professional group that has offered explanations and interventions other than those of psychiatry. British psychologists who followed the approach of behaviour modification have shared with psychiatrists the view that psychopathy has a genetic basis. According to them, when this inherited predisposition is coupled with positive reinforcement for asocial behaviour, it leads to psychopathy. Such psychologists have thus focused on developing techniques that would reduce the socially undesirable behaviour and increase acceptable behaviour.[47] In so far as these techniques seek to produce changes that are not wanted by the client, they deviate from the principle stated by the psychologists themselves – that of helping to change only what the client wants to change. Other professional groups who might have challenged these assumptions – social workers and nurses – have, by and large, trailed after psychiatrists and psychologists, and have not contributed significantly to the debate over the concept of psychopathy or to perspectives on how such problems should be practically managed.

The continuing impasse and disquiet over the definition of psychopathy and psychiatric intervention for people so labelled was expressed in two main ways. First, ordinary mental hospitals tended not to admit patients known as psychopaths, especially those of the aggressive type. Requests for the transfer of such patients from special hospitals were often refused.[48] Second, another psychiatric classification, that of 'personality disorder', was developed in the 1970s. This classification is based upon the assumption that no illness is present, but that certain personality traits are impaired or missing.[49] Let us consider whether this new terminology sorts out the difficulties involved in conceptualizing psychopathy and how to intervene in it.

First, it must be pointed out that the definition of personality disorder is no clearer than that of psychopathy. It does, perhaps, promote a view of such behaviour as more rooted in the physical make-up of the person, hence perhaps suggesting that investigations should proceed in the direction of a genetic aetiology, and interventions be biased towards physical methods.

Second, in so far as it clearly indicates a non-illness state, the classification of personality disorder signifies a reversal of the position embodied in the 1959 Act. Yet, whilst the condition is now considered not to be an illness, psychiatrists have not come forward to suggest that the category, and those falling under it, should no longer form a part of their responsibilities, or should fall outside the ambit of 'mental disorder' and the scope of mental-health legislation. In this context we should remember that this legislation does specify certain states that may be undesirable, such as alcoholism and promiscuity but that do not, on their own, justify psychiatric intervention.

Perhaps the major innovation is the idea of regional medium-secure units. This has come from administrators and criminologists working together, and was championed by the Committee chaired by Lord Butler that reported in 1975.[50] By this time, the impact of the de-designation of hospitals was acknowledged, and it was recognized that ordinary psychiatric hospitals could not do the job of confining this group of people who were not criminal enough to be processed through the criminal justice system into prolonged imprisonment, and yet not mentally ill enough to be effectively contained within the reformed psychiatric system. The solution of regional medium-secure units was an attempt to escape the dichotomies of prison vs hospital and criminal vs sick person. It proposed an institution that would incorporate both settings and both labels. These units were to make potential or actual dangerousness their main diagnostic criterion, yet, as the employment of nurses as the major staff group indicates, such dangerousness was to be understood firmly within the parameters of psychiatry.

In contrast to the fate of policies of community care, this policy option was not merely accepted verbally, but got the cash to back it up. The smallness of the units appealed: they appeared to resolve anxieties about the creation of yet more large and unwieldy institutions; they met worries about the costs incurred by large special hospitals; and they did not lend themselves to public fears of the concentration of large numbers of dangerous people in their midst. By 1977 it looked as if, in a few years, the prison system, the psychiatric hospitals and the psychiatric wards of general hospitals would be relieved of the burden of the psychopath. Simultaneously, it looked as if these individuals would at last receive what they required: construed as adequate interventions in the right setting – that is, amongst their own kind and in an institution combining both prison and hospital.

Yet in 1985 only 12 such units out of the projected 35 were in existence. The reasons for this shortfall lie not only in the difficulties that have been encountered in co-operation between the different authorities involved in the establishment of such hybrid institutions, but also in the reluctance of nurses to work in these settings and with these client groups.[51] The nurses' reluctance to work with this group – expressed in the demand to be paid 'danger money' – signifies not only a fear of violence, but also the tacit recognition that they are being put into a role that is primarily custodial, and one in which they have little to offer therapeutically. The reluctance of nurses to involve themselves in such institutions is intelligible, for the role they are offered runs quite contrary to the direction of development of the ideology of psychiatric nursing within the psychiatric system at large. This stresses the specialized therapeutic skills of the nurse, upon which the claims of this group to professional status are grounded.

However, although the policy of regional medium-secure units is clearly not meeting its original objective, the Ministry has not abandoned it. Perhaps this is because it can find no other way out of the mess in which it finds itself when it comes to governing psychopaths. Over and above the practical and professional problems, however, one important thing has been overlooked by the protagonists of the idea of the regional medium-secure unit. Such a policy, far from being a progressive solution to the problem of the psychopath, further marginalizes such people, almost makes outcasts of them, and it further criminalizes those of them who have, in fact, committed no offence.

The position of parliament and government

In the period after 1959, Members of Parliament no longer raised the issue of psychopathy. Instead, those with an interest in such issues pressed for better care for mentally ill offenders, especially for those in prison who should have been in hospital, and for those in special hospital who could have been in ordinary hospital.[52] Psychopathy had, it would appear, come to be taken for granted as a category of psychiatric disturbance.

The report of the Butler Committee in 1975 was the first official reconsideration of the issues involved in psychopathy since 1959. The Committee, whose mandate was to look at all the issues concerning mentally ill offenders, devoted a considerable part of its report to psychopathy. It formally confirmed what was common knowledge in psychiatric circles: 'Neither "psychopathic disorder" nor "subnormality" is a specific diagnosis: they are generic terms adopted for the purpose of legal categorisation and capable of covering a number of specific diagnoses, although in the case of psychopathic disorders reliable specific diagnoses have still to be developed'.[53] Indeed the Committee thought that there were strong arguments for the category to be deleted from the law on the grounds that there was a lack of inter-professional agreement, potential for abusing people's liberty, and that the concept itself was logically defective.[54]

The Committee felt that it was 'highly undesirable to label people as psychopaths', and that this was especially true for young people. Nonetheless, they hesitated to suggest that the category be withdrawn from the legislation, largely, it appears, because it had been there for sixteen years.[55] With bureaucratic logic winning out, they proposed instead to substitute the category of personality disorders, but without defining these.

And, as already discussed, the Committee, despite its awareness of the limitations of all methods of intervention, came
out strongly in favour of the creation of special units for
psychopaths.[56]

The 1978 Review of the Mental Health Act, published three
years after the Butler Committee had reported, stated clearly
that there were no plans to change the categorization of psychopaths, despite the doubts it expressed about the definition of
psychopathy and the likely 'recovery' of psychopaths.[57] It gave
no reasons for this decision, apart from stating that a change
in terminology from psychopathy to personality disorder would
not be useful.

Most recently, the document on reform of mental-health
legislation that formed the basis for the 1982 Mental Health
(Amendment) Act and hence for the Mental Health Act 1983,
stated the official view of the matter quite clearly:

> The government has considered whether psychopathic disorder
> should be excluded from the Act, the weight of current medical
> opinion is that most psychopaths are not likely to benefit from
> treatment in hospital and are for the penal system to deal with
> when they commit offences but that there are some persons suf-
> fering from psychopathic disorder who can be helped by detention
> in hospital. For this reason, the category is not excluded from the
> Act.[58]

The same reasoning is given for the decision to raise the age
limit for the compulsory admission of psychopaths, and to link
such detention to a notion of 'treatability'. The concept of
treatability is defined as the existence of an expectation of
further benefit from treatment.[59] This criterion of treatability
is noteworthy, for it is applicable to psychopathy, and is not
applied to the mentally ill or to the severely mentally handicapped. The lack of substance in the phrase 'expectation of
benefit' suggests that the criterion is aimed at fending off the
accusation that psychopaths and mildly mentally handicapped
people are detained in hospitals merely to keep them in confinement when they have not committed the offences that
might be expected of them.

It should be remembered that the Scottish Mental Health
Act of 1960 does not include psychopathy as a specific category
of mental disorder. No one has claimed that psychopaths in
Scotland have fared less well than their English counterparts,

or that the proportion of Scottish psychopaths who are dangerous exceeds that in England. One is left, therefore, to wonder why it is that the Scottish example is not followed south of the border: what is it about the system of social regulation in England that appears to make the category of psychopathy indispensable?

Conclusion

The main difference between the situation obtaining in 1959 and that today is that both the government and the psychiatric system recognize the incongruity of the concept of psychopathy. The lack of suitable methods of intervention was already acknowledged in 1959, and that has not changed since. Nevertheless, neither the government nor the professionals are averse to the continued existence of the category, or to the incorporation of those diagnosed under it within the umbrella of mental disorder. Perhaps this state of affairs, which can hardly be regarded as satisfactory, continues, because no other discipline has come up with a more coherent framework of analysis or technology of intervention. But perhaps, despite the contradictions in the concept of psychopathy and the repetitive failures of social and therapeutic interventions, the category persists because of what it makes possible.

The category of psychopathy, whatever its logical imperfections and therapeutic disappointments, arose out of the fundamental shifts in social policy that followed the Second World War. It sought to confer intelligibility upon the behaviours of a residual group who did not fit into any of the new stereotypes of the poor, the criminal or the ill. It accorded with the sectional interests of a faction within psychiatry who sought to use it for the advancement of the principles of therapeutic resocialization through the therapeutic-community movement. The concept of psychopathy did not, in fact, provide the base from which this section of psychiatry would successfully expand, although it has provided the therapeutic-community movement with a continued foothold within our society. Nor did the category offer effective solutions to the problems of overstretched prisons, to the unhappiness of those who were diagnosed, or to the problems of management encountered in the reformed psychiatric system. But it has a function nonetheless. It enables the state to accomplish the social management of a troublesome group of individuals, and it enables psychiatry to maintain and sustain its mandate over those whose conduct is socially undesirable yet who do not fall within the ambit of our system of criminal justice.

The rejection of the psychiatrization of the accused by the jury in the recent trials of Sutcliffe (1983) and Neilson (1984) suggests that lay people may be ready to re-examine issues like the classification of psychopathy. There is, however, no indication of such readiness by either psychiatrists or the government, or of any interest in doing so among MPs, demonstrating that the categorization still meets the requirement of being an effective smoke-screen.

8

Psychiatry in prisons: promises, premises, practices and politics

Pat Carlen

Forensic psychiatry is authoritatively charged with the legal, judicial and moral management of lawbreakers and others who, from time to time, come to the attention of the courts. Its immediate and formal licence to practise emanates from law and medicine and its overt and major sites of operation are the prison and the courtroom. Amongst forensic psychiatry's formidable array of technologies have been included brain surgery, electro-convulsive therapy, the injection and oral administration of drugs, deprivation of food, privileges and comfort as part of behaviour-modification programmes, aversion therapies, sensory deprivation and, most recently, 'therapeutic-community' type group work. The forever elusive subject of forensic psychiatry's inquiry has always been the putative legal subject – he or she, who having (or not) the capacity to know better, breaks the law. Forensic psychiatry's equally elusive objective has been to create a space of recognition wherein the legal subject who defies comprehension can be assessed, classified, controlled, transformed and, finally, (if in the meantime he or she has not been completely destroyed) recycled as a reconditioned and resigned citizen. This essay discusses the promises, premises, practices and politics of forensic psychiatry. The first section outlines and analyses the early history and modes of development of the prison psychiatric services; the second discusses some of the discourses within which present-day psychiatric penality is constituted; the third outlines and analyses the

contemporary uses of psychiatry in prisons; the essay concludes
by discussing the political dimensions of contemporary and
competing trends in the premises and practices of forensic
psychiatry and in the discourses of medical jurisprudence.[1]

The promise of psychiatry

> I believe that if we had, in conjunction with a scheme of control,
> a scientific clearing and sorting house for convicted persons with
> proper places of treatment . . . that the doctor's work would soon
> become all important and the gaoler, as we know him, be out of
> work . . . The prisoner should come to his trial bringing his dossier
> with him, so that he can be dealt with according to the findings of
> the skilled psychiatrists who have taken his measure and understood
> the treatment of his neurosis. These experts should be made
> entirely responsible for the disposal of the criminal or insane, or
> inebriate group.[2]

When Mary Gordon, a former Inspector of Prisons wrote those
words in 1922 there had already been over a century of concern
relating to the containment, assessment and classification of
insane or mentally abnormal offenders.[3] Yet it was not until
1808 that the County Asylum Act empowered 'local judges to
set up asylums for the care of the insane, including the insane
offender'[4] and not until 1836 that the Secretary of State was
'granted authority to transfer dangerous convicts to the County
Asylums'.[5] The 1843 'regulations for local gaols . . . required
the Governor to call the attention of the chaplain and the
medical officer without delay "to any prisoner whose state of
mind requires their attention".'[6] and by the middle of the
nineteenth century the prison doctor was not only giving evidence to the courts concerning the accused's state of mind
but was also charged with ensuring that prisoners undergoing
punishment received only as much physical and mental pain
as the doctor thought they could stand. From the start, therefore, the relationship between prison doctor and prisoner patient was totally different from the conventional doctor–patient
relationship. As Mary Gordon said, 'The prisoner does not
consult the doctor, the State pays the doctor and consults
him about the prisoner.'[7] Certainly, with regard to prison
psychiatric services, that is the relationship that still obtains

today – forensic psychiatry's primary task is still the assessment and classification of prisoners.

In addition to diagnosis and classification, the mid-nineteenth century prison-doctors had to force-feed recalcitrant prisoners, supervise corporal punishment, assess the mental effects of solitary confinement and the silent system, and witness executions. Thus they were already being used to fling a cloak of medical respectability over the whole penal system, though throughout the nineteenth century this veil was continually lifted by critics who not only drew repeated attention to the fact that large numbers of mentally abnormal people were being sent to prison, but also contended that imprisonment can, in itself, induce mentally abnormal states in previously normal people.[8] True, prisoners considered too mentally infirm to stand the rigours of imprisonment were supposed to be transferred to the County Asylums, but the asylums, employing the same argument as today's 'open-door' mental hospitals, more often than not pleaded lack of security as a reason for refusing admission to the mentally infirm criminal. As a result, in 1861, Bethlem Hospital opened a wing for insane persons charged with offences and in 1863 Broadmoor was opened as a Criminal Lunatic Asylum. Since then several institutions have been opened and a series of statutes have been enacted, all with the design of removing mentally abnormal offenders from the prisons. They have not succeeded in their aim, and for three major reasons. First, as quickly as one group of mentally abnormal offenders has been removed from the prisons, the prison authorities have identified a new group, one whose previously tolerated behaviour is now beyond the newly defined bounds of recognition and comprehension. Second, there has always already existed a group of prisoners who, though recognized by lay people as being crazy, stubbornly remain outside the definitions of recognizable mental illness that are forever being endowed with new meanings by the latest mental-health legislation. Third, by the beginning of the twentieth century the ideological, economic and political conditions were such that psychiatrists no longer had to choose whether or not to take into their asylums the rejects of the prison. By the 1920s psychiatry had ceased to be an alternatively sited system of moral management. Since 1895 when the Gladstone Committee had tentatively suggested that prison doctors should be recruited from those who had made a special study of lunacy, psychiatry had slowly inseminated the whole judicial and penal process and, within the prisons, the psychiatrically oriented medical officer was already usurping the office of the prison-chaplain as chief arbiter of morals and authorized technician of behavioural change. Prison had become a prime site for the practice of state-sponsored psychiatry. How had such a situation come about?

The premises of psychiatric penality

The eighteenth-century diminution of the medieval use of physical punishment engendering either death or pain, together with the simultaneous rise of the prison as a place of punishment, has been well-documented by Michel Foucault, Dario Melossi and Massimo Pavarini, and Michael Ignatieff.[9] However, although techniques of moral management involving the manipulating of emotions such as guilt, and the engendering of the mental and moral states of humility and dependence were practised in asylums, from the end of the eighteenth century (in Britain, for example, at Samuel Tuke's Retreat at York),[10] early attempts at moral management in the prisons depended much more on the manipulation of the spatial and temporal techniques of surveillance, together with moral instruction, than on techniques aimed directly at a scientifically conceived site of criminal motivation and/or consciousness.[11] The nineteenth-century silent and separate systems, for example, had been expected to put the prisoner in the *right frame of mind* for the receipt of moral instruction from the chaplain; by the early twentieth century the psychiatrist was expected to see into, and change, the *mind itself*. Moreover, whatever economic reasons there may have been behind the demands that prisoners should be returned to the (reserve) labour-force as rehabilitated rather than debilitated (potential) workers,[12] additional impetuses to psychiatric penality came not only from the prisons' omnipresent and diversified audience of 'humanitarian', or 'authoritarian' or 'libertarian' critics, but also from the exasperated prison administrators themselves. For, after a century and a half of experimentation, by the early 1920s it was patently obvious that a series of ever-changing prison regimes had spectacularly failed in their aims of promoting good order in the prisons and inducing penitence and the internalization of the work-ethic in the prisoners. The searchers after the perfect prison regime seemed to have reached an impasse. The silent and solitary systems (supported by the harsh physical punishments of flogging and birching which, we should recall, were not actually abandoned in prisons in England and Wales until 1962),[13] had produced either totally hardened or totally debilitated convicts.[14] Increased association, on the other hand, always seemed to result in a strengthening of the so-called 'prison subculture' that made prisoners even less amenable to the so-called 'reformative' influences. The positivistic project that had assumed that once the 'criminal mind' had been assessed it could be worked upon and reformed no longer seemed feasible. In any case, twentieth-century psychiatry promised something rather better. Psychiatry, especially that branch most influenced by a positivist reading of Freudian psychoanalysis, was not claiming that it would *reform*. Therapeutic forensic psychiatry would *transform*, and it would do so by kindling within the prisoner the guilt that had already been established by the court. This, then, was to be the miraculous triumph of twentieth-century medical jurisprudence: that psychiatry would realize what law had posited.

The promoters of pscychiatric penality were over-optimistic; they had reckoned without some of the other, older and extremely tenacious elements within penal discourse, without some of the problems which were always-already insoluble within classical medical jurisprudence. These archival discourses primarily revolved around the classical debate concerning the relative powers and rights of the individual and the state, though in penal discourse they usually surfaced as statements concerning punishment vs treatment and the scientifically correct classification of prisoners' mental states. Today these statements are themselves circumscribed by other discourses: older discourses predicated upon the positivistic demand and idealistic desire for a 'cure for crime'; newer discourses concerned (variously) with the development of pharmaceutical and electronic modes of control, the growth in power of the nursing profession and the prison officers, the peculiar position of the Prison Medical Service and, finally, with the politics of imprisonment itself.

The two major discourses that have obstructed the unimpeded growth of psychiatric power within the prisons have been those of retribution and of rights. Despite recent evidence that the British 'public' might not be as punitive as has always been claimed,[15] within the prison the effects of the former have usually been more in evidence than those of the latter. Whatever the official rhetoric, prison personnel have perenially insisted that prisons should be places for punishment,[16] and this view was enthusiastically embraced and endorsed by Leon Brittan, Tory Home Secretary until 1985, who almost daily proclaimed retribution to be a main concern of the Conservative Party's penal platform. Luckily (or not) the discourse of retribution that has circumscribed and/or inseminated the more medically or therapeutically oriented discourses of forensic psychiatry has, in its turn, constantly been denied full sway by the various discourses of individual rights.

As I have argued elsewhere, although within penal politics the substantive elements of the discourse of rights 'usually include, at the least, notions of state, society, the individual, humanity, God, freedom, and oppression, their meanings emerge contradictorily and with diverse effects as they combine in discourses that are either politically opposed, or just discursively asymmetrical, to each other.'[17] Even so, most proponents of punishment as opposed to treatment would agree on the following proposition: that the state has the right to impose *retributive* punishment and the individual to receive *expiatory* punishment. Most would then go on to support this proposition by arguing (according to their creed or politics) either that treatment reduces the essential humanity of the individual by denying to her or him the free-will to break the law, [18] or that it illegitimately encroaches upon that area of political action where the individual should remain free to oppose the state.[19]

Proponents of treatment, on the other hand, argue from positions of physiological, psychological or psycho-social determinism. First they argue that certain types (or syndromes) of lawbreaking are in themselves evidence of a diminution of free-will stemming from either physiological or mental abnormality. Then they argue one of two ways. *Either* for both the individual and/or the public good the person should be treated surgically, pharmaceutically or electronically so that some kind of behavioural change be effected;[20] *or* that in the name of both democracy *and* individual autonomy the damaged person should be therapeutically transformed so that, as a *newly autonomous* individual, he or she can *choose* to behave as a law-abiding citizen. If these arguments are accepted, then no issue of rights is involved other than the correct assessment and classification of the offender in the first place. As we shall see later in this essay, the accurate assessment and classification of offenders has been the constant (and, incidentally, most lucrative) chimera of forensic psychiatry.

In 1919 the punishment/treatment dichotomy was institutionalized when the Birmingham justices appointed a full-time prison medical officer to report to the courts on the mental state of remand prisoners and to recommend whether treatment might be more appropriate than punishment. The medical officer appointed was the psychoanalytically oriented Hamblin-Smith who wrote in the preface to his book *The Psychology of the Criminal* that it was only through increased investigation of the offender's mentality that 'we can hope to solve the problems which criminality presents.'[21] The Prison Report for 1919–20 also raised the question of the feasibility of treatment rather than punishment for some categories of offender,[22] whilst in 1932 The Departmental Persistent Offenders Committee asserted that 'there is reason to believe that certain delinquents may be amenable to psychological treatment.'[23] Thereafter, The Prison Medical Service, founded in 1774 by the Act for Preserving The Health of Prisoners in Gaol and Preventing Gaol Distemper rapidly expanded.[24] By 1972 there were 100 full-time prison medical officers, 96 per cent of whom were recognized under Section 28 of the 1959 Mental Health Act as having 'special experience in the diagnosis and/or treatment of mental disorders' and, with the founding of The Royal College of Psychiatrists in 1971 'no less than forty full-time [prison] medical officers were awarded fellowships or memberships'.[25]

In the meantime, major steps towards therapeutically treating offenders within the prison system (as opposed to merely classifying them) had been taken in 1933 when 'Dr W. H. Hubert . . . was . . . appointed to carry out psychological treatment of selected prisoners at Wormwood Scrubs,' and again in 1962 when Grendon Underwood psychiatric prison was opened.[26] Yet twenty-three years later, in 1985, the majority of prisoners who come into contact with psychiatrists in prison do so only for the purposes of assessment, categorization, and the prescription of drugs. The personnel of those psychiatric units that *are* engaging in therapeutic work consider themselves to be constantly under the threat of closure. This is not to argue that the institutionalized power of forensic psychiatry has diminished; it is to point out that amongst prison officials, prisoners, prison officers and criminologists there are many who believe not only that psychiatry has reneged on its promises to reform criminals and empty the prisons of mentally abnormal offenders, but also that prison psychiatry has contributed little towards bettering the lot of either prisoners or their gaolers.

The practice of psychiatry in prisons[27]

The most recent book on prison health care argues that with the decline in expectations of what psychiatry can achieve in prisons there is today less concern that full-time prison doctors should have qualifications in forensic psychiatry.[28] This decline in the positivist belief that psychiatry can cure crime has not been matched by any decline in the equally positivist belief that psychiatry can accurately assess and categorize the prisoner's mental state. Smith writes that:

> Almost half of the full time medical officer's time is taken up with writing reports . . . The main focus of these reports, particularly the court reports, is the prisoner's mental state, and , although the prison medical service currently wants to recruit experienced general practitioners rather than psychiatrists, for this part of the full time doctor's work experience of psychiatry is more useful than experience of general practice.[29]

Yet, despite the fact that there is 'a high proportion of qualified psychiatrists in the Prison Medical Service and among the visiting NHS consultants',[30] assessment and categorization is seldom followed by special psychiatric treatment within the prison:

> All prisoners are seen on reception, and this consultation is a key one: here the physically ill, the mentally-disturbed and the suicidal must be sorted out . . . These examinations are usually done at great speed and under great pressure. The idea that this might be an ideal opportunity for practising a little preventive medicine was quite laughable to many of the prison doctors to whom I spoke. They were doing well, they thought, if they could sort out the

suicidal from the non-suicidal or those who were going to develop delirium tremens from those who would sober up peacefully, and in the circumstances they were.[31]

The Senior Medical Officer at Wandsworth Prison described to me the procedure for treating disturbed prisoners:

> If a prisoner is, or becomes, mentally-ill, then the hospital officer [a prison officer who has had some nursing training] will first of all have him seen by one of the visiting G.Ps. If the visiting G.P. thinks that there is something that might be serious then he refers him to the full time doctor so that he can be admitted to the hospital here for hospital treatment. People who are acutely disturbed are kept on the Observation level. Even when we think that someone should go to the Special Hospital under the terms of the Mental Health Act [1983] we have great difficulty getting them transferred.[32]

Prison Medical Officers have few effective guidelines on how to proceed with prisoners who appear to them to be mentally ill because they know from experience, first, that their own diagnoses are often held to be at odds with the legally effective categories of mental illness as defined under 1983 Mental Health Act, and, second, that elastic as the concept of mental illness is in the world at large, within the prison there is a danger that it can be stretched to cover any and every kind of behaviour. Though, therefore, it is likely that many prison personnel would, in one sense, agree with the prison medical officer who told me that 'over 80 per cent of prisoners have some kind of mental illness, mostly personality disorders,' they would also know that whilst, speaking *literally*, the term personality disorder can be said to cover a multitude of *sins* (see chapter 7),[32] it does not cover many *treatable* forms of *mental illness*. The then Home Secretary Leon Brittan may have given comfort to some when, in February 1984, he told the Liverpool City Bench that the Home Office was 'conducting an exercise to try to assess more accurately how many offenders there are in prison who ought to be transferred to hospital',[34] but to others he would have been merely demonstrating his ignorance of the complexities of penal politics and psychiatric diagnosis. For, as Richard Smith has written, 'asking how many mentally abnormal people there are in prison is similar to asking how many people there are with drink problems in the community.'[35]

There have in fact already been several attempts to estimate the numbers of mentally abnormal people in prison though, given the interrelated definitional, diagnostic and methodological problems, it is not surprising that these attempts have proved to be somewhat inconclusive.[36] Perhaps, then, once one moves outside that very narrow definitional space where psychiatric diagnoses coincide with the categories authorized by the mental-health legislation as justifying a prisoner's removal to hospital, one cannot in medical jurisprudence go much beyond Lord Justice Lawton's phenomenological definition, that mental illness is nothing more nor less than what 'ordinary sensible people' think it is.[37]

Every prison medical officer to whom I spoke stressed that even when it is recommended that a prison inmate be transferred to a psychiatric hospital, and even when that inmate is perceived to be so dangerous that he or she warrants removal to a Special Hospital, there are several obstacles to surmount before he or she is actually removed (see the concluding section of this essay). The 1983 *Report on the Work of the Prison Department* records, however, a higher number of transfers being effected in 1983 than in previous years: 'The number of reports submitted recommending transfer to psychiatric hospitals under Section 72 or 73 of the 1959 Act or Section 47 or 48 of the Mental Health Act 1983 (140) and the number of transfers actually effected (110) were somewhat higher than the corresponding figures for 1982 (121 and 92 respectively).'[38] The Home Office keeps a record of the numbers of prisoners previously recommended for transfer to hospital and yet still in the prison and, though in November 1983 the penal establishments contained 220 sentenced prisoners (plus 180 remand prisoners) who came within the categories of the mental-health legislation, by November 1984 the figure for sentenced prisoners had fallen to 91.[39] Those inmates, together with those few who were removed to hospital, constitute only a tiny proportion of the much larger number of prisoners who to 'ordinary sensible' observers appear to be suffering from some abnormality that either might benefit from psychiatric treatment or that might have been considered as releasing them from full culpability for the offence for which they were convicted. Thus, in addition to psychotically disturbed people, there are many prisoners who define themselves as being chronically depressed and many others who at some time or other have been diagnosed by psychiatrists as suffering from neurosis, schizophrenia, alcoholism, drug-dependence or some kind of non-specific (and therefore non-treatable) personality disorder.[40] Furthermore, Coid concluded from his review of the best relevant studies that epileptics and the mentally handicapped are exposed to a higher risk of imprisonment than the general population.[41]

Now, even if all those above-mentioned categories of supposedly mentally abnormal prisoners are seen by a psychiatrist (and that is unlikely) few of them will receive any treatment other than increased observation (either in the hospital, on the wing, in seclusion in their own cells or in isolation in a stripped cell) and medication. Conversely, there is a strong belief amongst prisoners that many prisoners who are *not* abnormal are defined as such if they violently oppose the prison staff and that thereafter they can become prime candidates for excessive doses of drugs, forced injections, mechanical restraints, or even removal to one of the Special Hospitals.[42] So what *do* psychiatrists do in prisons, and what psychiatrically inspired or sanctioned treatments or disciplinary techniques are either administered or practised?

The average daily prison population for England and Wales in 1983 was 43,500,[42] and during that year 10,832 inmates were referred to visiting consultant psychiatrists. Prison medical staff prepared a total of 8,923 psychiatric reports for the courts (161 were for people remanded on bail) and 'in addition 3,778 inmates were visited by consultant psychiatrists to examine them and prepare reports at the request of their solicitors.'[44] Special facilities for prisoners with mental abnormalities are provided at Grendon Underwood Prison and in special wings at Holloway, Parkhurst, Wakefield, and in Wormwood Scrubs Prisons; also at Feltham and Glen Parva Youth Custody Centres. For the rest, prison doctors have to manage as best they can either on their own or with the help of drugs and/or visiting consultant psychiatrists. In some prisons they have the additional support of therapeutic groups run by probation officers or other specialist therapists. As for physical methods of psychiatric treatment, 'Brain surgery . . . is almost never used in British prisons,'[45] whilst the 1983 *Report of the work of the Prison Department* recorded that during the year: 'Seven inmates were offered and accepted electroconvulsive therapy for the treatment of their mental illness, 1 inmate received the treatment within the establishment and 7 [sic] as an outpatient in an NHS Hospital.'[46]

The Director of the Prison Medical Service has recently pointed out that 'prison medical officers do not have the statutory authority to give treatment without consent.'[47] Nonetheless, the fact remains that under the law 'tranquillising treatment may be given without consent in prisons by medical officers [when there is] a threat to life, or grievous harm to the individual, staff, or other inmates, or the likelihood of irreversible deterioration of the patient's condition.'[48] This legal provision has led to situations that have moved some informed observers to suggest that perhaps the circumstances licensing forced injections are too readily said to obtain wherever a prisoner's behaviour threatens to disrupt prison discipline. Be that as it may, even though many violent or self-mutilating prisoners fear the psychiatrist's formal (though seldom-used) power to recommend their removal to a Special Hospital, most inmates who come into contact with psychiatrists in prison do so solely for the purpose of assessment. Many will thereafter be prescribed psychotropic and other drugs that act on the central nervous system.[49] A very small proportion of all prisoners will be offered, and will accept, treatment in a therapeutic-community type setting within the penal system.

Although in 1975 the Butler Report claimed that 'there are now 43 establishments with psychiatric units, 36 prisons, six borstals and one remand centre,'[50] today the penal establishments best known for their therapeutic group work are Grendon Underwood Psychiatric Prison and the Annexe at Wormwood Scrubs.[51] Both are organized around what Dr W. J. Gray, the first Medical Superintendent of Grendon, called a 'group- and community oriented regime',[52] though the Butler Report reveals that between 1962 and 1975 other treatments at Grendon had included 'electro-convulsive therapy, insulin treatment, narcosis and other drug treatment, occupational therapy, physiotherapy and relaxation and speech therapy'.[53] At the time of Gunn's detailed study, however, he was able to report that in 1971–3 'the regime operating in Grendon . . . was that of a therapeutic community, modified to the extent that prison rules require.'[54] At a very general level, that describes the Grendon regime as it has persisted throughout the prison's 23-year existence. The psychiatric facilities at Wormwood Scrubs, on the other hand, have had a more chequered history. Between 1933 and 1939 (when war put a stop to the work) individual psychotherapy was begun as just one type of treatment on offer amongst a battery of others, e.g. electro-convulsive and aversion therapy, and it was not until 1972 that Dr Max Glatt founded the Annexe in its present form as a therapeutic community. There are differences in the populations and in some of the organizational features of the prison communities at Grendon and Wormwood Scrubs,[55] but both aim to develop 'insight'[56] in the prisoners through 'group counselling',[57] in a system 'in which all the resources of the institution – staff, patients and relations – are mobilised in the interests of treatment . . . Treatment takes place in small groups . . . and in larger community meetings of thirty or forty people living in the same wing.'[58] But, like every other aspect of penal history, the history of treatment based on therapeutic-community principles within the prisons has been one of controversy. The many functions of therapeutic groups within the penal system are as complex and controversial as are those of every other psychiatric practice undertaken at the behest of the courts or under the auspices of the Prison Medical Service. It is to the politics of psychiatric penal practice that I now turn.

The politics of penal psychiatry

Forensic psychiatry's failure to reform criminals and empty the prisons of mentally abnormal offenders has come as no surprise to some. From the beginning of the century many have criticized the notion that a population of law breakers is self-evidently a site of production for psychiatric problems, psychiatric diagnoses and psychiatric treatments. Even apart from questions of rights, some of the cynics have believed that imprisonment itself is responsible for most of the depressed or bizarre behaviour exhibited by inmates; others have argued that it is impossible to practice effective psychiatric treatment in a penal setting. Mary Gordon, for instance, writing about Borstal girls in 1922 stated that 'as far as [she] could ascertain, many of the girls had shown no signs of mental or emotional upset until they came under their long Borstal sentence.'[59] By

1934, Hamblin-Smith had realized that 'there are the gravest objections to combining the ideas of punishment and medical treatment.'[60] Today the claims of forensic psychiatry are deceptively modest. Most of the prison doctors to whom I spoke claimed that, as far as psychiatric treatment is concerned, their greatest hope is to alleviate prisoners' present psychiatric problems rather than to effect a complete change in their way of life outside the prison. Yet, despite the modesty of its present claims, psychiatry retains powerful interests in the penal industry, interests that, though circumscribed by a forever-changing penal politics, are deeply embedded in modern penality. What, then, *are* the functions of contemporary psychiatric penality? How appropriate is it to claim that imprisonment has been psychiatrized? In debating these questions let us examine separately the politics of therapeutic-community type treatment in prisons, the politics of pharmaceutical treatment in prisons, and the politics of the psychiatric diagnosis of offenders.

The politics of therapeutic-community type treatments

It is very difficult for anyone well-appraised of the generally disgusting and brutalizing conditions obtaining in British prisons to look other than favourably upon any penal innovation that permits prison officers to show a genuine concern for prisoners, and for prisoners to expect at least a minimal degree of courtesy from officers. At Grendon, (in 1976 and 1985) Wormwood Scrubs Annexe (1985) and at the Barlinnie Special Unit (1981) I met officers who were deeply involved with, and committed to, the principles of therapeutic groups, who were well aware of the limitations imposed by the prison setting but who felt, nonetheless, that if anything could be done to ease a prisoner's personality problems it should be attempted. The main concerns of the Annexe officers at Wormwood Scrubs were that they themselves had received no official training as group leaders (though several had voluntarily attended training sessions at the Henderson Hospital) and that, whatever progress prisoners might make whilst at the Annexe, the aftercare facilities for them were absolutely non-existent. At the Wormwood Scrubs Annexe (where I was able to observe officer–prisoner interaction for longer periods than when I visited Grendon) the usual hierarchical prisoner–officer relations had, at least on the surface, been modified in several ways. Prisoners were called by their first names, were invited to voice to the Principal Hospital Officer any criticisms they might have of his personal style towards them, and were encouraged to keep in touch with the Annexe officers after their release from prison. Ex-prisoners are already allowed to return to the Annexe and spend half a day with their group.[61] What the Principal Hospital Officer would like would be a hostel for ex-Annexe prisoners, and a drop-in centre outside the prison where, after their release, all ex-Annexe prisoners could maintain contact with other members of their group, including the officers. Prisoners I spoke to at the Annexe and ex-Grendon prisoners I have spoken to since their release, whilst expressing mixed feelings about the philosophy and methods of the therapeutic regimes, generally agreed that the Scrubs' Annexe and Grendon Prison provide more civilized forms of penal containment than are generally to be found in the rest of the prison system. Yet, whatever the perceptions and experiences of the officers and prisoners involved, an assessment of therapeutic group treatment has also to consider its wider implications: the contradictory elements embedded in the philosophy of therapeutic group counselling in general; and the amplification of the more coercive elements in group therapy, particularly when it is practised in prison.

Marc Schiffer has written that 'a major risk or side-effect of group psychotherapy is what Whitaker and Lieberman have referred to as "subversion of individuality". This . . . may be brought about by the operation of various psychological and group phenomena such as projection, splitting, scapegoating, contagion, the legitimisation of unanimous decisions and the pressure toward conformity.'[62] Certainly my own observation of group therapy in prisons has convinced me that one of the major techniques employed to provoke prisoners into 'opening themselves up' is the old prison-officer ploy of inducing in prisoners guilt about the plight of their families whilst they themselves are in prison. This may indeed make prisoners more amenable to group pressures but it is far from self-evident that it sends them back to their families better able to cope with the emotional and economic pressures confronting them therein. Futhermore, it seems odd that in a society based on individualism and a predatory competitiveness a penal therapy should be employed that, at first sight, demands the diminution of individualism. However, when psychotherapeutic group treatment is practised in prisons it does not aim at the destruction of *all* individualism. It aims only at the subversion of the prisoner's loyalty to the so-called prison subculture (or 'prisoners' code'). The ultimate aim is the regeneration of the prisoner as a non-'criminally contaminated' individual. The apparent opposition between individualism and group work obscures the promotion of individualism that is the aim of such groups. The technology works *via the mechanism of the group* upon the individual.

The therapeutic community's aim of subverting the prison 'subculture' was made quite explicit by Grendon's first medical superintendent who asserted that, 'the prisoners' code is socially unacceptable and quite hostile to ordinary social standards.[63] The inmate subculture is grossly anti-therapeutic.'[64] Maybe so, but it does involve values (such as loyalty) that are lauded in the world at large, though it is true to say that these values are at odds with some of the operative principles of therapeutic groups. Thus Whitely, Briggs and Turner had reservations about the setting-up of therapeutic groups in prisons. 'We needed to know how convicted felons in prison would take to a culture which required "feedback" to operate. Would they see this as "snitching"? Would they be able to violate the well-established inmate "code of ethics" and feed incidences of delinquent behaviour publicly into meetings?'[65] These reservations were echoed by prisoners at Grendon in 1984 who said, 'Here you get ex-crooks talking like policemen and that's just not right,' and 'Here they rely a lot on what *they* call "therapeutic feedback" . . . What *we* usually call "grassing"!'

The language of regeneration is used again and again as prisoners who refuse to accept the group's viewpoint are reproved with comments like, 'I think we're seeing the "old" Maurice now,' or 'I wonder about your motivation for being in the group,' or, 'When you say things like that I wonder how much you've *really* changed.' (Remember that sometimes these comments are by officers who will soon be doing a cell search, writing a prisoner's parole report). Verbal coercion is finely wielded to ensure that participation in the group is at the appropriate level for the gaining of insight. Being *too* articulate or *too* intellectual is frowned upon. Consider the following exchange:

Prisoner 1   Have you ever thought about what you're doing to your wife?
        If you *really* loved her you wouldn't keep coming back here.
Prisoner 2   I do love her. We have a good relationship.
Prisoner 3   I don't think you do, otherwise you wouldn't go out fighting people.
Prisoner 2   Why can't I love my wife *and* have a short temper?
Officer   Now you're playing with words.[65]
Prisoner 2   But I don't see it like that.
Prisoner 1   Isn't that the point of the groups, to make you see things you wouldn't otherwise see?
Prisoner 2   But that's not my problem, whether I love my wife. My problem is my temper.
Prisoner 3   If you knew what your problem is you wouldn't be here.

And so on. Called 'moral management' when occuring in a therapeutic group, the foregoing conversation is similar to many others I have heard between prisoners and prison officers in conventional prison settings, where such exchanges are usually referred to as 'wind-ups'. The difference is that in prison settings modelled on therapeutic communities the prisoners are voluntary parties to such conversations and the exchanges tend to be contained without violence. Why, then, are there not more such regimes in prisons? The reasons inhere in a complex of prisoner, prison-officer and penal ideologies.

A prisoner's agreement is necessary before he or she can be transferred to a therapeutic-community regime and many prisoners refuse the offer of such transfers because they have a generalized fear of being psychiatrized or because they have a specific fear of being labelled 'nut cases' or 'nonces' (sex offenders). Furthermore, in men's prisons the macho ethic of being 'able to take prison' can sometimes militate against any attempts by 'do-gooders' to find ways of making the general atmosphere less tense. Certainly, prisoners make a strong point when they claim that if the authorities really wished to reduce tension in order to better the lot of prisoners (rather than for organizational-control purposes) they could do so by reducing prison overcrowding and the monotony and rigidity of the prison regimes. It appears, therefore, that until some serious attempt is made by the authorities to improve conditions in *all prisons*, prisoners will continue to view with suspicion the authorities' half-hearted and haphazard attempts to change *them*.

The supposedly democratic ethos of therapeutic communities is seen by many prison officers as being antithetical to the fundamental tenets of an hierarchically organized prison discipline. The contempt in which therapy (of any kind) is held by many prison officers was summed up for me by the prison officer who explained that the main functions of therapeutic-community settings in prisons have little to do with prisoners' psychiatric problems at all. According to him they exist: 'to contain those officers who are not happy in the main prison because they think we should be helping prisoners; to keep sex-offenders where they'll cause least trouble; and to let "do-gooders" think that prisoners who want to give up drugs and drink really can get help in prison.' An examination of contemporary penal rhetoric, ideology and practice makes me suspect that he is right.

The history of psychiatric penality has been one of unfulfilled promise, and this has been a continuing source of its power. For the need in a democracy to justify the state's power to punish has resulted in a perennial demand for future panaceas for present penal ills. For some time past the promise of 'small units' including 'specialized' therapeutic units has been the official answer to that demand. The official answer can be viewed with scepticism for several interrelated reasons.

First, there is still a strongly held belief in Home Office and prison circles that there is a popular and political demand that any prison regime which is not overwhelmingly punitive should justify its existence by providing statistical proof that it contributes to crime reduction. There is no such statistical evidence. Second, there has also been no evidence that any government is prepared to pay for the specialist prison-officer training and other specialist facilities that such units would demand. Third, the diagnostic problems relating to that group of offenders (defined as having 'personality disorders') who are presently seen as being the most likely candidates for such units means that there is not effective support for therapeutic regimes from prison psychiatrists. Fourth, it is not official policy to give to prison officers the type of specialist training that those involved in existing therapeutic-community regimes are already requesting in vain. Finally, many psychiatrists and prison personnel (even those committed to therapeutic-community regimes) will admit in private that the gaining of insight will do little to help those prisoners whose behaviour may indeed be very disturbed but who, nonetheless, are in prison mainly because they have fallen through the welfare net and who, upon release, will once more have to face homelessness, social isolation, poverty and blatent government indifference to their desperate situations.

Therapeutic-community type regimes at present cater for only a very small proportion of prison inmates. They function to contain the humanitarian impulse of a minority of prison officers and to ease some of the pains of imprisonment of those inmates who, in return for a superficially more democratic regime are prepared to demonstrate publicly a willingness 'to work at their problems'.[67] Additionally, they serve to contain those prisoners whose unacceptable behaviour has persisted undeterred by the system's more physical attempts to contain them. The Barlinnie Special Unit was set up 'in an attempt to find a better way of dealing with a group of violent and difficult prisoners who were proving unmanageable within the Scottish Prison System'.[68] A medical officer at Feltham Youth Custody Centre told me that in addition 'to those with a specific psychiatric disorder we also take those who have been "wrongly allocated" in other words, ones who've worn out the staff in other places, ones who've been down the block all the time in other prisons.' And, although I would not want to give the impression that Holloway's C1 Unit for the highly disturbed is a therapeutic unit, a recent description of it suggests that *any* specialized psychiatric unit is likely also to have a disciplinary function:

> When it was first opened in 1977 C1 had the primary function of holding and caring for the most disturbed women received into Holloway. The phrase 'disturbed' was double-edged. It was seen as referring to both psychiatrically ill women AND those whose behaviour or mental state was clearly disturbed, as evidenced by the difficulties they presented the prison in the management of their persistently disruptive behaviour, but who were not considered to be suffering from mental illness.[69]

For the reasons outlined above, any future development of small units (a development likely for control purposes)[70] will not necessarily result in an increase in the number of therapeutic-community type regimes. In the meantime, it appears that, both for treatment and control purposes, prison doctors, prison officers and prisoners alike have greater faith in the pharmaceutical fix.

The politics of pharmaceutical treatment in prisons

'One of the commonest accusations levelled against prison doctors is that they drug prisoners as a method of control.'[71] Prison doctors are the first to admit that the 'accusation' has some substance. Within prisons 'control' is not loaded with the emotive and negative meanings given to it by some of the prisons' more libertarian critics. Incidents can occur that are terrifying to staff and inmates alike and, on those occasions, staff, knowing that some prisoners have previously been in mental hospitals where they have been kept permanently sedated, resent being criticized for using drugs to control violent behaviour 'from which every other agency is copping out' (Deputy Governor).[72] In fact, many prisoners demand drugs and one prisoner told me that in retrospect she is glad that she was forcibly injected when, distraught to learn that the man she had stabbed had died, she began to lash out at prisoners and at prison officers. Other prisoners, as I have already mentioned, are convinced that forced injections are too readily used to control unruly (but not dangerous) prisoners.

Obviously, the issue of forced injections in prisons, as well as that of drug prescriptions in general, must be closely monitored. What Smith has called the popular press's 'prurient interest' in prisons has, nonetheless, had good effect in relation to prison medication . . . as he himself admits: 'These accusations [of controlling prisoners by the use of drugs] have had such an impact that in the last few years the prison department has taken to publishing figures on the amount of psychotropic drugs prescribed in various prisons.'[73] And here we touch on one of the central issues of penal politics – the extreme secrecy of the Home Office on matters of prison administration. Of course the issue of drugs in prison is a contentious one. Prison doctors are in an impossible position. Many of their prisoner-patients (especially women) will have been prescribed massive doses of drugs for years before they arrive at the prison. If the prison doctor continues the prescription there is the suspicion that the medicine is now being given *solely* for control purposes; if he or she discontinues it there is the accusation that the prisoner is being denied the medication that was legitimately prescribed outside. Furthermore, many prisoners put enormous pressure on doctors to prescribe drugs to ease the pains of imprisonment. Yet, all that being recognized, whilst the Home Office continues to cloak prison administration in an almost impenetrable secrecy, whilst some Prison Department officials continue to treat requests for information in a way that provokes thinking people into believing that they must have something to hide, prison doctors can expect to have all kinds of accusations levelled at them as concerned parties try to force the Home Office into a greater accountability for its administration of the prisons.[74]

The politics of the psychiatric diagnosis of offenders

Speaking in 1973 about the role of medical care in Norwegian prisons Nils Christie, a Norwegian criminologist, said, 'Recently there has been over-emphasis on using medical personnel for the diagnostic stage. A maximum of energy is used for giving advice to the courts and little is left for treatment.'[75] This sums up well the contemporary practise of psychiatry in British prisons. That the psychiatric diagnosis of offenders functions mainly to endow judicial proceedings with a spurious scientificity and prisons with an equally spurious element of rehabilitative treatment is not entirely the fault of psychiatrists. In addition to the limitations of psychiatric knowledge itself, there are also economic and political reasons why psychiatric diagnosis is seldom followed by psychiatric treatment.

Although there has been a steady increase in the numbers of defendants remanded for medical reports over the years, the majority of those who finally receive a prison sentence are assessed as having personality disorders that are untreatable under the terms of the Mental Health Act 1983. A hospital officer at Feltham Youth Custody Centre described the young men there: 'We have the boys who are too disturbed to go into a normal hospital and not disturbed enough for a Special Hospital. They are very sad, very damaged, most of our boys. By the time we get them, many of them have been through Care, Special Schools. And many are homeless.' Again and again I have spoken to prison officers who have argued that they should be specially trained to look after the 'sad' but, as I have argued elsewhere, in its simultaneous identification of 'personality disorder' *and* its refusal to recognise it as a category of treatable 'mental illness' psychiatry has succeeded in a masterly stroke of professional imperialism. Psychiatry has placed 'personality disorder' under a continuous erasure which ensures that at present there is neither a place whence it can be *ex*propriated nor a place to which it can be *a*ppropriated by any other intending 'experts' or professionals: 'We say, "If prison officers have to deal with them, prison officers need the training." Back comes the answer, "What kind of training, if psychiatrists can't do anything? " ' [75]

Some psychiatrists do believe that they could provide some help for offenders defined as having personality disorders but they cannot get them transferred to a hospital because 'open-door' mental hospitals are no longer secure enough to hold them.[77] The Senior Medical Officer at Wandsworth Prison described how this situation affects prisoners:

> Psychiatrists come here, assesses them, take the fee and then turn round and say 'Sorry, we can't take them under the terms of the Act.' Or even if they agree that they *should* take them they'll jump through all kinds of hoops to put off admitting them. Sometimes a psychiatrist will bring a nurse with him and then it depends more on the nurse than the doctor. The unions are so strong that if the nurse doesn't want the patient then he can't be transferred.

Even if an offender-patient is transferred to a Special Hospital, government financial cuts may mean that the actual treatment he or she receives is minimal.

In addition to psychiatry's continuing inability to offer treatment for a whole range of perceived behavioural abnormalities, forensic psychiatrists themselves have increasingly come to doubt that psychiatric diagnosis can be followed by effective treatment of the imprisoned patient. The physical conditions in some prisons make it impossible for the prison authorities to act on even the most basic psychiatric diagnosis, for example, that a prisoner has suicidal tendencies. The hospital wing at Wormwood Scrubs as it was in March 1985 is a case in point. It had no wards and could only hold 20 patients in individual cells. Any patient who was depressed or suicidal would be put in an ordinary non-protected cell, with springs on the door and a hot water pipe running up the wall on all of which he could injure himself. Staff shortages caused by the government's economic policy further aggravated the situation, as a hospital officer explained:

> There is nowhere for the patients to have association except on the landing. We let them out as often as the staffing situation will allow but they can't do anything except walk round and round this landing. It is totally unnecessary to hold prisoners in these conditions and totally irresponsible in those cases where we've already been told that the prisoner is depressed or suicidal.

Psychiatrists have also increasingly come to suspect that in the disciplinary conditions obtaining in prisons it is difficult to be sure that the cause of violent or other abnormal behaviour is not to be found in the prison itself. Mary Gordon believed that to be the case in 1922: 'I believe that 111 cases of violence, of which 33 ended by restraint of the girl by handcuffs last year, were not due to any other cause than a pathological state induced by the character of the disciplinary conditions which we impose in our prisons.'[78] More and more psychiatrists have since come to hold that view.[79]

Others have gone further. They believe that psychiatry has little to offer prison inmates since those with 'personality disorders' are not in prison primarily because they are essentially either bad, mad or sad but because they are the people that no other agency wants. This view, put to me by many people working in prisons, was most recently summed up by the Senior Medical Officer at Wandsworth Prison. In November 1984, I asked him, 'What can you do here for disturbed prisoners? ' He replied: 'The present government's cuts mean that they cut down on geriatric, drug centres and other facilities and the people who need those facilities now come to prison. All we can do for them is try to give them a change of scenery by moving them round to different prisons every now and again.' The humanitarianism and common sense of some prison officers lead them also to suggest that the disciplinary regimes of most prisons are inimical to the needs of the prisoners defined as having personality disorders but the prison officers know, even better than the psychiatrists, that modification of the present discipline code would not be acceptable to most of their colleagues. For, it is not some latter-day anomaly that brings the 'sad' and the 'dispossessed' into prisons. At least since the seventeenth-century prisons, asylums and workhouses have been *consistently* used to confine and discipline the poor, the unemployed, the unemployable and the socially inept. And while offical reports have consistently deplored this situation,[80] prison personnel have recognized that the mentally abnormal offender fulfils a useful function within the prison. In conversation with me several prison staff have echoed the words of Dr Dorothy Speed who said at a 1973 conference: 'If we have to have prisons it seems that we need the sad to help us manage the population inside.'[81]

Given, then, that the diagnosis of convicted offenders as being 'mentally abnormal' has only a minimal likelihood of resulting in their receiving any treatment either in a hospital or a prison, why do courts continue to remand for medical reports? Apart from the fact that many judges and magistrates are ignorant of the actual situation in the prisons and the mental hospitals, the medical remand has both a punitive and a legitimating function.

The punitive function of the psychiatric remand is best illustrated in relation to women's imprisonment. A former governor of Holloway Prison, Dr Bull, told the House of Commons Expenditure Committee in 1978 that remand in custody is 'simply a device to put women in prison for three weeks – perhaps just as a punitive way'.[82] An analysis of the sentences of women remanded to Holloway's C1 unit for the highly disturbed from November 1982 to May 1983 found as follows:

> Of all those on C1 for medical reports 25.6% went to court and were bailed, 32.9% went to court and were given a variety of non-custodial awards (ranging from case dismissed to probation), and 25% were given hospital orders. The remaining women went to normal location (11%), to another prison (1.2%) or were discharged (3.7%). *One must wonder if the 58% who were bailed or given non-custodial awards, together with the 25% given hospital orders could have been remanded to hospitals for medical reports or seen on bail.*[83]

Yet, though they occur, punitive medical remands are frowned upon by the Home Office. Principally and legitimately, the major function of the psychiatric remand is the legitimation of the court's final decision according to the canons of culpability and rights enshrined in medical jurisprudence.

The limits to psychiatric penality

The historical and contemporary practices and politics of forensic psychiatry as described in this essay suggest that whilst psychiatry has developed and retained an all-powerful grip on the assessment and diagnosis of criminals, its powers within the prisons have been limited. Within the prisons psychiatry has only been able to engage in practices that have either the ideological function of appearing to answer the continuing (though nowadays muted) demand that imprisonment should mean more than the locking up of prisoners, or the function of legitimating the mechanical, physical or pharmaceutical control of prisoners whose behaviour threatens to disrupt prison discipline. Many psychiatrists would like to do more for prisoners than present prison conditions allow.

Disenchanted with previous psychiatric attempts at rehabilitation many argue that they would be content to contribute merely towards a more 'humane containment' of prisoners. It is unlikely that they will be given the chance. On the one hand, commentators as far apart as Boyle and Butler argue that special therapeutic units do *not* necessarily require psychiatric supervision[84] whilst, on the other hand, the ideological tenacity of the 'cure for crime' myth was displayed in the last major inquiry into British prisons where May argued that ' "humane containment" suffers from the fatal defect that it is a means without an end.'[85] What May did not foresee was that, under the present government with its emphasis on retribution, it has at last become respectable official policy to proclaim publicly what has often been expressed privately – that imprisonment never has been anything more than an end in itself.

In conclusion, it is argued that although *the criminal* has been psychiatrized in the name of medical jurisprudence, *the prison* has withstood psychiatrization. The promises of forensic psychiatry, the humanitarian urges of liberal reformers, the triumph of medicine over religion – all were insufficient to establish psychiatry as the dominant power within the prison. The penal site that forensic psychiatry sought to conquer was always-already occupied by a phalanx of competing discourses too powerful to dislodge. The triumph of penality is that by continual discursive realignments, the meanings of criminality and the aims of imprisonment forever reside in a definitional void. Into this void forensic psychiatry has itself been drawn. In return for prestige and limited powers, psychiatry has been assimilated by modern penality and medical jurisprudence, and, within the prisons, it has been refashioned as one more weapon in the prison's never-ending quest for ideological justification of its power to punish.

9

Psychiatry as a problem of democracy

Colin Gordon

Some of the most powerful critics of psychiatry have been psychiatrists or psychotherapists: R. D. Laing and David Cooper in Britain, Thomas Szasz in the USA, Franco Basaglia in Italy, Felix Guattari in France. Others have been sociologists: Erving Goffman and, later, Andrew Scull in the USA and Robert Castel in France. Others, again, have approached psychiatry from other disciplines or from none: Michel Foucault was classified, at least in his own country, principally as a philosopher; a number of recent British contributors to the debate have backgrounds in branches of theoretical and applied psychology. A considerable impetus for enquiry and criticism has, of course, also come from the experiences and dissatisfactions not only of the working personnel of psychiatric services but of their clients and patients as well.

I should like to begin here with a look at the sociologists. How far, and in what ways, can sociology be expected to throw light on the problems of psychiatry? Some examples suggest that the answer is by bringing to bear a faculty of detachment, a fresh gaze, rather than an authoritative expertise. Goffman's *Asylums* is a work of great conceptual sophistication, but (although of course this is not really a paradox) its classic value consists in its achievement as a *description*: Goffman devised and put to work a way of describing the structures of everyday existence in an asylum.[1] Although Robert Castel's work has a different direction, it shares something of the spirit of

Goffman's. Castel's enterprise might be called an attempt at a descriptive macrosociology of the formation and trans-formation of psychiatric practices.[2] Among other things, his books are contributions to modern and contemporary history, general histories of a particular problem – like some of the classic sociological writings, and also those of Foucault, to which they acknowledge a substantial debt. It is customary now to look back with complacency on a vanished past when histories of psychiatry were hagiographies compiled for self-serving corporate ends by members of the profession itself. But it is also true that today the most valuable extant studies of the field are the work of others than professional historians.

But can one speak of a sociological perspective on psychiatry in the sense of a set of particular sociological theses that adjudicate on those issues that have been contested with such public vigour and asperity since the coming of anti-psychiatry: the nature, function and value of psychiatric knowledge and practice; the nature, origin and appropriate treatment of the phenomena psychiatry diagnoses and treats as mental illness? We might be tempted to say that the main contribution of sociology in this context is to permit a more analytical dis-crimination between these several points of contention. An account of the social forces that shape the public vocation entrusted to psychiatry may perfectly well be undertaken with-out, for example, a prior obligation to adjudicate whether the past or present descriptions by psychiatry of those consigned to its care constitute an act of diagnosis or merely one of labelling. The results of such an analysis might, in turn, con-ceivably help to clarify our ideas as to what political or ethical criteria can most relevantly be brought to bear on the latter argument.

But a rather stronger set of results – or of worthwhile hypotheses – might also be envisaged. This would be a char-acterization of the distinctive features of those societies in which there occur the specific practices we identify under the name psychiatry. Such a characterization would consist of two elements. First, it would entail an evaluation of the extent to which psychiatry's existence corresponds to specific structures of demand, particular modes of individual and collective con-duct, forms of social stratification, kinds of prevalent power-relations, etc. Second, it would be an appraisal not only of the various problems of societies to which it is the overt or effective *raison d'être* of psychiatry to minister, but also of the extent to which the problems posed in or by psychiatry itself are, in a more general sense, problems of and for a certain general type of society – problems that reflect, implicate or call in question a society's nature and its future. In this essay I should like to review our existing resources and materials for the treatment of these questions. I shall suggest that despite, or because of, the polemical animus of recent psycho-political arguments, these lines of analysis have not been pursued as fully or thoroughly as might be wished. This is not, however, to say that the controversies conducted since the appearance of anti-psychiatry have been a long history of error. Perhaps some recent misconceptions have still not been fully disposed of: I shall air some opinions on this below. But I shall also try to show where the recent literature remains rich in perspectives and insights whose value is far from exhausted. It may be that, contrary to appearances, the present politico-intellectual climate – one more marked by the recognition of uncertainty than by triumphs of critical conviction – is becoming more propitious to a search for new ways of configuring questions about psychiatry within the wider framework of our social and political reflection. It is to the extent that we are disposed to reappraise the problems of democracy that we may be able to find a fresh viewpoint on psychiatry, as one among such problems.

One of the ways left sociology came into confluence with the ideas of anti-psychiatry was through its interest in the notion of deviancy. This was also one of sociology's most ambitious attempts to comment not only on the existence of psychiatry as a sociological fact, but on the inner validity of psychiatric thought and activity. Psychiatric judgments could be exposed as a theoretical transcription of culturally arbitrary sanctions against conduct stigmatized within a given society as 'deviant'. The deviancy theorists who thought Foucault supported their positions were in fact inverting his argument. As early as in his *Maladie mentale et personnalité* (1954), Foucault places the concept of deviance as part of the problem, not part of the answer, for a history of madness. One of the two key questions that book proposed for examination was, 'How did our culture come to give mental illness the meaning of deviancy, and to the patient a status that excludes him? '[3] In 1961 his *Histoire de la folie* documented his argument for the view that 'the fact that we can find a resemblance between the internees of the eighteenth century and our own contemporary figure of the asocial individual is indeed a fact, but probably one that belongs to the order of results: for that figure was brought into being as an effect of the act of internment itself.'[4]

To view 'deviancy' as the developed, culturally specific product of a collective apparatus of perception and manipulation, rather than as its malleable raw material, can be a step towards enhancing the ambit of sociological reflection concerning psychiatry. To concede the existence of 'madness' as an anthropological quasi-universal arguably makes it easier to allow proper weight to the immensely variable character and effect of what Foucault called the 'experience of madness', a term intended here to mean principally the social experience of others' madness and, in a larger sense, the relation between the treatment of madness within a society and corresponding structures of general social experience.

Foucault's *Histoire de la Folie* has an especially percipient treatment of the way psychiatry's beginnings are interlinked with a kind of reflexive intensification of that relationship, a development that is, in turn, one of the phenomena characteristically associated with a *consciousness of modernity*. Foucault's ideas have been taken up in a highly interesting book by the German social psychiatrist Klaus Dörner, *Bürger und Irre*, and developed by him as the thesis that the appearance in the different European nations of a fully fledged psychiatry has in each case been conditional on the existence of a culture capable of critically diagnosing its own ills – including the incidence of mental disorders – as symptoms of its own modernity.[5] The formation of this new kind of reflexive social time-consciousness, itself conditional on the presence of a certain range of cultural and political practices (a literary and political press, a public space of argument and critique, and the other political rudiments of a 'civil society') nurtures the social sensibility to the social ill of insanity that, in Dörner's view, is the true historic basis of psychiatry.

One of the interesting features of this hypothesis is its connection both to anti-psychiatric ideas of the present and to an ultimately benign view of the mission of psychiatry. The idea of madness as an ill of civilization and modernity leads, in one direction, to the idea of madness as a social creation and of the 'mad' as society's casualties, if not its victims. In another direction, it institutes psychiatry as the work of Enlightenment. Psychiatry is cast here as society's critical consciousness of its own self and its present, its task the restitution of injuries suffered in the adventure of its modernity. Dörner, who draws so heavily here on Foucault's earlier achievement, criticizes him in this regard as an unmitigated debunker of the Enlightenment aspiration. This is surely a mistake; in later years Foucault appears to have convinced even so severe an exponent of this accusation as Jürgen Habermas of its falsity. Esteem for the Enlightenment idea is one thing; unwillingness to scrutinize its sequels is, on the other hand, itself a pious betrayal of its real meaning. A more consistent path is to extend critical reflection to cover the phenomena of society's psychiatric sensibility and their effects as a further and intrinsic problem of modernity. A critical psychiatry has often been supposed to demand a deeper anthropological doctrine capable of denouncing the distortions inflicted upon true humanity by society, distortions that manifest themselves under the appearances of psychiatric illness. The alternative possibility, towards which the present remarks are intended to point, is that the most pragmatically effective direction for anthropological reflection concerning the problem of psychiatry might actually be provided by a political sociology.

The beginnings of psychiatry are bound up not only with the cultural ethos of Enlightenment but also with the political roots of modern liberalism and democracy, and their basis in the shaping of distinctive norms of political citizenship. From its outset the new mental medicine is grounded in the forms of opinion, judgment, scandal and sanction proper to a public political consciousness. In the French case, where the therapeutic internment of the insane is preceded and prepared by the revolutionary suppression of the administrative internment of other categories of 'deviance', Foucault notes how the ordinary citizen is attributed under the Revolution a dual role previously held by the police: 'at once "man of the law" and "man of government" '. The treatment of derangement or disorder becomes at once a civic duty and an affair of state.

It is as a citizen that the individual may be subjected to a specifically medical regime of constraint, and it is to the qualities of a citizen that mental medicine undertakes to restore the incapacitated subject. The known historic deficiencies of this regime – the rigour of its tutelage, the lesser certainty of its medications – need in turn to be seen in relation to the limits and ambiguities of the corresponding model of social citizenship. Broadly speaking, in the early liberal period, not everyone is a member of society – not necessarily or simply on account of qualifications of status or property, but because the social body is itself conceived as confronted by an amorphous, asocial population, a pauperized mass deficient in the fundamental habits of sociality: order, industry, providence, the pursuit of betterment. Citizenship similarly connotes not the automatic fact of universal equality but a model of integrated economic and political conduct that social policy strives to propagate, teach and enforce. This strategic configuration has another and harsher side that figures largely in the history of psychiatry. Psychiatry functions, not indeed as a centrepiece, but as one wing of a nineteenth-century strategy of transcribing problems of collective order, social, political and economic, into problems of morality; that sector of the population that cannot be assimilated to society by methods of improvement must be neutralized as a social danger. The meaning of psychiatry as a social medicine undergoes here a profound modification of its sometime Enlightenment principles.

By the mid-nineteenth century, psychiatry had acquired a new way of connecting mental illness, society and history. At one time luxury and idle wealth had been identified as principal pathogenic factors in the modern environment. In the nineteenth century the accent shifts towards squalor and idle poverty. The insane degenerate pauper is no longer a casualty of progress, but rather the detritus of evolution. Madness now becomes the

> stigmata of a class which has abandoned the forms of bourgeois ethics; and at the very moment when the philosophical concept of alienation acquired a historical meaning through the economic analysis of labour, the medical and psychological concept of alienation frees itself totally from history, to become instead a moral critique in the name of the compromised salvation of the species.[6]

Contemporary neo-liberalism is not a revived form of social Darwinism; the whole strategic basis of social order and normalization has been transformed too fundamentally in the present century for these past expedients to be cited merely as a basis for an extrapolation of present dangers. But it may not be impossible to identify equivalents of the *form* of ambiguity pinpointed by Foucault, within the terms of our present prospects, in modern political postures towards the psychiatrized: more subtle methodologies of security, new ways of index-linking citizenship to social obligation.

One way in which to draw together the current problems of public policy in relation to psychiatry might be through an appraisal of the latter's linkage with two values or principles: community and citizenship. The former term is itself notorious for the multiplicity and polyvalence of the uses to which it is put in the present domain of reflections on social policy. Most or all of these ambiguities need to be vigilantly registered where one is dealing with psychiatry; indeed, psychiatry has itself been a major original contributor to the language of community. A rapid inventory of these inflections of vocabulary may help to clarify some corresponding questions of strategy.

Psychiatric care located and conducted 'in the community' is now an ideal shared perhaps by a majority consensus of interested opinion. It is also, not insignificantly, the habitual mode of formulation of a negative demand: the demand for a psychiatry that is, by common consent, no longer to be principally domiciled in specialized psychiatric hospitals. 'The community' is a term that can connote a (politically variable) multiplicity of values and virtues; this multiplicity can, in turn, amount to a convenient indeterminacy. The prevailing public consensus around the principle of relocating psychiatric services into 'the community' arguably depends to a considerable degree on the way in which the labile suggestiveness of the latter term serves to obscure the component of incoherence, indefinition or sheer wishful thinking in existing specifications of the institutions, practices and professional–administrative structures that are proposed.

But this status of the term 'community' as a polyvalent positive counterposed to the uncontroversial negative of asylum psychiatry perhaps only unfolds its full complexity when we consider that the institution of the asylum itself and the ideal of community are by no means historical strangers to one another; on the contrary. The 'miraculous coincidence' that harmonized the carceral powers of the alienists with their therapeutic vocation – the imperative medical demand for the separation of the mentally ill from their previous social environment – did not, in general, correspond to a habit of medical indifference to the interpersonal social determinants of mental health. The method of moral treatment in the asylum involved, at least among its intentions, the principle of a restitution of the patient as social being through immersion in an artificial environment that would be a kind of super-community, a milieu supercharged with restitutive moral influences. Even the authoritarian, not to say punitive measures often espoused by the alienists were a reflection, rather than a contradiction, of this conception of therapy and community. In differing forms, something like this idea of an organized (clarified, simplified) intensification of community has been and no doubt remains one of the most esteemed remedies of psychiatric therapy. The anti-psychiatric movement itself had its beginnings in Laing's post-war experience of the 'therapeutic community' methods developed by Maxwell Jones – methods that were also taken up as a model by Basaglia and the *Psichiatria Democratica* movement in Italy, among others.[7] While these ideas developed, on the one hand, into the practical core of the anti-psychiatric enterprises pursued, in precarious and isolated circumstances, by Laing and others, the majority of extant therapeutic communities have existed and perhaps continue to exist as local enclaves within already existing psychiatric hospitals.

There is no particular occasion here for irony at anyone's expense, and it would be highly misleading to suggest any general affinity between the principles of the therapeutic community and the character of actually existing asylums throughout the history of modern psychiatry. But it may be relevant to note in this context the extent to which a great variety of at least temporarily prestigious innovations in psychiatric therapy have been linked, albeit in a tangential or inadvertent manner, to some kind of 'community effect' within the asylum, that is, to the creation among medical personnel and patients alike of a collective atmosphere of enthusiasm, optimism and purpose, an atmosphere to which it may well be plausible to credit some remarkable, if transitory improvements in the institutions' levels of therapeutic success. In some cases this appears to have been the unplanned effect and the cause of the supposed clinical efficacy of somatic therapies that inspired intense professional enthusiasm in their day and are now entirely discredited, such as the technique of insulin-shock therapy. As an opposite extreme, but still as an instance relevant to our theme, one might cite the work of Franco Basaglia and his associates in reforming, transforming and, in some cases, actually closing down the psychiatric hospitals under their authority, a process centred around an intense and continuous practice of collective discussion involving personnel and patients alike.[8] The possibility of such an achievement undoubtedly derived from the existence at the time of a wider climate of political mobilization that, in many parts of Italy, corresponded to a kind of social revolution. At the same time, one of its most interesting and impressive features was the positive quality of the new connections established between the medical and politico-communal registers: patients in these institutions perceived their own political protest and struggle against repressive and carceral treatments as an endeavour mutually bound up with their struggle to recover their own health. The singular and more-or-less transitory character of each of these episodes does not detract from their instructive value. Indeed, one might well further extend the scope of these reflections to make mention of a related phenomenon, the well-attested tendency for recorded levels of psychiatric illness to fall during times of war, a phenomenon that may not implausibly be taken, at least in part, as the by-product of a concerted mobilization and intensification of solidarity within 'the community'.

One must underline that none of these considerations justify cynicism about the prospects for future kinds of community such as are currently being proposed. One can merely note that, while some of the ideas enshrined in the idea of 'community' have an honourable and credible place among available therapeutic options, they are not in themselves unknown to the psychiatry of past and present, and their efficacy, while often real, has not often been sustainable: the asylum and the community are alike at least in the sense that both ideas have been objects at times imaginarily invested with extravagant virtues and powers. The notion of an ethical-topological opposition between asylum and 'community' – between, respectively, a closed space of repression and internment and an open space of liberty and solidarity – is, in some respects, both paradoxical and unreal. The asylum has sometimes harboured a 'community': the 'community' into which policies of decarceration may propose to decant the populations of the interned is not necessarily likely to be a recognizable incarnation of the highest values evoked by its name.

Such a lesson has been demonstrated through the effects of some American policies of psychiatric reform that have transformed the former populations of closed hospitals into an oppressed underclass of semi-vagrants. This particular adverse precedent does not, of course, prove that all policies for a community psychiatry must lead to such results. But it underlines, at least, a minimal and fairly uncontroversial cautionary consideration, namely that the diminution of public fear and intolerance of psychiatry's clientele that (in combination with developments in medication) has probably been one of the conditions of feasibility of a dismantling of the asylum system, can reasonably be expected to disperse and relocate, but not of itself to do away with all the previous abuses, injustices and servitudes undergone by the psychiatrically disturbed. Asylum walls are not the only means of social invisibility. These problems can be illustrated from the remarkable and historically venerable case of the Flemish village of Geel, whose lay inhabitants accomodate in their homes, under a minimum of formal constraint, psychiatric patients who might under other circumstances have been expected to be hospitalized. Not all accounts of Geel testify without reservation to the libertarian qualities of such a solution in which the population of civil society takes upon itself with a will (and for a remuneration) the tutelary duties of the collectivity.

Few reformers today would believe that a mere attempt to set up the most unmediated custodial relationship between society at large and 'its' psychiatric patients will lead to the most satisfactory results in either political or medical terms. A more plausible and serious eventuality may be guessed at if, on the other hand, one takes into consideration some further meanings and tactics invested in the term 'community'. It is probably a significant indicator of the political conjunction of our time that the currency of this term is now so equivocally shared between, on the one hand, projects and practices of collective solidarity, mobilization and mutuality and, on the other, policies of specialized security and pacification. A 'community psychiatry' might develop in the future that owed more to the latter series of precedents than the former: 'community psychiatry' might come to assume a meaning analogous – *mutatis mutandis* – with that of 'community policing'. Recalling the American example mentioned above, it might not be extravagant to envisage a psychiatric version of 'community' that amounted to a kind of institutionalized semi-ghettoization: an assimilation of the management of the disturbed into the repertoire of special measures and techniques deployed to govern those problem-regions of the social body distinguished by special concentrations of risk and handicap. For the ethnic minorities, it has been suggested that something like such a 'community psychiatry' already exists (see chapter 4).

The language of 'community' deserves, in psychiatric discussion as elsewhere, to be taken both seriously and vigilantly. The kind of attention it most demands involves more than the routine procedures of ideological critique, the unmasking of politically culpable mystification and manoeuvre. It is rather that, as was noted above in regard to the various dimensions of the 'social' in psychiatry, the vocabulary of community expresses – in its distinctive and politically non-reducible terms – the ways in which the intrinsic dilemmas and hazards of psychiatric policy choices implicate a diverse range of current scenarios and potentialities affecting what may be termed, for want of a better formula, the orientation of the communal constitution of society. 'Community psychiatry', like psychiatry in general, encounters in its own terms a modern equivalent of the historical options described by Foucault in his remarks on the notion of alienation, between a paradigm of enlightenment and a paradigm of prophylaxis.

Analysis of the notion of community can be supplemented here by re-evaluation of another term we have seen to be fundamental to psychiatric politics – that of citizenship. The historical studies of Foucault and Castel draw attention to the fact that psychiatry has, virtually since its inception, been entrusted by society with a wider mandate than might have been deduced solely from a sober appraisal of its medical capabilities, and that this vocation converged with a set of epistemological changes that established the specific psychiatric conception of mental illness through a process that at the same time had the effect of detaching psychiatry from an older tradition of continuities between mental and general medicine. Their analyses, which offer us the most convincing extant interpretation of these developments, are linked to a hypothesis concering the new and specific form of social demand that the new mental medicine was called upon to satisfy; and it would not be inaccurate to describe this new demand as amounting, in its essence, to a problem of citizenship. In a bourgeois polity committed to the principles of legality and liberty, the public significations of insanity, in its dual aspect of political and legal incompetence, and social disorder or scandal, have demanded a regime of treatment capable of simultaneously and harmoniously satisfying society's demand, on its own behalf, for constitutionally acceptable measures for the preservation of norms of order and conduct, and its demand, on behalf of the individual affected, for measures of treatment capable of the restitution of his/her status and faculties as subject and citizen.

It has always been true of psychiatry that it functions as a political technology, and of Western liberal societies that they utilize psychiatry as such a technology, but these truths are only half of the story. What is really constitutive both of psychiatry and, correspondingly, of the specific form of liberal society that is still our own, is the inseparable superposition of the dual demands of order and restitution. It is by no means implicit in the kinds of analysis proposed by Foucault or Castel that the demand for civil restitution operates in reality only as a palatable cover for an imperative of political order. Such a supposition does not really offer the best possible guide to an understanding of how the problems concerning the functioning of psychiatry that pose themselves in our society are also, in a deeper sense, problems that touch on the constitution of our societies themselves. The basic duality of the demand our society addresses to psychiatry is fundamental for psychiatry and characteristic of our society.

The ways in which these demands are conjoined in the specific terms of psychiatry's mandate and its methods have indeed been historically realized in highly variable ways, with significant corresponding repercussions for society as a whole. At one extreme, a prophylactic philosophy of 'social defence' can bind the medical salvation of society to a rigorous segregation of the unfit; at another, a therapeutic activism can collaborate with an egalitarian recasting of structures of collective organization; and it is far from uncommon for actual practice to hybridize these seemingly contrary strategies. But, across all these possible combinations and variations, it remains necessary to recognize that each of these basic demands for and on psychiatry – the demand society makes specifically in terms of the self-interest of the collectivity, and the demand it makes on behalf of its incapacitated individual citizen – always retains its separate and irreducible force. *This* circumstance is unlikely to be altered by the realization of even the most radical transformations currently within the compass of our political imagination.

To see psychiatric affairs as thus inscribed within an inherently strained and ambiguous, highly mobile but ultimately inescapable constellation of forces, to recognize that society's confrontation with psychiatry and the psychiatrized is also, in more than a platitudinous sense, a confrontation with itself, may help clarify, among other things, the often tortuous ways in which psychiatry impinges on the public sensibility. It illuminates the trade-offs and feedbacks between the scandal of madness and the scandals of psychiatric internment, or between fear or intolerance of the disturbed and deviant, and fear and mistrust of professional power. Scapegoating, complicity and authentic disquiet are apt to commingle here in a dubious cocktail. Perhaps one salutary step forward in this area of discussion would be a reassessment of the connections between citizenship and expertise. One of the important strengths of Castel's work is its accent on the character of psychiatry as an expertise, as a special knowledge that confers special powers: psychiatric expertise as a tutelage legitimated by knowledge. A feature of the anti-psychiatric period that has perhaps not had sufficient notice is that criticisms of psychiatric expertise have by no means generally been conceived as criticisms of medical/therapeutic expertise in general. Some of the fiercest salvoes directed at the strictly medical pretensions of psychiatry have originated from exponents of rival expertises with unsatisfied demands for professional authority. Indeed, while it is always legitimate and necessary to insist on inspection of both the knowledge-claims and the power-claims of particular expertises, there is no immediately obvious case for seeking the radical elimination of expertise, or (more loosely) specialized professional competence from the field of activity currently occupied by psychiatry and its competitors. Only an extravagantly credulous faith in the Rousseauist virtues of 'the community', or 'civil society', could license such a move. A more rational course might be to explore ways of answering society's need, relative to psychiatric expertise or its aspiring substitutes, on the one hand for *resources alternative and complementary to expertise as such* and, on the other, for norms of professional conduct that recognize the requirement for inner qualitative constraints on the exercise of expertise: more precisely, for a critical consciousness of *the citizenship of expertise.*

One main way towards meeting these demands will surely be through the further pursuit of the valuable initiatives developed in recent years for the safeguard or restoration of the civil rights of the psychiatrized. 'Community psychiatry' ought thus be made to mean, at least, that the principle of citizenship is not merely a component in the ideal terms of specification of therapeutic objectives, but a continuous criterion of therapeutic action. A further and complementary means towards meeting the double need formulated above would be a broader examination of the empirical modalities of collective demand for psychiatry, the social 'surfaces of emergence' (in Foucault's phrase) of psychiatric need. This kind of analysis need not, and indeed should not be predicated on partisan convictions about the validity of psychiatric diagnosis or, conversely, the necessity of preventive intervention within the social body by psychiatric or other expert agencies. Restriction of therapeutic intervention or of access to therapy need not be a ruling motive here; on the other hand, it should arguably be a significant part of the work of any future community psychiatry to put at the disposal of the community a more thorough and detailed knowledge of the social pathways to psychiatrization. Where this has already been done, notably for example in the study of depression among housewives, the results have been significant both therapeutically and politically. There is still much work remaining to be done by a sociology of psychiatric affairs.

Notes

1 Critiques of psychiatry and critical sociologies of madness

1 Foucault's classic study is of course his *Histoire de la folie* (Paris, Gallimard, 1972) which is still only available in English in a drastically abridged edition published as *Madness and Civilization – a history of insanity in the age of reason* (London, Tavistock, 1967). The most stimulating of Castel's studies is his *L'Ordre psychiatrique* (Paris, Editions de Minuit, 1976); see also the study of American psychiatry by F. Castel, R. Castel and A. Lovell, *The Psychiatric Society* (New York, Columbia University Press, 1982).

2 Castel, *L'Ordre psychiatrique*.

3 On psychiatry in France, in addition to Castel's *L'Ordre psychiatrique* see his *La Gestion des risques* (Paris, Editions de Minuit, 1981). On psychiatry in the USA, see D. J. Rothman, *The Discovery of the Asylum: social order and disorder in the New Republic* (Boston, Little, Brown & Co., 1971) and *Conscience and Convenience: the asylum and its alternatives in Progressive America* (Boston, Little, Brown & Co., 1980).

4 Castel, *L'Ordre psychiatrique*, p. 271.

5 There is a useful discussion of the model of the Gheel colony in William Ll, Parry-Jones, 'The model of the Geel Lunatic Colony and its influence on the nineteenth-century asylum system in Britain', in Andrew Scull (ed.), *Madhouses, Mad-Doctors and Madmen: the social history of psychiatry in the Victorian era* (London, The Athlone Press, 1981).

6 See, for instance, the views expressed in Anthony Clare, *Psychiatry in Dissent*, 2nd edn (London, Tavistock, 1980).

7 See the discussions of moral treatment in Michael Donnelly, *Managing the Mind: a study of medical psychology in early nineteenth-century*

Britain (London, Tavistock, 1983); and Nikolas Rose, *The Psychological Complex: psychology, politics and society in England 1869–1939* (London: Routledge & Kegan Paul, 1985).

8 The expression comes from Castel, *L'Ordre psychiatrique*, p. 278.

9 On these issues see the discussion by Nikolas Rose in chapter 6 of this volume.

10 On these issues in France see Castel, *L'Ordre psychiatrique*, and my discussion of his book in 'The territory of the psychiatrist', *I & C* (Autumn 1980), 63–105.

11 See, for instance, G. Baruch and A. Treacher, *Psychiatry Observed* (London, Routledge & Kegan Paul, 1978), as well as A. Treacher and G. Baruch 'Towards a critical history of the psychiatric profession', in D. Ingleby (ed.), *Critical Psychiatry* (Harmondsworth, Penguin, 1981). See also the account by Andrew Scull in *Museums of Madness: the social organization of insanity in nineteeth-century England* (London, Allen Lane, 1979).

12 See Scull, *Museums of Madness*.

13 B. Morel, *Traité des dégénérescences physiques, intellectuelles, et morales de l'espèce humaine* (Paris, 1857).

14 Cited in Castel, *L'Ordre psychiatrique*, p. 280.

15 See Andrew Scull, *Decarceration: community treatment and the deviant – a radical view*, 2nd edn (Cambridge, Polity Press, 1984).

16 See the remarks on this subject in Castel, *La Gestion*.

17 See, for instance, on this question M. Jones, *Social Psychiatry* (London, Tavistock, 1952); R. D. Hinshelwood and N. Manning, *Therapeutic Communities: reflections and progress* (London, Routledge & Kegan Paul, 1979).

18 See W. R. Barton, *Institutional Neurosis* (Bristol, John Wright & Sons, 1959).

19 Unfortunately there is little of Basaglia's writings translated into English. See, however his 'Problems of law and psychiatry: the Italian experience', *International Journal of Law and Psychiatry*, 3 (1) (1980), 17–36. See also F. Basaglia and F. Basaglia (eds), *Les Criminels de paix* (Paris, Presses Universitaires de France, 1980). There is a forthcoming edition of Franco Basaglia's writings, edited by Anne Lovell and Nancy Scheper-Hughes, *Psychiatry Inside Out: Selected Writings of Franco Basaglia* (New York, Columbia University Press, 1986).

20 See E. Goffman, *Asylums: essays on the social situation of mental patients and other inmates* (New York, Doubleday, 1962).

21 See the views of John Wing in *Reasoning about Madness* (Oxford, Oxford University Press, 1978).

22 Clare, *Psychiatry in Dissent*, p. 161.

23 See, in particular, the arguments in Treacher and Baruch, 'Towards a critical history'.

24 See D. Armstrong, *Political Anatomy of the Body: medical knowledge in Britain in the twentieth century* (Cambridge, Cambridge University Press, 1983); see also Rose, *Psychological Complex*.

25 Castel's *La Gestion* has some interesting remarks on this issue.

26 Castel, *La Gestion*, pp. 9–17.

27 T. J. Scheff, *Being Mentally Ill* (Chicago, Aldine, 1966); D. L. Rosenhan, 'On being sane in insane places', *Science*, 179 (1973) 250–8.

28 S. Cohen and A. Scull (eds), *Social Control and the State* (Oxford, Martin Robertson, 1983).

29 There is a useful discussion of the notion of 'revisionist' history in M. Ignatieff, 'State, civil society and total institutions; a critique of recent social histories of punishment', in Cohen and Scull, *Social Control and the State*.

30 Scull, *Museums of Madness*.

31 Ibid., p. 17.

32 N. Kittrie, *The Right to be Different* (Baltimore, Johns Hopkins University Press, 1971); Scull, *Museums of Madness*.

33 Treacher and Baruch, 'Towards a critical history'.

34 See G. Rosen, 'Cameralism and the concept of medical police', *Bulletin for the History of Medicine* 27 (1953), 21–42; 'The philosophy of ideology and the emergence of modern medicine in France', *Bulletin for the History of Medicine* 20 (1946), 328–39.

35 Armstrong, *Political Anatomy of the Body*.

36 See the remarks by David Armstrong on the notion of coping in *Political Anatomy of the Body*.

37 Cohen and Scull, *Social Control and the State*.

38 See the discussion of the notion of social control in M. Janowitz, *The Last Half Century* (Chicago, 1978).

39 A. Scull, 'Humanitarianism or control? Some observations on the historiography of Anglo-American psychiatry', in Cohen and Scull, *Social Control and the State*.

40 See David Ingleby's useful discussion of the literature in 'Mental health and social order', in Cohen and Scull, *Social Control and the State*.

41 The main texts from which the following discussion is drawn are: Foucault, *Histoire de la folie*; Castel, *L'Ordre psychiatrique*; and M. Foucault, *Mental Illness and Psychology* (New York, Harper & Row, 1976).

42 Foucault, *Histoire de la folie*, pp. 126–31.

43 Ibid., pp. 404–5.

44 See my review of *L'Ordre psychiatrique*, 'The territory of the psychiatrist'.

45 Castel, Castel and Lovell, *The Psychiatric Society*.

46 Rose, *Psychological Complex*.

47 K. Döerner, *Madmen and the Bourgeoisie* (Oxford, Basil Blackwell, 1981).

48 Scull, *Decarceration*.

49 This notion of 'surfaces of emergence' is drawn from M. Foucault, *The Archaeology of Knowledge* (London, Tavistock, 1972), p. 41.

50 On these different issues see, respectively, J. Donzelot, *The Policing of Families* (London, Hutchinson, 1980); Castel, Castel and Lovell,

The Psychiatric Society; Rose, *Psychological Complex*; M. Foucault, 'About the concept of the "dangerous individual" in 19th-century legal psychiatry', *International Journal of Law and Psychiatry*, 1 (1978), 1–18; and my discussion of the interrelations of mental health and employment in chapter 5 of this volume.

51 M. Foucault, *The History of Sexuality* (Harmondsworth, Penguin, 1981), vol. 1, *An Introduction*.

52 The most recent acute example of such a misunderstanding is to be found in K. Jones and A. J. Fowles, *Ideas on Institutions: analysing the literature on long-term care and custody* (London, Routledge & Kegan Paul, 1984), chapter 2.

53 On the notion of 'technologies of the self ', See M. Foucault, *L'Usage des plaisirs* (Paris, Gallimard, 1984) and *Le Souci de soi* (Paris, Gallimard, 1984). These are volumes two and three, respectively, of the French edition of Foucault's *History of Sexuality*.

54 M. Foucault, *Discipline and Punish – the birth of the prison* (London, Allen Lane, 1977).

2   Psychiatry: the discipline of mental health

1 I use the term 'psychiatry' here to refer to all those disciplines concerned with the troubles and disorders of conduct, emotion and thought and the conditions for mental health. It thus has a wider reference than the medical specialism.

2 This literature is extensively discussed and referenced by Peter Miller in chapter 1 of this volume.

3 Whilst nineteenth-century psychiatry has been much analysed (see the discussion and references in chapter 1 of this volume), there are few adequate accounts of developments in psychiatry in Britain during this century. In an essay of this sort it is not appropriate to provide an extensive bibliographic apparatus referring to primary sources; by and large I have confined myself to referencing more detailed secondary sources on particular topics. Each of these provides references to primary material that the interested reader may follow up.

4 This material is discussed in detail in Nikolas Rose, *The Psychological Complex: psychology, politics and society in England 1869–1939* (London, Routledge & Kegan Paul, 1985), esp. ch. 6. See also David Armstrong, *Political Anatomy of the Body: medical knowledge in Britain in the twentieth century* (Cambridge, Cambridge University Press, 1983).

5 Rose, *Psychological Complex*, pp. 131–5, 146–58. See also Armstrong, *Political Anatomy*.

6 Rose, *Psychological Complex*, esp. pp. 177–9. See also George Rosen, 'Social stress and mental disease from the 18th century to the present: some origins of social psychiatry', *Millbank Memorial Fund Quarterly*, 37 (5) 1959.

7 Rose, *Psychological Complex*.

8 Ibid., pp. 164–6, 180–91. See also Armstrong, *Political Anatomy*, pp. 19–31.

9 Rose, *Psychological Complex*, pp. 182–3. See L. S. Hearnshaw, *A Short History of British Psychology, 1840–1940* (London, Methuen, 1964), pp. 245–6 for a concise account of the debate.

10 Rose, *Psychological Complex*, pp. 197–209.

11 Royal Commission on Lunacy and Mental Disorder, *Report* (London, HMSO, 1926) Cmd 2700, pp. 16–22.

12 See John R. Rees, *The Shaping of Psychiatry by War* (London, Chapman and Hall, 1945), p. 29.

13 See Kathleen Jones, *A History of the Mental Health Services* (London, Routledge & Kegan Paul, 1972), pp. 235–6.

14 Elizabeth Barnes (ed.), *Psychosocial nursing: studies from the Cassel Hospital* (London, Tavistock, 1968), pp. 10–15.

15 Rose, *Psychological Complex*, pp. 158–63.

16 Ibid., pp. 163–75.

17 See, for example, Jones, *Mental Health Services*, pp. 226–61 and 283–305.

18 M. Lomax, *Experiences of an Asylum Doctor* (London, George Allen & Unwin, 1921); W. R. Barton, *Institutional Neurosis*, (Bristol, John Wright & Sons, 1959); E. Goffman, *Asylums: essays on the social situation of mental patients and other inmates* (New York, Doubleday, 1961); J. Wing, 'Institutionalism in mental hospitals', *British Journal of Social and Clinical Psychology*, 1 (1962), 38–51.

19 A. Scull, *Decarceration: community treatment and the deviant – a radical view*, 2nd edn (Cambridge, Polity Press, 1984); G. Baruch and A. Treacher, *Psychiatry Observed* (London, Routledge & Kegan Paul, 1978); A. Treacher and G. Baruch, 'Towards a critical history of the psychiatric profession' in D. Ingleby (ed.), *Critical Psychiatry* (Harmondsworth, Penguin, 1981), pp. 120–59.

20 This argument is made most strongly by Treacher and Baruch, 'Towards a critical history'.

21 This argument is put forward most clearly in Scull, *Decarceration*.

22 See P. Sedgwick, *Psychopolitics* (Pluto Press, London, 1982), pp. 201–6.

23 The Minister is quoted in Jones, *Mental Health Services*, p. 307, which also gives details of the various publications mentioned above.

24 The descriptions ins from D. H. Clark, *Administrative Psychiatry* (London, Tavistock, 1964).

25 Baruch and Treacher, *Psychiatry Observed*, give a useful account of this period.

26 In the following paragraphs I have drawn upon J. R. Rees, 'Three years of military psychiatry in the United Kingdom', *British Medical Journal*, 1 (1943), 1–6, and *The Shaping of Psychiatry by War*; R. H. Ahrenfeld, *Psychiatry in the British Army in the Second World War*

(London, Routledge & Kegan Paul, 1958); H. V. Dicks, *Fifty Years of the Tavistock Clinic* (London, Routledge & Kegan Paul, 1970).

27 For details of the various incarnations and offshoots of the Tavistock Institute, see Dicks, *Fifty Years*. Three key early publications by Elliot Jacques are 'Interpretive group discussion as a method of facilitating social change. A progress report on the use of group methods in the investigation and resolution of social problems', *Human Relations*, 1 (1947), 533–49; 'Studies in the social development of an industrial community (The Glacier Project 1.) ', *Human Relations*. 3 (1950), 223–49; *The Changing Culture of a Factory* (London, Tavistock, 1950).

28 Rees, *Shaping of Psychiatry*, p. 46.

29 See the material presented in Jones, *Mental Health Services*, pp. 262–82.

30 The issues in the following paragraph are discussed at length in Rose, *Psychological Complex*.

31 Ibid. esp. pp. 176–219.

32 See Office of Strategic Services Assessment Staff, *Assessment of Men*(New York, Reinhart, 1948); P. E. Vernon and J. B. Parry, *Personnel Selection in the British Forces* (London, London University Press, 1949); B. S. Morris, 'Officer selection in the British Army', *Occupational Psychology*, 23 (1949), 219–34. Excerpts from this material are presented in B. Semeonoff (ed.), *Personality Assessment* (Harmondsworth, Penguin, 1966).

33 See, for example, the papers collected together in H. J. Eysenck (ed., *Behaviour Therapy and the Neuroses* (Oxford, Pergamon, 1960).

34 The best overview is E. Younghusband, *Social Work in Britain: 1950–1975*(London, George Allen & Unwin, 1978). See also N. Timms, *Psychiatric Social Work in Great Britain, 1939–1962* (London, Routledge & Kegan Paul, 1964).

35 See Jones, *Mental Health Services*, pp. 321–34.

36 The most developed argument along these lines is Baruch and Treacher, *Psychiatry Observed*. For further discussion, see chapter 1 of this volume.

37 These figures are from R. Lacey and S. Woodward, *That's Life Survey on Tranquillisers* (London, British Broadcasting Corporation in association with National Association for Mental Health, 1985).

38 For this account I have drawn on M. Jones, *Social Psychiatry* (London, Tavistock, 1952); F. Kräupl Taylor, 'A history of group and administrative therapy in Great Britain', *British Journal of Medical Psychology*, 31 (1958), 153–73; N. P. Manning, 'Innovation in social policy – the case of the therapeutic community', *Journal of Social Policy*, 5 (1976), pp. 265–79.

39 M. Jones, 'Therapeutic communities past, present and future', in M. Pines and L. Rafelson (eds), *The Individual and the Group* (London, Plenum Press, 1982), vol. 1, p. 519.

40 T. Main, 'The hospital as a therapeutic institution', *Bulletin of the Menninger Clinic*, 10 (1946), 67.

41 T. Main develops these aspects in his riveting paper of 1957 entitled 'The ailment', *British Journal of Medical Psychology*, 30 (1957), 129–45.

42 Jones, *Social Psychiatry*.

43 See, for example, A. T. Wilson, M. Doyle and J. Kelnar, 'Group techniques in a transitional community', *The Lancet*, 1 (1947), 735–8; A. Curle, 'Transitional communities and social reconnection. A follow-up study of the civil resettlement of British prisoners of war', *Human Relations*, 1 (1947), 42–68. Cf. Kräupl Taylor, 'A history of group and administrative therapy'.

44 Jones, *Social Psychiatry*, Introduction.

45 Kräupl Taylor, 'A history of group and administrative therapy', p. 158.

46 Cf. R. N. Rapoport, *Community as Doctor* (London, Tavistock, 1960), pp. 51–78.

47 For example, A. H. Stanton and M. S. Schwartz, *The Mental Hospital* (London, Tavistock, 1954); W. Caudill, *The Psychiatric Hospital as a Small Society* (Cambridge, Mass., Harvard University Press, 1958).

48 D. Martin, *Adventure in Psychiatry* (Oxford, Cassirer, 1962); Clark, *Administrative Psychiatry*; on Main see E. Barnes (ed.), *Psychosocial Nursing: studies from the Cassel Hospital* (London, Tavistock, 1968), esp. pp. 4–15.

49 Details are in Kräupl Taylor, 'A history of group and administrative therapy', p. 155–6.

50 Developments in nursing can be traced through the articles and letters in *Nursing Mirror* and *Nursing Times* over this period. See also M. Meacher (ed.), *New Methods of Mental Health Care* (Oxford, Pergamon, 1979). For nursing and administrative therapy, see Barnes, *Psychosocial Nursing*, esp. part II. These developments in nursing are consonant with the shift in medical perception noted in D. Armstrong, 'The patient's view', (unpublished paper, London, Guys Hospital Medical School, 1984).

51 See the discussion by Peter Miller in chapter 5 of this volume.

52 For the development of therapeutic communities, see D. H. Clark, 'The therapeutic community: concept, practice, future', *British Journal of Psychiatry*, 117 (1970), 375–88, and Jones, 'Therapeutic communities'. An idea of the current state of play can be gained from the papers collected in N. Manning and R. Hinshelwood (eds), *The Therapeutic Community: Reflections and Progress* (London, Routledge & Kegan Paul, 1979).

53 See M. Yelloly, *Social Work Theory and Psychoanalysis* (Wokingham, Van Nostrand Reinhold, 1980). The pre-war developments are discussed in Rose, *Psychological Complex*.

54 The work of H. J. Eysenck was crucial; see, for example, 'Learning theory and behaviour therapy', *Journal of Mental Science*, 105 (1959), 61–75, and the papers collected in Eysenck, *Behaviour Therapy*.

55 The proliferation of these techniques in Britain rather lags behind

developments in the USA.R. Herink (ed.), *The Psychotherapy Hand-book* (New York, Meridian, 1980) lists more than 250 dfferent ther-apies from Active Analytic Therapy to the Zaraleya Psychoenergetic Technique. See also F. Castel, R. Castel and A. Lovell, *The Psy-chiatric Society* (New York, Columbia University Press, 1982).

3   Psychiatry and the construction of the feminine

1 DHSS Statistics. For critical discussions of such statistical findings see J. Busfield, 'Gender, mental illness and psychiatry', in M. Evans and C. Ungerson (eds), *Sexual Divisions: Patterns & Processes*, (London, Tavistock, 1983); and D. Smith, 'The statistics on mental illness: what they will not tell us about women and why', in D. Smith (ed.), *Women Look at Psychiatry*, (Toronto, Press Gang Publishers, 1975).
2 P. Chesler, *Women and Madness*, (London, Allen Lane, 1974).
3 For example, *Phoenix Rising*, 5, (1) (Feb. 1985), special issue on women & psychiatry; J. Rohrbaugh, *Women, Psychology's Puzzle*, (Brighton, Harvester, 1985); C. Mowbray, S. Lanir, and M. Hulce (eds), *Women and Mental Health*, (New York, Harrington Park Press, 1984). See also contributions by D. Smith, E. King, M. Kimball, and E. Rubin in Smith, *Women Look at Psychiatry*.
4 For example, I. Al-Issa, *The Psychopathology of Women*, (Englewood Cliffs, New Jersey, Prentice Hall, 1980);, E. Howell and M. Bayes, *Women and Mental Health*, (New York, Basic Books, 1981), esp. chapters 14–18.
5 Al-Issa, *Psychopathology*, back cover.
6 R. Seidenberg and K. DeCrow. *Women Who Marry Houses*, (New York, McGraw Hill, 1983), pp. 40–1.
7 E. Howell, 'Women: from Freud to the present', in Howell and Bayes, *Women & Mental Health*.
8 Ibid., p. 6.
9 G. Brown and T. Harris, *Social Origins of Depression*, (London, Tavistock, 1978).
10 For example, W. Gove and J. Tudor, 'Adult sex roles and mental illness', *American Journal of Sociology*, 78 (1973), 812f. For a general discussion of work in this area, see J. Bernard, *The Future of Marriage*, (New York, World Publishing Co., 1972).
11 J. Ryan, *Feminism and Therapy*, (London, Polytechnic of North London, 1983), The Pam Smith Memorial Lecture, p. 16.
12 Chesler quotes such notables as Ellen West, Zelda Fitzgerald and Sylvia Plath.
13 F. Cheek, 'A serendipitous finding: sex role and schizophrenia', *Journal of Abnormal & Social Psychology*, 69 (1964), 4.
14 D. McClelland and N. Watt, 'Sex role alienation and schizophrenia', *Journal of Abnormal Psychology*, 73 (1964), 3.
15 Chesler, *Women and Madness*, pp. 53–4; emphasis in original.

16 Sexual abuses are discussed in V. Davidson's 'Psychiatry's problem with no name', in Howell and Bayes, *Women and Mental Health*. See also Sylvia Plath, *The Bell Jar*, (London, Faber & Faber, 1963); Chesler, *Women and Madness*, chapters 5 and 6; and 'Women against psychiatric assault', *Off Our Backs*, 12 and 13. (1982).

17 I. Broverman, D. Broverman, F. Clarkson, P. Rosenkrantz, and S. Vogel, 'Sex role stereotypes and mental health', *Journal of Consulting & Clinical Psychology*, 34 (1970), 1f.

18 Both cases might be regarded as a historical residue from an earlier psychiatric discourse in which gender categories did play a constitutive role. In each case they retain a place only at the boundaries of the modern psychiatric system.

19 See H. Allen, 'At the mercy of her hormones: premenstrual tension and the law', *mf* 9 (1984), 19f; K. Dalton, *The Premenstrual Syndrome*, (London, Heinemann, 1964).

20 See I. Brockington and R. Kumar, *Motherhood and Mental Illness*, (London, Academic Press, 1982).

21 See P. Weideger, *Female Cycles* (London, Women's Press, 1978).

22 See D. Armstrong, 'Madness and coping', *Sociology of Health & Illness*, 2 (1980), 195f.

23 For example, E. Nickerson, K. O'Laughlin and L. Hirschman. 'Learned helplessness and depression in women', *International Journal of Women's Studies*, 2 (1979) 340f; M. Seligman, *Helplessness*, (San Francisco, Freeman & Co., 1975).

24 For example, L. Eichenbaum and S. Orbach, *Outside In, Inside Out*, (Harmondsworth, Penguin, 1982). See also articles on feminist therapy in Mowbray et al. *Women Look at Psychiatry*.

25 This centre, established in 1976, provides the focus for feminist therapy in Britain, and I shall be referring to their work throughout this discussion.

26 Eichenbaum and Orbach, *Outside Inside*, 11f.

27 Ibid., p. 105f.

28 Ryan, *Feminism and Therapy*, pp. 9–10.

29 See Eichenbaum and Orbach, *Outside Inside*, chapter 1 and 2.

30 Ibid., p. 27f.

31 Ibid., p. 119.

4 Racism and transcultural psychiatry

1 R. Cochrane, 'Mental illness in immigrants to England and Wales: an analysis of mental hospital admissions', *Social Psychiatry*, 12 (1977), p. 22.

2 O. Ødergaard, 'Emigration and insanity', *Acta Psychiatria et Neurologica* (1932), supplement 4.

3 G. Dean, H. Walsh, H. Dowing and E. Shelly, 'First admissions of

native born and immigrants to psychiatric hospitals in south east England, 1976', *British Journal of Psychiatry*, 139 (1981), 506–12.

4 S. Ramon, 'The logic of pragmatism in mental health policy', *Critical Social Policy*, 2 (2) (1982).

5 R. Littlewood and M. Lipsedge, *Aliens and Alienists: Ethnic Minorities and Psychiatry* (Harmondsworth, Penguin, 1982).

6 P. Hitch and P. Clegg, 'Modes of referral of overseas immigrant and native born first admissions to psychiatric hospital', *Social Science and Medicine*, 11 (1980), 369–74.

7 Black Health Workers and Patients Group, 'Psychiatry and the corporate state', *Race and Class*, XXV (2) (1983); see also their 'Black communities experience of psychiatric services', *International Journal of Social Psychiatry*, 30–1 (1/2) (1984).

8 It is in this 'circuit of control' that psychiatry has played a part in events that have lead to the deaths of many black people: of Richard 'Cartoon' Campbell at Ashford Remand Centre in 1979, Winston Rose in 1981, Paul Worrel in 1982 and Michael Martin in 1984. Together with the enforced detention and use of psychotropic drugs in the cases of Steve Thompson at Gartree Prison in 1979 and Abena Simba-Tola at Holloway Prison in 1982 these all point to the repressive, violent and coercive potential of the powers of psychiatry as encountered by black people. See T. Hercules, 'I hereby sentence you . . .', *City Limits (Dec, 1982)*; 'Thatcher's Britain' (on Paul Worrel), *Fight Racism, Fight Imperialism* (May 1983); and E. Francis, 'How did Michael Martin die? ' in *Openmind* (MIND) (Jan. 1985) and *Voice* (March 1985).

9 G. I. Tewfik and A. Okasha, 'Psychosis and immigration', *Postgraduate Medical Journal*, 41 (1965) 603–12, and Chandresa, cited in 'Mental health and racism – background paper', *Runnymede Trust Bulletin*, 158 (1983).

10 Cochrane, 'Mental illness in immigrants', p. 22.

11 R. Littlewood and S. Cross, 'Ethnic minorities and psychiatric services', *Sociology of Health and Illness*, 2 (2) (1980), 194–201.

12 On the 'prehistory' or 'archive' of contemporary transcultural discourse in psychiatry, see G. M. Foster and B. G. Anderson, *Medical Anthropology* (New York, John Wiley, 1978) esp. chapter on Ethnopsychiatry. Although not addressed to the subject of psychiatric research in the colonial context, essays in T. Asad (ed.) *Anthropology and the Colonial Encounter* (London, Ithaca Press, 1975), part 1, offer a relevant method for a possible historical archeology of transculturalism as a discursive formation.

13 Tewfik and Okasha, 'Psychosis and immigration', E. B. Gordon 'Mentally ill West Indian immigrants', *British Journal of Psychiatry*, 111 (1965), 877–87, A. Kiev, 'Beliefs and delusions of West Indian immigrants to London', *British Journal of Psychiatry, 109 (1963), 356–63*; 'Psychotherapeutic aspects of pentecostal sects among West Indian immigrants to England', *British Journal of Sociology*, 15 (1964), 129–38; 'Psychiatric morbidity of West Indian immigrants in

an urban group practice', *British Journal of Psychiatry*, 111 (1965), 51–6; 'Psychiatric disorders in minority groups' in *'Psychology and Race'*, ed. P. Watson (Harmondsworth, Penguin, 1973) and A. Kiev, *Transcultural Psychiatry*, (Harmondsworth, Penguin, 1972).

14 C. Bagley, 'Mental illness in immigrant minorities in London', *Journal of Biosocial Science* 3, (1971), 449–59; and 'The social aetiology of schizophrenia in immigrant groups', *International Journal of Social Psychiatry*, 17 (1971), 292–304. R. Cochrane, et al, 'Measuring psychological disturbance in Asian immigrants to Britain', *Social Science and Medicine*, 11, (1977), 157–64; and 'Psychological and behavioural disturbance in West Indians, Indians and Pakistanis in Britain', *British Journal of Psychiatry*, 134 (1979), 201–10. See also P. Rack, 'Review of the psychiatric literature', in Community Relations Commission, *Mental Health in a Multi-Racial Society*, (London, CRC, 1976), appendex 1.

15 An account of the unit is given in P. Rack, *Race, Culture and Mental Disorder*, (London, Tavistock, 1982), appendix 4, pp. 266–9.

16 J. Cox, 'Culture and medical management', *Bulletin of the Transcultural Psychiatry Society*, 6 (Sept. 1983).

17 Littlewood and Lipsedge, *Aliens and Alienists*, p. 9.

18 J. Leff, 'Psychiatry Around the Globe – a Transcultural View' (London, John Wiley, 1980); A. Leighton and J. M. Murphy 'Cross-cultural psychiatry', in A. H. Leighton and D. C. Leighton (eds), *Approaches to Cross-Cultural Psychiatry* (New York, Basic Books, 1958).

19 A. Burke, 'The consequences of unplanned repatriation', *British Journal of Psychiatry*, 123 (1973), 102–11; and 'Transcultural Psychiatry – Racism and Mental Illness', *International Journal of Social Psychiatry*, 30–1 (1/2) (1984).

20 From the constitution of the Transcultural Psychiatry Society (UK), circa 1976; for information on TCPS contact, The Secretary, Suman Fernando, Chase Farm Hospital, Enfield, Middlesex.

20 R. Littlewood and M. Lipsedge, 'Some social and phenomenological characteristics of psychotic immigrants', *Psychological Medicine*, 11 (1981), 289.

22 R. Littlewood and M. Lipsedge, 'Acute psychotic reactions in Caribbean born patients', *Psychological Medicine*, 11 (1981), p. 318.

23 Littlewood and Lipsedge, 'Acute psychotic reactions', pp. 307–9.

24 Community Relations Commission, *Mental Health in a Multi-Racial Society*, pp. 28–9.

25 Ibid., p. 29.

26 Littlewood and Lipsedge, 'Social and phenomenological characteristics', p. 287.

27 Littlewood and Lipsedge, 'Acute psychotic reactions', p. 315, emphasis added.

28 Despite the fact that the women's movement and psychiatric research have drawn attention to the disproportionate number of women diagnosed as 'depressive', which is often seen as a response to the stresses

of women's dual role as workers and wives/mothers, *gender* is conspicuous by its absence from the transcultural perspective. At no point do the authors discuss the gender composition of their sample of Caribbean and African patients. See G. Brown and T. Harris, *Social Origins of Depression* (London, Tavistock Books, 1978).

29 David Armstrong, *Political Anatomy of the Body: medical knowledge in Britain in the twentieth century*, (Cambridge, Cambridge University Press, 1983), esp pp. 19–31, 64–72.

30 Littlewood and Lipsedge, 'Acute psychotic reactions', p. 316.

31 Ibid.

32 Littlewood and Cross, 'Ethnic minorities and psychiatric services'.

33 This case study appears in Littlewood and Lipsedge, *Aliens and Alienists*, pp. 218–32; and in R. Littlewood, 'Anthropology and psychiatry – an alternative approach', *British Journal of Medical Psychology* 53 (1980), 213–25.

34 Littlewood and Lipsedge, *Aliens and Alienists*, p. 28.

35 Rack, *Race, Culture & Mental Disorder*, pp. 4–5.

36 Littlewood and Cross, 'Ethnic minorities and psychiatric services', p. 200.

37 Littlewood and Lipsedge, *Aliens and Alienists*, pp. 128–32.

38 P. Rack, 'Diagnosing mental illness in Asian patients', in V. S. Khan, (ed), *Minority Families in Britain: Stress and Support* (London, Macmillan, 1979), p. 176.

39 Tewfik and Okasha, 'Psychoses and Immigration' p. 603.

40 A critical examination of the policy investment in 'psychological' techniques in the discourse of multi-cultural education is offered by M. Stone, *The Education of the Black Child in Britain* (London, Fontana, 1977).

41 R. Ballard, 'Ethnic minorities and the social services: what type of service? ', *Minority Families in Britain*, p. 149, emphases added.

42 Ibid., pp. 159 and 164, emphasis added.

43 Ibid., pp. 148 and 162, emphasis added.

44 Ibid., p. 157, emphasis added.

45 Ibid., p. 160.

46 Examples of the discourse on 'ethnicity' in policy-oriented texts are, J. Triseloitis, (ed.), *Social Work with Coloured Immigrants and their Families* (Oxford, Oxford University Press for the Institute of Race Relations, 1969); Khan, *Minority Families in Britain*; J. Cheetham, *Social Work and Ethnicity* (London, Allen & Unwin, 1982), National Institute of Social Services, Library, 43, and M. Loney et al., *Social and Community Work in a Multi-Racial Society* (London, Harper & Row, 1983).

47 Ballard, 'Ethnic minorities and the social services', p. 162, emphasis added.

48 Rack, *Race, Culture and Mental Disorder*, pp. 101–49.

49 Littlewood and Lipsedge, *Aliens and Alienists*, pp. 13–17, 28–36.

50 Armstrong, *Political Anatomy*, pp. 69–72, 110–12.

51 Cited in Armstrong, *Political Anatomy*, p. 102.

52 Rack, *Race, Culture and Mental Disorder*, p. 4–5, emphasis added.
53 Armstrong, *Political Anatomy*, pp. 69–72, 110–12.
54 The marked psychological emphasis in 'ethnicity' studies is most apparent in research on children, such as D. Milner, *Children and Race* (Harmondsworth, Penguin, 1975), and in research on the cultural practices of Afro-Caribbean youth in particular, such as E. Cashmore and B. Troyna (eds), *Black Youth in Crisis* (London, Allen & Unwin, 1983). The orthodox sociological notion of 'alienation' as used in this context is so pervasive (see Roy Kerridge, 'Why these blacks of Brixton hate the police', *Daily Mail*, 13 April 1981; and 'Myths that poison the minds of Britain's blacks', *Daily Mail*, 1 July 1983), that Lord Scarman's official report finds it necessary to cite evidence that this notion is not applicable, *The Scarman Report* (Harmondsworth, Penguin, 1982), p. 29. The research in question is G. Gaskell and P. Smith, 'Race and "Alienated Youth" : A Conceptual and Empirical Inquiry', Dept. of Social Psychology, London School of Economics, April 1981, who found that, against the orthodox sociological definition of 'alienation', black youth were *not* alienated; see also, Gaskell and Smith, Are young blacks really alienated?, *New Society*, 14 May 1981.
55 Littlewood and Lipsedge, *Aliens and Alienists*, p. 23. The use of Durkheim's concept is made explicit in the authors' prediction that, 'The diagnosis of schizophrenia will probably become less common (in the future) . . . They (Afro-Caribbeans) will perhaps be seen as having a "situational reaction". Such situational reactions are themselves likely to become less common, to be replaced by drug overdoses. It is probable that suicide among Afro-Britons [sic] will become more frequent: in the United States Southern blacks who plan to move north have initially a low suicide rate which goes up some time after they have moved' *Aliens and Alienists*, (p. 241). The matrix for their reasoning is, E. Durkheim, *Suicide*, (London, Routledge, Kegan & Paul, 1952.)
56 Littlewood and Lipsedge, *Aliens and Alienists*, p. 236.
57 Alternative approaches to such 'psychologistic' readings of the importance of religion in Caribbean societies and cultures are offered by R. Bastide, *African Civilisations in the New World* (London, Hurst & Co., 1971); C. L. R. James, *The Black Jacobins* (London, Allison & Busby, 1980); and S. Hall, 'Religious Cults and Social Movements', (unpublished paper, presented at Centre for Caribbean Studies, London University, 10 May 1985).
58 M. Foucault, *Discipline and Punish – the birth of the prison* (London, Allen Lane, 1977), p. 192; see also his *Madness and Civilisation – a history of insanity in the age of reason*, (London, Tavistock, 1967) and *The Birth of the Clinic*, (London, Tavistock, 1973).
59 Armstrong, *Political Anatomy*, p. 72.
60 Littlewood and Lipsedge, *Aliens and Alienists*, p. 8.
61 F. Fanon, *Black Skin White Mask*, (London, Paladin Books, 1970), p. 29.

62 F. Fanon, *The Wretched of the Earth* (Harmondsworth, Penguin, 1967), esp. 'Colonial war and mental disorder' (pp. 200–50), and 'Medicine and colonialism' in *A Dying Colonialism*, (Harmondsworth, Penguin, 1970), offer the most explicit of his political viewpoints on race, racism and health care.

63 See D. Ingelby (ed.), *Critical Psychiatry* (Harmondsworth, Penguin, 1982) and P. Sedgwick, *Psycho-politics* (London, Pluto Press, 1981). Neither substantively addresses the issue of race for an agenda of politics in psychiatry.

64 E. Lawrence, 'White sociology/black struggle', *Multiracial Education* (NAME [National Association for Multi-Racial Education] journal), 9 (3) (1981) and 'In the abundance of water the fool is thirsty: sociology and black pathology', in *The Empire Strikes Back*, CCCS [Centre for Contemporary Cultural Studies] (London, Hutchinson, 1982). P. Parmar, 'Young Asian women: a critique of the pathological approach', *Multiracial Education*, 9 (3) (1981). Aside from Khan's *Minority Families in Britain*, Lawrence and Parmar's critiques also cover, S. Wallman (ed), *Ethnicity At Work* (London, Macmillan, 1979). Other relevant critiques of ethnicity can be found in M. Barker, *The New Racism* (London, Junction Books, 1982) and M. Duffield, 'New Racism . . . new realism: two sides of the same coin', *Radical Philosophy*, 37 (Summer 1984).

65 The phenomenon of 'pathologisation' described by Lawrence has also been critically assessed as the 'cultural deprivation' or 'culture of poverty' argument in social policy discourse. A key text presenting this argument is O. Lewis, *The Children of Sanchez* (Harmondsworth, Penguin, 1983). The culturalist system of representation offered by these arguments was embraced by US Senator Patrick Moynihan's report, *The Negro Family – The Case For National Action*, (Office of Policy Planning and Research, US Department of Labor, Washington, 1965); reprinted in L. Rainwater and W. Yancey (eds), *The Moynihan Report and the Politics of Controversy*, (London, MIT Press, 1967). The Moynihan Report gave official endorsement to the view that Afro-American's 'culture' or way of life, as instituted in family organisation, was a 'pathological' entity responsible for social disadvantages in a market society.

In Britain, during the 'rediscovery of poverty' in the late 1960s, similar culturalist arguments informed policy discourses on 'deprivation' and 'disadvantage' in, *Report of the Committee on Housing in Greater London* (Milner-Holland Report), (Ministry of Housing and Local Government, HMSO, 1965); *Children and Their Primary Schools*, Vol 2 (Plowden Report), (Central Advisory Council for Education (England), Department of Education and Science, 1967), HMSO; *Report of the Committee on Local Authority and Allied Personal Social Services* (Seebhom Report), (HMSO, 1968); and actual legislation, the 'Urban Programme', *Local Government Grants (Social Need) Act* 1969.

Useful critiques of the relations between sociological research and social policy formation around 'cultural deprivationist' arguments can be found in, C. Valentine (ed.) *Culture and Poverty*, University of Chicago Press, Chicago 1968 and W. Ryan *Blaming the Victim*, Orbach and Chambers, London, 1971.

66 On non-medical criteria in compulsory admissions procedures, see P. Bean *Compulsory Admissions to Mental Hospitals* (London, John Wiley, 1980). On the use of the concept of 'dangerousness' in the history of mental health law, see M. Foucault, 'About the concept of the "dangerous individual" in 19th-century legal psychiatry', *International Journal of Law and Psychiatry*, (1978), 1–19.

67 J. Wing, *Reasoning About Madness* (Oxford University Press, 1978) and A. Clare, *Psychiatry in Dissent* (London, Tavistock, 1980).

68 Thanks are due to Graham Burchell for comments on this essay, and to Errol Francis, Buddy Larrier and Dr Sashi Sashidarahan for previous collaborative work and discussions on the issues addressed here.

5 Psychotherapy of work and unemployment

1 The concept 'surfaces of emergence' is outlined in M. Foucault, *The Archaeology of Knowledge* (London, Tavistock, 1972), p. 41.

2 I owe this formulation to R. Castel, *La Gestion des risques* (Paris, Editions de Minuit, 1981).

3 See F. Guery and D. Deleule, *Le corps productif* (Paris, Maison Mame, 1972); see also J. Donzelot, "Pleasure in work", in G. Burchell, C. Gordon, P. Miller (eds.), *The Foucault Effect* (Brighton, Harvester Press, forthcoming). On the relations between the economic machine and the human organism see G. Canguilhem, 'Machine et organisme' in his *La Connaissance de la vie*, 2nd edn, (Paris, Vrin, 1980).

4 On this subject see D. Armstrong, *Political Anatomy of the Body: medical knowledge in Britain in the twentieth century* (Cambridge, Cambridge University Press, 1983), see also N. Rose, *The Psychological Complex* (London, Routledge & Kegan Paul, 1985). The child and the home are prominent figures here.

5 F. W. Taylor, *The Principles of Scientific Management* (New York, Harper & Brothers, 1913).

6 On this question see P. Miller and T. O'Leary, 'Accounting and the construction of the governable person', *Accounting, Organizations and Society* (in press).

7 This was an application of a psychology of individual differences to the 'practical' concerns of the war industry. An excellent discussion of these issues in the USA is contained in M. S. Viteles, *Industrial Psychology* (New York, Norton & Co., 1932), in particular section two. See also H. Munsterberg, *Psychology and Industrial Efficiency* (London, Constable, 1913).

8 Myers was one of the central figures in Britain. See H. J. Welch and

C. S. Myers, *Ten Years of Industrial Psychology: an account of the first decade of the National Institute of Industrial Psychology* (London, Pitman & Sons, 1932); C. S. Myers, *Industrial Psychology in Great Britain* (London, Jonathan Cape, 1926).

9 This was the concern, first of the Health of Munition Workers' Committee of 1915–17, then of the Industrial Fatigue Research Board founded in 1918, which subsequently changed its title to the Industrial Health Research Board in 1929. For an overview of the concerns of these bodies see M. Rose, *Industrial Behaviour: theoretical developments since Taylor* (Harmondsworth, Penguin, 1978). See also E. Farmer, 'Early days in industrial psychology: an autobiographical note', *Occupational Psychology*, 32 (1958), 264–7.

10 Farmer, 'Early days in industrial psychology'. See also the excellent discussion of accident-proneness as a characteristic of the individual in Viteles, *Industrial Psychology*.

11 Myers, cited in C. Sofer, *Organizations in Theory and Practice* (London, Heinemann Educational Books, 1972). p. 47.

12 Welch and Myers, *Ten Years of Industrial Psychology*, p. 4.

13 See E. Mayo, *The Human Problems of an Industrial Civilization* (New York, Macmillan, 1933).

14 The best discussions are L. Baritz, *The Servants of Power: a history of the use of social science in American industry* (Middletown, Connecticut, Wesleyan University Press, 1960); J. A. C. Brown, *The Social Psychology of Industry* (Harmondsworth, Penguin, 1980); and Rose, *Industrial Behaviour*.

15 Mayo, *The Human Problems*, p. 52.

16 Mayo, *The Human Problems*.

17 The 'appraisal' interview is one important technique through which such principles were to be developed. See for instance the views expressed in N. R. F. Maier, 'Three types of appraisal interview', *Personnel*, 34 (1958), 27–40. See also Mayo, *The Human Problems* on the more general question of interviews.

18 E. Durkheim, *The Division of Labour in Society* (New York, Macmillan, 1933), p. 28.

19 Durkheim, *Division of Labour*, p. 28.

20 Mayo, *The Human Problems*.

21 See Viteles, *Industrial Psychology*, chapter 26. See also V. E. Fisher and J. V. Hanna, *The Dissatisfied Worker* (New York, 1931).

22 Fisher and Hanna, *The Dissatisfied Worker*, pp. vii–viii.

23 Ibid.

24 M. C. Jarrett, 'The mental hygiene of industry', *Mental Hygiene*, 4 (1920), 367–84.

25 V. V. Anderson, 'Psychiatry in industry', in H. Elkind (ed.), *Preventive Management* (New York, 1931).

26 Anderson, 'Psychiatry in industry'.

27 M. Smith, M. Culpin and E. Farmer, 'A study of telegraphists' cramp', *Industrial Fatigue Research Board* (1927) Report No. 43.

28 Ibid., p. 20.

29 See J. A. Garraty, *Unemployment in History* (New York, Harper & Row, 1978); J. Harris, *Unemployment and Politics: a study in English social policy 1886–1914* (Oxford, Clarendon Press, 1972).
30 See J. Tomlinson, *Problems of British Economic Policy 1870–1945* (London, Methuen, 1981).
31 A useful account of these is to be found in J. Horne, 'Youth unemployment programmes: a historical account of the development of "dole colleges" ' in D. Gleeson (ed.), *Youth Training and the Search for Work* (London, Routledge & Kegan Paul, 1983). See also G. Rees and T. L. Rees, 'Juvenile unemployment and the state between the wars', in T. L. Rees and P. Atkinson, *Youth Unemployment and State Intervention* (London, Routledge & Kegan Paul, 1982).
32 Rees and Rees, 'Juvenile unemployment and the state', p. 18.
33 Ibid., p. 19.
34 This term is taken from M. Foucault, *L'Usage des plaisirs* (Paris, Gallimard, 1984).
35 V. A. Bell, *Junior Instruction Centres and their Future* (Edinburgh, 1935), cited in Horne, 'Youth unemployment programmes', p. 320.
36 Ibid., p. 321.
37 See, for instance, E. W. Bakke, *The Unemployed Man* (London, Nisbet, 1933); H. L. Beales and R. S. Lambert (eds), *Memoirs of the Unemployed* (London, Victor Gollancz, 1934); M. Jahoda, P. F. Lazarsfeld and H. Zeisel, *Marienthal: the sociography of an unemployed community* (London, Tavistock, 1972); M. Komarovsky, *The Unemployed Man and his Family* (New York, Arno Press, 1971); *Pilgrim Trust, Men Without Work* (Cambridge, Cambridge University Press, 1938).
38 See P. Eisenberg and P. F. Lazarsfeld, 'The psychological effects of unemployment', *Psychological Bulletin* 35 (1938), 358–90.
39 See Bakke, *Unemployed Man*.
40 See Jahoda, Lazarsfeld and Zeisel, *Marienthal*.
41 The following is based principally on J. R. Rees, *The Shaping of Psychiatry by War* (London, Chapman & Hall, 1945); and R. H. Ahrenfeld, *Psychiatry in the British Army in the Second World War* (London, Routledge & Kegan Paul, 1958). See also the *Report of the Expert Committee on the Work of Psychologists and Psychiatrists in the Services* (London, HMSO, 1947).
42 Rees, *The Shaping of Psychiatry by War*, p. 48.
43 Ibid., p. 57.
44 See T. F. Rodger, 'Personnel selection', in N. G. Harris (ed.), *Modern Trends in Psychological Medicine* (London, Butterworth & Co., 1948).
45 Rees, *The Shaping of Psychiatry by War*, p. 53.
46 See S. A. Stouffer et al., *The American Soldier* (Princeton, Princeton University Press, 1949), four volumes.
47 Stouffer, *The American Soldier, volume II, combat and its aftermath*, p. 207.

48 For further details on this see Stouffer, *The American Soldier*, vol. II, chapter 9.
49 H. S. Sullivan, *The Fusion of Psychiatry and Social Science*, (New York, Norton & Co., 1971), p. 133.
50 Rees, *The Shaping of Psychiatry by War*, p. 65. On the question of officer selection see also B. S. Morris, 'Officer selection in the British Army, 1942–1945', *Occupational Psychology* (October 1949).
51 Ibid., p. 89.
52 Ibid., p. 83.
53 Stouffer, *The American Soldier*.
54 Ibid., vol. II, pp. 130–1.
55 E. A. Shils, 'Primary groups in the American army', in R. K. Merton and P. F. Lazarsfeld (eds), *Continuities in Social Research: studies in the scope and method of the American soldier* (New York, The Free Press, 1950), p. 22.
56 E. A. Shils, 'The study of the primary group' in H. D. Lasswell and D. Lerner (eds), *The Policy Sciences: recent developments in scope and methods* (Palo Alto, Stanford University Press, 1951), p. 64.
57 R. F. Tredgold, *Human Relations in Modern Industry* (London, Methuen, 1965), pp. 26–9.
58 Ibid., p. 28.
59 Ibid.
60 Mayo, *The Human Problems*. This is an important topic which I can do no more than point to in the space of this essay.
61 J. M. M. Hill and E. L. Trist, *Industrial Accidents, Sickness and Other Absences* (London, Tavistock, 1962) provides a useful discussion of the relationship between absenteeism and industrial accidents in the two decades following the Second World War.
62 H. V. Dicks, 'Principles of mental hygiene', in N. G. Harris (ed.), *Modern Trends in Psychological Medicine* (London, Butterworth & Co., 1948). p. 310.
63 Ibid., p. 311.
64 Ibid., p. 330.
65 Ibid., p. 331.
66 R. F. Tredgold, 'Mental hygiene in industry', in Harris, *Modern Trends in Psychological Medicine*.
67 Ibid., p. 364.
68 R. Fraser, *The Incidence of Neurosis among Factory Workers* (London, HMSO, 1947), Industrial Health Research Board Report No. 90, p. 9.
69 Tredgold, 'Mental hygiene in industry', p. 367.
70 Mayo, *The Human Problems*. See also F. J. Roethlisberger and W. J. Dickson, *Management and the Worker* (Cambridge, Mass., Harvard University Press, 1939).
71 Rees, *The Shaping of the Psychiatry by War*, p. 70.
72 W. R. Bion, 'The leaderless group project', *Bulletin of the Menninger Clinic*, 10 (May 1946), 77.
73 On this see Sofer, *Organizations*, pp. 199–202.

74 Hill and Trist, *Industrial Accidents*. See also the more general discussion of the issue in Viteles, *Industrial Psychology*, chapter 17.
75 Hill and Trist, *Industrial Accidents*, p. 3.
76 See M. Argyle, 'Explorations in the treatment of personality disorders
and neuroses by social skills training', *British Journal of Medical
Psychology*, 47 (1974) 63–72; see also his *Social Skills and Work*
(London, Methuen, 1980).
77 I. Illich, *The Right to Usful Unemployment and its Professional Enem-
ies* (London, Marion Boyars, 1978).
78 See L. Fagin and M. Little, *The Forsaken Families* (Harmondsworth,
Penguin, 1984).

6 Law, rights and psychiatry

1 I have made some of the arguments in this essay elsewhere. A
shortened version was given at the Conference of the Socio-Legal
Group at Oxford in March 1985, and published, in amended form,
as 'Unreasonable rights: mental illness and the limits of the law',
Journal of Law and Society, 12 (1985), 199–219. I would like to thank
Phil Jones and Hilary Lim for discussing issues of rights with me, and
Clive Unsworth for his comments on an earlier draft and for letting
me see draft chapters of his forthcoming book, *The Politics of Mental
Health Legislation* (Oxford, Oxford University Press, 1986). Thanks
also to Hilary Allen, Rob Baldwin, David Freedman, Barr Hindess
and Carol Stephens for critical comments on an earlier draft.
2 Analagous arguments were also made concerning the role of psychiatry in the criminal justice system. See L. Gostin, 'Human rights,
judicial review and the mentally disordered offender', *Criminal Law
Review*, (1982), 779, and'Psychiatric detention without limit of time:
the Broadmoor cases', in P. Scratton and P. Gordon (eds), *Causes
for Concern* (Harmondsworth, Penguin, 1984), pp. 273–87. I do not
deal with these directly in this essay.
3 These are most clearly summarized in L. Gostin, 'The ideology of
entitlement: the application of contemporary legal approaches to
psychiatry', in P. Bean (ed.), *Mental Illness: changes and trends*
(London, John Wiley, 1983), pp. 27–54, and 'Contemporary social
historical perspectives on mental health reform', *Journal of Law and
Society*, 10 (1983), 47–70.
4 See J. S. Mill, *On Liberty (London, Parker, 1859)*. See also Monahan,
'John Stuart Mill on the liberty of the mentally ill', *American Journal
of Psychiatry*, 134 (1977), 1428–9.
5 See, for example, N. Kittrie, *The Right to be Different* (Baltimore,
Johns Hopkins University Press, 1971) and T. Szasz, *Law, Liberty
and Psychiatry* (New York, Macmillan, 1963). Note that Mill explicitly
excluded from these considerations those in a state to require being
taken care of by others, lacking the ordinary amount of understanding

or not in the maturity of their faculties. Hence the provenance of this argument against compulsory detention is questionable. See Monahan, 'Mill on the liberty of the mentally ill', p. 1429.

6 For a good discussion of the anti-psychiatry of Szasz, Laing and Goffman, see P. Sedgwick, *Psychopolitics* (London, Pluto Press, 1982). Recent uses of the notion of medicalization of social control in relation to psychiatry can be found in D. Ingleby (ed.), *Critical Psychiatry* (Harmondsworth, Penguin, 1981). See also the discussion by Peter Miller in chapter 1 of this volume.

7 Classically in F. von Hayek, *The Road to Serfdom* (London, Routledge & Kegan Paul, 1944).

8 Especially A. V. Dicey, *Law of the Constitution* (London, Macmillan, 1885) and *Law and Opinion in England* (London, Macmillan, 1905). See W. A. Robson, *Justice and Administrative Law* (London, Stevens, 1951).

9 For a discussion in the context of psychiatry see J. Murphy, 'Criminal punishment and psychiatric fallacies', *Law and Society Review*, 4 (1969), 111. See also Kittrie, *The Right to be Different*.

10 The terms are from J. Jowell, 'The legal control of administrative discretion', *Public Law* (1973), 178–220. A good collection of materials on these debates is in M. Adler and S. Asquith (eds), *Discretion and Welfare* (London, Heinemann, 1981).

11 Such arguments based upon entitlements are usually dated from the writings of Charles Reich, 'The new property', *Yale Law Journal*, 733 (1964) 73, and 'Individual rights and social welfare', *Yale Law Journal*, 74 (1964) 1245.

12 Section 136 of the Mental Health Act 1959. See L. O. Gostin, *A Human Condition* (London, National Association for Mental Health, 1975), vol. 1, pp. 31–3. See also Lord Percy, *Report of the Royal Commission on the Law relating to Mental Illness and Mental Deficiency 1954–1957* (London, HMSO, 1957), para 169, 412; and D. Wexler, *Mental Health Law* (New York, Plenum Press, 1981), pp. 36–7.

13 *Baxstrom* v. *Herald*, see H. Wiley, 'Operation Baxstrom after one year', *American Journal of Psychiatry*, 124 (1968).

14 Discussed in R. Castel, F. Castel and A. Lovell *The Psychiatric Society* (New York, Columbia University Press, 1982), pp. 99–100.

15 Criteria and procedures varied, and still vary, from state to state. See Wexler, *Mental Health Law*.

16 Ibid., esp. pp. 71–113.

17 These cases are summarized and discussed in P. M. Wald and P. R. Friedman, 'The politics of mental health advocacy in the United States', *International Journal of Law and Psychiatry*, 1 (1978), 137–52. See also L. H. Roth, 'Involuntary civil commitment: the right to treatment and the right to refuse treatment', *Psychiatric Annals*, 7 (1977) 244–57.

18 The best source of information on these rulings is the *Mental Disability Law Reporter*.

19 See M. S. Lottman, 'Enforcement of judicial decrees: now comes the hard part', *Mental Disability Law Reporter*, (1976), 69–76.

20 Gostin, *Human Condition*, vol. 1, p. 15.

21 The Act is discussed in detail in K. Jones, *A History of the Mental Health Services* (London, Routledge & Kegan Paul, 1972), pp. 176–8.

22 For the debate see Unsworth, *Mental Health Legislation*, chapter 9 and Jones, *Mental Health Services*, pp. 306–20.

23 Mental Health Act 1959, Sections 25 and 26.

24 Mental Health Act 1959, Sections 122, 123 and 124.

25 See, for example, the papers collected in the *Millbank Memorial Fund Quarterly, Health and Society*, 57 (1979), part 4.

26 B. Wootton, *Social Science and Social Pathology* (London, George Allen & Unwin, 1959) and C. Greenland, *Mental Illness and Civil Liberty* (London, Bell, 1970).

27 The major text was Gostin, *Human Condition*. See also MIND, *Evidence to the Royal Commission on the NHS with Regard to Services for Mentally Ill People* (London, National Association for Mental Health, 1977). The main offical responses were DHSS, *A Review of the Mental Health Act 1959* (London, HMSO, 1976); *Review of the Mental Health Act 1959* (London, HMSO, Cmnd. 732, 1978), *Reform of Mental Health Legislation* (London, HMSO, 1981), Cmnd. 8405. H. J. Steadman discusses the differences between the official approach and that of MIND in 'Attempting to protect patients rights under a medical model', *International Journal of Law and Psychiatry*, 2 (1979) 185–97.

28 Gostin, 'Contemporary perspectives' and 'The ideology of entitlement'.

29 Gostin, *Human Condition*, vol. 1, pp. 3–4.

30 Ibid., pp. 19–43.

31 Ibid., chapter 6.

32 Ibid., chapters 5–7.

33 Ibid., chapter 10. Whilst the notion of such contracts might appear outlandish, similar systems are advocated in developments that seek to 'professionalize' nursing, such as 'primary nursing' and 'the nursing process', and are used in many residential institutions for disturbed adults and children under social-work authority.

34 Ibid., pp. 115–25.

35 Ibid., pp. 36–7.

36 Gostin, 'Contemporary perspectives', p.50

37 Gostin, *Human Condition*, vol. 1, pp. 101–14.

38 Mental Health Act 1959, Section 141.

39 See *Pountney* v. *Griffiths*, 1975, discussed in Gostin, *Human Condition*, vol. 1, pp. 106–9.

40 See C. A. Johnson and B. C. Canon, *Judicial Policies, Implementation and Impact* (Washington, Congressional Quarterly Inc., 1984).

41 For two different perspectives on the American rights movements see S. Scheingold, *The Politics of Rights*, (Yale University Press, New

Haven, 1974) and E. Sparer, 'Fundamental human rights, legal entitlements and the social struggle', *Stanford Law Review*, 36 (1984), pp. 509–574.

42 The advent of the European Court of Human Rights changed this to some extent, and MIND made use of this court, and the language of rights it used, as a means of forcing the British Government to change its policies and regulations. These cases are discussed in B. Hoggett, *Mental Health Law*, 2nd edn. (Sweet and Maxwell, London, 1984), passim.

43 T. H. Marshall, *The Right to Welfare*, (Hutchinson, London, 1981).

44 The classic argument is R. M. Titmuss, 'Welfare "rights", law and discretion', *Political Quarterly*, 42 (1971), pp. 113–132.

45 Jones, *Mental Health Services*, chapter 7.

46 This movement is discussed in the papers collected in Adler and Asquith, *Discretion and Welfare*.

47 For the key cases, see Hoggett, *Mental Health Law*, passim.

48 The best general account is Hoggett, *Mental Health Law*.

49 Mental Health Act 1983, Sections 13 and 14.

50 Ibid., Part V.

51 Ibid., Sections 56–64.

52 Ibid., Section 121.

53 E.g. J. Shapland and T. Williams, 'Legalism revived: new mental health legislation in England', *International Journal of Law and Psychiatry*, 6 (1983), pp. 351–369.

54 E.g. K. Jones, 'The limitations of the legal approach to mental health', *International Journal of Law and Psychiatry*, 3 (1980), 1–15; A. Clare, 'Can the law reform psychiatric care?', *Mind Out*, 48 (1981), 17; D. Carson, 'Mental processes: the Mental Health Act 1983', *Journal of Social Welfare Law* (1985), 195–211.

55 L. Gostin, 'Ideology of entitlement', pp. 37–8 and 'Contemporary perspectives', p. 55. See also S. Morse, 'Crazy behaviour, morals and science: an analysis of mental health law', *California Law Review*, 51 (1978), 527–654.

56 See, for example, A. L. Caplan et al., *Concept of Health and Disease* (New York, Addison Wesley, 1981).

57 See I. Zola, 'Pathways to the doctor', *Social Science and Medicine* 7 (1973), 677–89, for one influential statement of this.

58 These issues are discussed clearly in Sedgwick, *Psychopolitics*, chapter 1, and P. Hirst and P. Woolley, *Social Relations and Human Attributes* (London, Tavistock, 1982).

59 For a recent collection of papers, see H. T. Englehardt Jr et al. (eds), *Clinical Judgment: A Critical Appraisal* (Dordrecht, Reidel, 1979).

60 The best account of clinical medicine as a theory and practice is M. Foucault, *Birth of the Clinic* (London, Tavistock, 1973). A clear account of this argument is in M. Cousins and A. Hussain, *Michel Foucault* (London, Macmillan, 1984).

61 Gostin, *Human Condition*, vol. 1, pp. 37–9 and 48–51. For a rather more sophisticated discussion of psychiatric diagnosis, see R. E.

Kendell, *The Role of Diagnosis in Psychiatry* (Oxford, Basil Blackwell, 1975).

62 A selection of these studies are cited in A. Clare, *Psychiatry in Dissent*, 2nd edn (London, Tavistock, 1980), pp. 138–9. Some other studies and their implications are discussed in T. J. Scheff, 'Decision rules, types of error and their consequences in medical diagnosis', *Behavioural Science*, 8 (1963), 97–107. D. Rosenhan, whose study 'On being sane in insane places' (*Science*, 179 (1973), 250–8) is ritually cited in the critique of psychiatric diagnosis, does not himself interpret his work as showing a problem in principle about diagnoses in psychiatry; see 'When does a diagnosis become a clinical judgment? ', in Englhardt, *Clinical Judgment*.

63 See J. Cocozza and H. Steadman, 'The failure of psychiatric predictions of dangerousness: clear and convincing evidence', *Rutgers Law Review*, 29 (1976), 1084–101, and the other studies by the same researchers cited in Steadman, 'Attempting to protect patients rights'.

64 Ibid.

65 See N. Walker, 'Dangerous people', *International Journal of Law and Psychiatry*, 1 (1978), 37–50.

66 See P. W. H. Fennell, 'The Mental Health Review Tribunal: a question of imbalance', *British Journal of Law and Society*, 2 (1976), 186–219; J. Peay, 'Mental Health Review Tribunals', *Law and Human Behaviour*, 5 (1981), 161–86 and 'Mental Health Review Tribunals and the Mental (Amendment) Act', *Criminal Law Review*, (1982), 794–808.

67 This is particularly stressed in the work of the American legal realists such as Roscoe Pound and Karl Llewellyn, and in the recent developments of this work by the authors in the Critical Legal Studies movement in the USA. See D. Trubek, 'Toward a social theory of law', *Yale Law Journal*, 82 (1972), 1–50; and the papers gathered in D. Kairys (ed.), *The Politics of Law* (New York, Pantheon, 1982).

68 For an interesting discussion see Anon., 'The role of council in the civil commitment process – a theoretical framework', *Yale Law Journal*, 84 (1975), 1540–63.

69 See J. Jacob, 'The right of the mental patient to his psychosis', *Modern Law Review*, 39 (1976), 17–42; L. Gostin, 'The merger of incompetency and certification: the illustration of unauthorised medical contact in the psychiatric context', *International Journal of Law and Psychiatry*, 2 (1979), 127–67; N. Milner, 'Models of rationality and mental health rights', *International Journal of Law and Psychiatry* , 4 (1981), 32–52.

70 Sedgwick, *Psychopolitics*, pp. 214–24.

71 See Roth, 'Involuntary civil commitment'.

72 For evidence on reasons for drug refusal by psychiatric patients see P. S. Applebaum and T. G. Gutheil, ' "Rotting with their rights on" : constitutional theory and clinical reality in drug refusal by psychiatric patients', *Bulletin of the American Journal of Psychiatry and the Law*, 7 (1979), 306–15.

73 See M. Foucault, *Discipline and Punish – the birth of the prison* (London, Allen Lane, 1977), esp. pp. 190–4.

74 This issue is well discussed in Hirst and Woolley, *Social Relations*.

75 See M. Foucault (ed.), *I, Pierre Rivierre . . .* (Harmondsworth, Penguin, 1978); R. Smith, *Trial By Medicine* (Edinburgh, Edinburgh University Press, 1981), and 'Expertise and causal attribution in deciding between crime and mental disorder', *Social Studies of Science*, 15 (1985), 67–98. On the debates in the recent English trial of Peter Sutcliffe (the so-called Yorkshire Ripper) over these issues, see H. Prins, 'Diminished responsibility and the Sutcliffe case: legal, psychiatric and social aspects (a "layman's" view) ', *Medicine, Science and the Law*, 20 (1980), 276–82.

76 See Unsworth, *Mental Health Legislation*, esp. chapter 1.

77 M. Weber, *The Theory of Social and Economic Organizations* (New York, Oxford University Press, 1947), p. 340, cited in Jowell, 'Legal control', p. 191. See also Unsworth, *Mental Health Legislation*, chapters 1 and 4.

78 See P. Carlen *Women's Imprisonment* (London, Routledge & Kegan Paul, 1983), chapters 6–8.

79 Gostin, 'Ideology of entitlement'.

80 See P. M. Wald and P. R. Friedman, 'The politics of mental health advocacy in the United States', *International Journal of Law and Psychiatry*, 1 (1978), 137–52.

81 Gostin now seems to recognize this: see 'Ideology of entitlement', p. 36. See also M. S. Lottman, 'Enforcement of judicial decrees: now comes the hard part', *Mental Disability Law Reporter*, 1 (1976), 69–76.

82 For some analyses of de-institutionalization in the USA see Castel, Castel and Lovell, *The Psychiatric Society*, A. Scull, *Decarceration: community treatment and the deviant – a radical view*, 2nd edn (Cambridge, Polity Press, 1984) and the papers gathered together in *Millbank Memorial Fund Quarterly, Health and Society*.

83 Gostin discusses some of the cases in 'Ideology of entitlement', pp. 31–4.

84 For example *R v Secretary of State for Social Services, West Midlands Regional Health Authority and Birmingham AHA (Teaching) ex parte Hincks and Others* reported in *The Lancet*, 8413 (1984), 1224.

85 For example, 'Bedsit despair of the mental hospital outcasts', *The Sunday Times*, 20 November 1983; 'Taunted man's death fall', *The Times*, 9 January 1984; 'Mental health', *The London Programme*, London Weekend Television, 15 June 1984. See also Social Services Committee, Second Report, *Community Care With Special Reference to Adult Mentally Ill and Mentally Handicapped People* (London, HMSO, 1985), vol. 1.

86 The best discussion of these issues is in A. MacIntyre, *After Virtue* (London, Duckworth, 1981).

87 For criticisms of professional discretion in social work see, for example, the contributions to H. Geach and E. Szwed, *Providing*

Civil Justice for Children (London, Arnold, 1983). A useful discussion of problems with the notion of community care' is P. Abrams, 'Community care', *Policy and Politics*, 6 (1977), 125–51. S. Cohen, in 'The punitive city: notes on the dispersal of social control' (*Contempoary Crises*, 3 (1979), 39–60) analyses analagous trends towards community alternatives to imprisonment' in terms of a widening of the net of social control, thinning the mesh and blurring the boundaries between the normal and the abnormal, and between the institution and society. These issues are discussed further in chapter 2 in this volume.

88 T. Cambell, *The Left and Rights*, (London, Routledge & Kegan Paul, 1983) provides a useful overview of these criticisms, whilst trying himself to refute them.

89 See Macintyre, *After Virtue*.

90 On Geel, see Sedgwick, *Psychopolitics*, pp. 241–56. I discuss therapeutic communities in chapter 2 in this volume.

7 The category of psychopathy

1 J. C. Pritchard, *A Treatise on Insanity and other Disorders affecting the Mind* (London, Sherwood, Gilbert & Piper, 1835).

2 D. K. Henderson and R. D. Gillespie, *A Textbook of Psychiatry* (Oxford, Oxford University Press, 1956). D. Henderson, *Psychopathic States* (New York, Norton, 1939).

3 W. Mayer-Gross, E. Slater and M. Roth, *Clinical Psychiatry* (London, Cassell, 1954).

4 Henderson, *Psychopathic States*; H. M. Cleckley, *The Mask of Sanity*, 2nd edn (London, Kimpton, 1950).

5 D. Curran and P. Mallinson, 'Psychopathic personality', *Journal of Mental Science*, 90 (1944), 266.

6 Cleckley, *The Mask* and the fifth edition of this book, which appeared in 1976.

7 O. Fenichel, *The Psychoanalytic Theory of Neurosis* (New York, Norton, 1945).

8 R. D. Hare, *Psychopathy: Theory and Research* (London, John Wiley, 1970).

9 L. N. Robins, *Deviant Children Grown Up: A Sociological and Psychiatric Study of Sociopathic Personality* (Baltimore, Williams & Williams, 1969).

10 Ibid.

11 H. Prins, *Offenders, Deviants of Patients* (London, Routledge & Kegan Paul, 1980), chapter 5.

12 D. J. West, 'Psychopaths: An Introductory Comment', in D. J. West (ed.), *Psychopathic Offenders* (Cambridge, Cambridge University Institute of Criminology, 1968), pp. 7–12.

13. DHSS, *Personal and Health Statistics* (London, HMSO, 1982) table 9.4.

14 For statistics related to prisons and special hospitals, see L. Gostin, *Secure Provision* (London, Tavistock, 1985).

15 S. B. Guze, *Criminality and Psychiatric Disorders* (Oxford, Oxford University Press, 1976).

16 See, for example, A. Scull, *Museums of Madness: the social organization of insanity in nineteenth century England* (London: Allen Lane, 1979).

17 R. D. Laing, *The Divided Self*, (London, Tavistock, 1961).

18 See Scull, *Museums*.

19 T. F. Main, 'The hospital as a therapeutic institution', *Bulletin of the Menninger Clinic*, 10 (1946), 66–70; M. Jones, *Social Psychiatry* (London, Tavistock, 1952). See also R. H. Ahrenfeldt, *Psychiatry in the British Army in the Second World War* (London, Routledge & Kegan Paul, 1958).

20 On the development of the 'national efficiency', approach, see B. Semmel, *Imperialism and Social Reform* (London, Allen & Unwin, 1960). The development of Taylorism is charted in D. Ralph, *Community and Madness* (Montreal, Black Rose, 1983).

21 E. Erickson, *Childhood and Society* (New York, Basic Books, 1950), part 2.

22 S. Freud, 'Beyond the pleasure principle' (1920), in *Collected Papers* (London, Hogarth Press, 1959).

23 D. Burlingham and A. Freud, *Young Children in Wartime* (London, Allen & Unwin, 1942).

24 See the British parliamentary debates on mental disorder and psychopathy in 1954, 1957 and 1959.

25 J. Busfield, 'The historical antecedents of decarceration: the mentally ill', paper given at the conference on the History of British Psychiatry, London School of Economics, 15 May 1982.

26 Editorial, 'Unlocked doors', *The Lancet*, 2 (1954).

27 For further discussion of these issues see A. Scull, *Decarceration: community treatment and the deviant – a radical view* (2nd edn., Cambridge, Polity Press, 1984) and S. Ramon, *Psychiatry in Britain: meaning and policy*, (London, Croom Helm, 1985), chapters 5 and 6.

28 'Unlocked doors', *The Lancet*, 1 (1954), 1117.

29 See DHSS, *Statistics* and Gostin, *Secure Provision*.

30 See articles in *The Lancet*: 'Unlocked doors'; 1 (1954) 1117; and 2 (1959), 117.

31 See Hare, *Psychopathy*, and Prins, *Offenders*.

32 E. S. Myers, 'The Royal Commission and the psychopath', *British Journal of Psychiatric Social Work*, 4 (1958), 27–33.

33 H. J. Eysenck, 'The inheritance of extraversion and introversion', *Acta psychologica*, 12 (1956), 95–110.

34 *Report of the Royal Commission on Mental Illness and Mental Deficiency* (London, HMSO, 1957), Cmnd. 169.

35 E. Goffman, *Stigma* (Harmondsworth, Penguin, 1961).

36 Mental Health Act 1959, Section 4 (4).

37 Ibid., Section 4 (1).
38 *Hansard*, vol. 573, p. 49.
39 Ibid., pp. 550–1.
40 Ibid., vol. 605, p. 430.
41 Ibid., p. 423.
42 J. S. Whitley, 'The psychopath and his treatment', *British Journal of Psychiatry*, (1973), reprinted in E. Silverstone (ed.), *Recommended Readings on Psychiatry* (London, Royal College of Psychiatrists, 1976), pp. 159–69.
43 Ibid., p. 159.
44 P. D. Scott, 'Psychopathic States: their prevention', and N. Walker et al., 'Hospital orders and psychopathic disorders', both in West, *Psychopathic Offenders*, pp. 82–7 and 13–22 respectively.
45 W. M. McCord and J. McCord, *Psychopathy and Delinquency* (New York, Grune & Stratton, 1956), p. 164.
46 Whitley, 'The psychopath', p. 166.
47 M. Gelder et al., *Oxford Textbook of Psychiatry* (Oxford, Oxford University Press, 1984); B. Sheldon, *Behaviour Modification: Theory, Practice and Philosophy* (London, Tavistock, 1982).
48 Gostin, *Secure Provision*.
49 Ibid.
50 *Report of the Committee on Mentally Abnormal Offenders* (Butler Report) (London, HMSO, 1975), Cmnd. 6244.
51 Gostin, *Secure Provision*, and A. P. Lewis, 'The Regional Secure Unit policy as a case of the spread of psychiatry in the 20th century', paper given at the conference on the History of British Psychiatry, London School of Economics, 15 May 1982.
52 *Hansard*, vol. 43, pp. 951–2.
53 Butler Report, p. 81.
54 Ibid., p. 849.
55 Ibid., pp. 85–6.
56 Ibid., pp. 89–93.
57 DHSS, *Review of the Mental Health Act 1959* (London, HMSO, 1978), Cmnd. 6233.
58 DHSS, *Reform of Mental Health Legislation* (London, HMSO, 1981), Cmnd. 8405, p. 4.
59 Ibid., p. 7.

8   Psychiatry in prisons

1 I should like to thank the following for the help they gave me whilst I was preparing this essay: Dr John Kilgour, Director of the Prison Medical Service; Dr Chiang, Dr Cruikshank, Dr B. W. Oakley and Dr Jeremy Coid; Principal Hospital Officer Mr D. Strong and all other staff and prisoners who talked with me at Wormwood Scrubs Annexe; the hospital officer who had a long talk with me at Feltham

Youth Custody Centre; the Governor, doctors and prisoners of Grendon Underwood Prison; and for their positive responses to my requests to visit their establishments, Dr Gooch (at Feltham) Dr Barret (at Wormwood Scrubs) and the Governor of Wandsworth Prison. The specific form and substance of this essay's arguments are in no way attributable to any of the aforementioned individuals.

2 M. Gordon, *Penal Discipline* (London, Routledge & Kegan Paul, 1922), p. 277.

3 In an essay of this length it is impossible to give a detailed history of the Prison Medical Service. The detailed and authoritative accounts of changing attitudes towards the relationship between crime, culpability and mental impairment are Nigel Walker, *Crime and Insanity in England* (Edinburgh, Edinburgh University Press, 1968) vol. 1, and Nigel Walker and Sarah McCabe, *Crime and Insanity in England* (Edinburgh, Edinburgh University Press, 1973) vol. 2. Good shorter accounts are to be found in J. Gunn et al., *Psychiatric Aspects of Imprisonment* (London, Academic Press, 1978) and W. J. Gray, 'The English Prison Medical Service: its historical background and recent developments', in G. Wolstenholme and M. J. O'Connor (eds), *The Medical Care of Prisoners and other Detainees* (Amsterdam, Elsevier, 1973), Ciba Foundation Symposium.

4 Gunn, *Psychiatric Aspects*, p. 4.

5 Gray, 'English Prison Medical Service', p. 132.

6 Walker and McCabe, *Crime and Insanity*, p. 50.

7 Gordon, *Penal Discipline*, p. 234.

8 Bally, in *Report of the Directors of Convict Prisons for 1851*, (London, HMSO, 1852), quoted in Gunn, *Psychiatric Aspects*, p. 6. See also H. Gladstone, *Report from the Departmental Committee on Prisons* (London, HMSO, 1895), C 7702. Walker and McCabe, *Crime and Insanity*, p. 51, also make the point that, during the last decade of the nineteenth century, prison medical officers consistently denied accusations that the high incidence of insanity in their prisons resulted from imprisonment itself.

9 M. Foucault, *Discipline and Punish – the birth of the prison* (London, Allen Lane, 1977); D. Melossi and M. Pavarini, *The Prison and the Factory Origins of the Penitentiary System* (London, Macmillan, 1981); M. Ignatieff, *A Just Measure of Pain* (London, Macmillan, 1978).

10 M. Foucault, *Mental Illness and Psychology* (London, Harper & Row, 1976); A. Scull, *Museums of Madness: the social organization of insanity in nineteenth century England* (London, Allen Lane, 1979).

11 J. Bentham, *Collected Works*, ed. J. Browning (Edinburgh, William Tait, 1843), 'Panopticon Papers' reprinted in M. P. Mack (ed.), *A Bentham Reader* (New York, Pegasus, 1969).

12 G. Rusche and O. Kirchheimer, *Punishment and Social Structure* (New York, Columbia University Press, 1939); Melossi and Pavarini, *Prison and Factory*.

13 M. Fitzgerald and J. Sim, *British Prisons* (Oxford, Basil Blackwell, 1982), p. 108.

14 G. Playfair, *The Punitive Obsession* (London, Gollancz, 1971).
15 M. Maguire, *Burglary in a Dwelling* (London, Heinemann, 1982); S. Shaw, *The People's Justice* (London, Prison Reform Trust, 1982); M. Hough and P. Mahew, *The British Crime Survey* (London, HMSO, 1983).
16 Playfair, *Punitive Obsession*; P. Carlen, *Women's Imprisonment* (London, Routledge & Kegan Paul, 1983).
17 P. Carlen, 'On rights and powers: some notes on penal politics', in D. Garland and P. Young (eds), *The Power to Punish* (London, Heinemann, 1983).
18 For example, T. Szasz, *The Second Sin* (London, Routledge & Kegan Paul, 1974).
19 For example, N. Kittrie, *The Right to be Different: Deviance and Enforced Therapy* (Baltimore, Johns Hopkins University Press, 1971).
20 H. J. Eysenck, *Crime and Personality* (London, Paladin, 1964).
21 M. Hamblin-Smith, *The Psychology of the Criminal* (London, Methuen, 1922).
22 Gunn, *Psychiatric Aspects*, p. 16.
23 Quoted in Gray, 'English Prison Medical Service', p. 130.
24 R. Smith, *Prison Health Care* (London, British Medical Association, 1984), esp. pp. 69–70.
25 Gray, 'English Prison Medical Service', p. 131.
26 Gunn, *Psychiatric Aspects*, p. 19.
27 I know of no sociological studies of the actual working of the Prison Medical Service, whilst the official secrecy surrounding the prisons and the treatent of prisoners (as documented, for example, in S. Cohen and L. Taylor, *Prison Secrets* (London, NCCL and Radical Alternatives to Prison, 1978) and S. Coggan and M. Walker, *Frightened for my Life: an Account of Deaths in British Prisons* (London, Fontana, 1982)) has previously been such that it is still very difficult to gain a complete picture of prison health care. However, the present Director of the Prison Medical Service, Dr John Kilgour, believes that it is in the public interest for more information to be available and, accordingly, he looked favourably upon my requests to visit some of the few prisons that have special psychiatric facilities. I was, therefore, able to visit Grendon Underwood Prison, the Annexe at Wormwood Scrubs Prison, and Feltham Youth Custody Centre. Additionally I was granted interviews specifically on the uses of psychiatry in the penal system by the following: the Medical Officer at Wandsworth Prison; a doctor from Broadmoor Hospital; several ex-prisoners; and Dr Kilgour himself. At all of the institutions named, and from all of the individuals interviewed, I received a great deal of information, with many prison personnel going out of their way to ensure that I was fully appraised of the complexities of their working situations. Regrettably, the authorities at Wakefield Prison refused to allow me to visit their Psychiatric Centre and, because of administrative difficulties at Holloway Prison at the time (winter 1984–5) I thought it advisable not to visit their C1 wing for the highly disturbed.

In this essay I am also drawing on information gained from eleven years' work with various prison-reform bodies, on information informally gained from numerous visits to a variety of penal establishments, and from official research done at the Scottish institution for women offenders during 1980–1 (see Carlen, *Women's Imprisonment*).

28 Smith, *Prison Health Care*.

29 Ibid., pp. 86–7.

30 J. Kilgour, 'The Prison Medical Service in England and Wales: a commentary from the Director of the Prison Medical Service', *British Medical Journal*, 288 (1984), 1603–5.

31 Smith, *Prison Health Care*, p. 88.

32 Senior Medical Officer, Wandsworth Prison, 16 November 1984.

33 For instance, the General Register Office's *Glossary of Mental Disorders* (London, HMSO, 1968), Studies on Medical and Population Subjects No. 22, p. 17, defined anti-social personality disorder thus: 'This term should be confined to those individuals who offend against society, who show a lack of sympathetic feeling and whose behaviour is not readily modifiable by experience including punishment. They may tend to abnormally aggressive and seriously irresponsible conduct.' The American Psychiatric Association's *Diagnostic and Statisical Manual of Mental Disorders* (New York, American Psychiatric Association, 1968), p. 43, gives a definition of anti-social personality disorder that encapsulates many of the phrases I have heard used again and again by the personnel of prisons, courts, hostels and common-lodging houses:

> This term is reserved for individuals who are basically unsocialised and whose behaviour pattern brings them repeatedly into conflict with society. They are incapable of significant loyalty to individuals, groups or social values. They are grossly selfish, callous, irresponsible, impulsive and unable to feel guilt or to learn from experience or punishment . . . They tend to blame others or offer plausible rationalisations for their behaviour.

34 L. Brittan, 'Working together in the criminal justice system', Address to the Liverpool City Bench, 10 February 1984, *Nacro News Digest*, 28 (March, 1984).

35 Smith, *Prison Health Care*, pp. 44–5.

36 Reviews of some of the better ones can be found in Smith, *Prison Health Care*, and J. Coid, 'How many psychiatric patients in prison? ', *British Journal of Psychiatry*, 145 (1984), 78–86.

37 Lawton [L. J.], *Weekly Law Reports*, (1973), pp. 857–83.

38 HMSO, *Report of the Work of the Prison Department, 1983* (London, HMSO, 1984), Cmnd 9306, p. 61. The figures given here refer to both sentenced and unsentenced inmates and the recommendations were actually made under Sections 72 (sentenced inmates) and 73 (unsentenced inmates) of the Mental Health Act 1959, prior to September 1983, and after that date under Sections 47 (sentenced inmates) and 48 (unsentenced inmates) of the Mental Health Act 1983. Under Section 47

the Home Secretary must be satisfied that the prisoner is (a) suffering from mental illness, psychopathic disorder, severe mental impairment or mental impairment; and (b) the mental disorder is of a nature or a degree which makes it appropriate for him to be detained in a hospital for medical treatment; and (c) in the case of psychopathic disorder or mental impairment, treatment 'is likely to alleviate or prevent a deterioration of his condition'. (L. Gostin, *A Practical Guide to Mental Health Law* (London, National Association for Mental Health, 1983), p. 38).

The criterion under Section 48 is that 'a person is suffering from mental illness or severe mental impairment "of a nature or degree which makes it appropriate for him to be detained for medical treatment" and "he is in urgent need of such treatment" ' (ibid., p. 39). The optimism expressed in the *1983 Prison Report* seems better supported in *Prison Statistics for England and Wales 1983* (London, HMSO, 1984), Cmnd 9363, where it is stated that 'in 1983 109 males and 6 females were removed to psychiatric hospitals under Sections 47 and 48 of the Mental Health Act 1983 or before 30 September 1983 under Sections 72 and 73 of the Mental Health Act 1959. This was the highest number of males in the past decade but for females it was around the average for recent years' (p. 157).

39 Information obtained at my interview with Dr Kilgour, the Director of the Prison Medical Service on 22 November 1984.

40 See A. Clare, *Psychiatry in Dissent*, 2nd edn (London, Tavistock, 1980), p. 20. See also P. Carlen, *Women's Imprisonment* and 'Law, psychiatry and women's imprisonment', *British Journal of Psychiatry*, (June 1985).

41 Coid, 'How many psychiatric patients', p. 84.

42 The number of prisoners 'restrained' is given in the *Prison Statistics*. In England and Wales in 1983, 759 men and 78 women were restrained. 49 of the men were restrained on medical grounds under Rule 46 (6) Prison Rules 1964, under Rule 49 (6) Detention Centre Rules and Rule 49 (6) Youth Custody Centre Rules 1983. The main means of restraint was by use of 'protected rooms for temporary confinement' but other means include the loose canvas jacket, handcuffs, the bodybelt and ankle straps (*Prison Statistics for 1983*). For a fuller description of the use of 'restraints' see Prison Reform Trust, *Beyond Restraint: the use of body belts, special stripped and padded cells in Britain's prisons* (London, Prison Reform Trust, 1984). See also J. O'Dwyer and P. Carlen, 'Josie: surviving Holloway and other women's prisons', in P. Carlen et al., *Criminal Women* (Cambridge, Polity Press, 1985).

43 HMSO, *Report of Prison Department 1983*, p. 7.

44 Ibid., p. 94.

45 Gunn, *Psychiatric Aspects*, p. 257, citing R. R. Prewer, 'Prison medicine', in L. Blom-Cooper (ed.), *Progress in Prison Reform* (Oxford, Clarendon Press, 1974).

46 HMSO, *1983 Prison Report*, p. 97.

47 Kilgour, 'Prison Medical Service', p. 1604.
48 Ibid.
49 See HMSO, *1983 Report*, pp. 98–101 for the number of doses actually dispensed and administered in various prison establishments in 1983.
50 HMSO, *Report of the Committee on Mentally Abnormal Offenders* (Butler Report) (London, HMSO, 1975), Cmnd. 6244.
51 Scotland's most well-known prison therapeutic community is the Barlinnie Special Unit, for descriptions of which see J. Boyle, *A Sense of Freedom* (London, Fontana, 1977) and R. Macdonald and J. Sim, *Scottish Prisons and the Special Unit* (Glasgow, Scottish Council for Civil Liberties, 1978).
52 Gray, 'English Prison Medical Service', p. 129.
53 Butler Report, p. 95.
54 Gunn, *Psychiatric Aspects*, p. 100.
55 For instance, the Annexe at Wormwood Scrubs caters mainly for prisoners who have the more easily identifiable problems related to sex offences, addiction offences and offences of violence. Grendon will take any prisoner who is not psychotic and can be loosely described as having a personality disorder. At Wormwood Scrubs, groups tend to be homogeneous with regards to types of offender, i.e. there are 'addictions' groups and 'sexual-offender' groups; at Grendon the groups are heterogeneous.
56 M. Schiffer, in *Psychiatry Behind Bars (Toronto, Butterworth, 1982)*, quotes L. R. Wolberg, *The Technique of Psychotherapy* (New York, Grune and Stratton, 1954), as dividing insight therapy into two subcategories: that with re-educative goals (i.e. those therapies concerned with the resolution of conscious conflicts) and that with reconstructive goals (i.e. those therapies concerned with achieving changes in characterthrough resolution of conscious conflicts). The groups I observed seemed to aim at the former (re-education), though the claims of some of the staff often seemed optimistically to imply that the groups could somehow magically achieve the latter (reconstruction). At the more mundane level, my observations led me to agree with some of the prisoners who told me that 'having insight means that you agree with everything that the "group" (meaning either the majority or the loudest method) says about you.'
57 Walker and McCabe, in *Crime and Insanity*, pp. 47–8, write:
'closely connected with penal systems is the development known as "group counselling" . . . This can be traced to California . . . where group psychotherapy was popularised in the nineteen forties. By the end of the 1939–45 war those responsible for the State Penitentiaries . . . were looking for psychiatrists and psychologists to form groups of long term prisoners for psychotherapy. Qualified psychotherapists, however, were already in demand for other work, with higher pay and prestige, and few were willing to spend much time in penitentiaries. The climate was thus favourable for the formation of groups which did not relay on the presence of a trained psychotherapist. [In Britain] in the early sixties [group counselling] was in operation in eight Borstals and nine prisons.

58 Gray, 'English Prison Medical Service'.
59 Gordon, *Penal Discipline*, p. 192
60 Hamblin-Smith, *Psychology of the Criminal*, p. 71.
61 At both Grendon and Wormwood Scrubs this procedure was obstructed by some prison officers on the grounds that it was against prison rules. Also see J. Gunn and D. Farrington (eds), *Abnormal Offenders, Delinquency and the Criminal Justice System* (London, John Wiley, 1982), p. 303, where the authors write:

> Some Grendon officers spend some of their spare time trying to help ex-inmates who have telephoned them because they are in difficulties within the community. These links are outside the responsibility of prison officers; indeed they are against the rules of the service. It was our impression that the relationships established within the prison are of considerable therapeutic value and can only be capitalised upon effectively if the Home Office were to allow some more flexible follow-up system for this group of men . . . It would not be impossible to allow Grendon men to be readmitted to the institution for short periods at time of major crisis.

62 Schiffer, *Psychiatry Behind Bars*. He is referring to D. S. Whittaker and M. A. Lieberman, *Psychotherapy through the Group Process* (London, Tavistock, 1965).
63 An assertion that is at odds with the experience of some women prisoners who say that is was mainly through discussion with other women prisoners that they gained insight into the circumstances that landed them in prison. See J. Hicks and P. Carlen, 'Jenny: in a criminal business', in Carlen, *Criminal Women*, where the experiences of Jenny Hicks leads one to wonder whether prison discussion groups led by people not in the employment of the Home Office would more nearly achieve the aims of therapeutic groups.
64 Gray, 'English Prison Medical Service'.
65 J. S. Whitely, D. Briggs and M. Turner, *Dealing with Deviants* (London, Hogarth Press, 1972), quoted in D, Kennard and J. Roberts, *An Introduction to Therapeutic Communities* (London, Routledge & Kegan Paul, 1983), p. 57.
66 It was stressed to me again and again that 'prisoners will try all kinds of things to avoid facing their problems. Concentrating on getting educational qualifications is one trick; intellectualising things is another' (prison officer, 1985). One Grendon ex-prisoner told me: 'If you always blamed youself for everything, that was "having insight". If you took a more sociological view, that was being "too intellectual".'
67 This is not to imply that I doubt the sincerity of the therapeutic-community officers' expressed commitment to the democratic ideology of prison therapeutic-community groups. It is only to stress that independently of any genuine desire to help prisoners, all prison officers are charged with maintaining prison discipline. Both prison officers and prisoners in therapeutic-community groups are well aware of the structural power differences that, in the last resort, will allow

prison officers to have unco-operative prisoners transferred to a more conventional regime.

68 Smith, *Prison Health Care*, p. 107.
69 C. Stewart and S. Shine, 'Disturbed women in Holloway' (unpublished paper, HMP Holloway, Psychology Unit, 1984), pp. 1–2.
70 Carlen, *Women's Imprisonment*, pp. 214–5.
71 Smith, *Prison Health Care*, p. 52.
72 Carlen. *Women's Imprisonment*, p. 207.
73 Smith, *Prison Health Care*, p. 53.
74 Doctors and others working in the prisons are well aware that the Prison Department's secrecy might do them a disservice. Many told me that, 'having nothing to hide', they welcomed outside investigators. Dr X's comment was typical of many others:

As a doctor I have nothing to hide. I go in for no outlandish treatments like ECT and I most likely prescribe fewer drugs than the patients could get outside. On the few occasions when I've been sked to forcibly inject I am clear in my mind that I did the best for the prisoner, and I could stand up and justify it in a court of law. Of course I wouldn't be so sure of myself if I were in a position where I had to justify the conditions in the rest of this place'.

(He waved vaguely towards the rest of the Victorian prison in which his hospital is situated.)
75 Wolstenholme and O'Connor, *Medical Care of Prisoners*, p. 27.
76 Carlen, *Women's Imprisonment*, p. 208. The comment is from the General Secretary of the Scottish Prison Officer's Association.
77 See the May Report: HMSO, *Report of a Committee of Inquiry into the United Kingdom Prison Service* (London, HMSO, 1979), Cmnd 7673, p. 49.
78 Gordon, *Penal Discipline*, p. 187.
79 See T: C: N: Gibbons, 'Female Offenders', *British Journal of Hospital Medicine*, (September 1971).
80 See, for example, the Butler Report; House of Commons, *The Reduction of Pressure on the Penal System: fifteenth report of the House of Commons Expenditure Committee* (London, HMSO, 1978); the May Report; Parliamentary All-Party Penal Affairs Group, *Too Many Prisoners.* (Chichester, Barry Rose, 1980).
81 Wolstenholme and O'Connor, *Medical Care of Prisoners*. See also Carlen, 'Law, psychiatry and women's imprisonment'.
82 F. Heidensohn, 'Women and the Penal System', in A. Morris (ed.), *Women and Crime* (Cambridge, University of Cambridge Institute of Criminology, 1981), Cropwood Conference Series No. 13,p. 127.
83 Stewart and Shine, *Disturbed Women*, p. 4, emphasis added.
84 J. Boyle, *Sense of Freedom*, p.264; Butler Report, p. 99.
85 May Report, para. 4.24.

9 Psychiatry as a problem of democracy

1 E. Goffman, *Asylums: Essays on the Social Situation of Mental Patients* (New York, Doubleday, 1961).
2 See, for example, R. Castel, *L'Ordre psychiatrique*, (Paris, Editions de Minuit, 1976); F. Castel, R. Castel and A. Lovell, *The Psychiatric Society* (New York, Columbia University Press, 1982).
3 M. Foucault, *Maladie mentale et personnalité* (Paris, Presses Universitaires de France, 1954) translated as *Mental Illness and Psychology* (New York, Harper & Row, 1976), p. 63.
4 M. Foucault, *Histoire de la folie*, (Paris, Gallimard, 1972), pp. 93–4, omitted from abridged English translation published as *Madness and Civilization: a history of insanity in the age of reason* (London, Tavistock, 1967).
5 K. Dörner, *Burger und Irre* (Frankfurt, Fischer, 1975), translated as *Madmen and the Bourgeoisie* (Oxford, Basil Blackwell, 1981).
6 Foucault, *Histoire de la folie*, p. 399, omitted from English edition.
7 On *Psichiatria Democratica*, see the forthcoming English edition of Franco Basaglia's writings, edited by Anne Lovell and Nancy Scheper-Hughes, *Psychiatry Inside Out. Selected Writings of Franco Basaglia* (New York, Columbia University, 1986); and Jean-Luc Metge, *Psichiatria Democratica (Paris, Editions du Scarabée, 1980).*
8 Ibid. On citizenship and the 'social question' see also G. Procacci, 'Social economy and the government of poverty', in G. Burchell et al. (eds), *The Foucault Effect* (Brighton, Harvester, 1986).

Index